# Chassin's Operative Strategy in Colon and Rectal Surgery

Carol E.H. Scott-Conner, MD, PhD
Professor of Surgery
University of Iowa Carver College of Medicine
Iowa City, Iowa
Editor

# Chassin's Operative Strategy in Colon and Rectal Surgery

Illustrations by Casper Henselmann

Springer

Carol E.H. Scott-Conner, MD, PhD
Professor of Surgery
University of Iowa Carver College of Medicine
Iowa City, IA 52242
USA

ISBN-10: 0-387-33043-7
ISBN-13: 978-1-4419-2200-7 e-ISBN-13: 978-0-387-68370-6

Printed on acid-free paper.


Softcover reprint of the hardcover 1st edition 2006
Reprinted from Carol E.H. Scott-Conner: *Chassin's Operative Strategy in General Surgery*, third edition, copyright 2002 Springer Science+Business Media, LLC.



9 8 7 6 5 4 3 2 1

springer.com

*To Harry*

*Carol E.H. Scott-Conner*

*To Charlotte*

*Jameson L. Chassin*

# Preface

More than half of the first volume of *Chassin's Operative Strategy in General Surgery*, introduced in 1980, was devoted to surgery of the small and large intestine and anorectum. This unusually rich and detailed coverage was maintained and even expanded in subsequent editions. The "big" Chassin's has become an invaluable resource for the surgical community.

In recent years, colorectal surgery has become a specialty unto itself, practiced by both colorectal and general surgeons. This volume, *Chassin's Operative Strategy in Colon and Rectal Surgery*, seek to provide the gold standard content of the large volume with the focus and specificity needed by colorectal surgeons. Practiced clinicians, fellows, and residents will all find valuable clinical guidance in these chapters.

Colorectal surgery is a rapidly-evolving surgical field. Since the last edition of the full volume of Chassin's, laparoscopic colon surgery has become the new standard of care for many patients. Thus, we have added four new, previously unpublished chapters to this new volume:

- laparoscopic right hemicolectomy
- laparoscopic left hemicolectomy
- laparoscopic abdominoperineal resection and total proctocolectomy with end ileostomy
- laparoscopic stoma construction and closure

Written by Steven D. Wexner, these new chapters provide the reader with the latest techniques in colorectal surgery. In addition to the clear, comprehensive text, these new chapters are enhanced by 52 lavish new illustrations by Caspar Henselmann, the skilled artist whose work has illuminated every edition of this text.

It is our hope that the reader will find *Chassin's Operative Strategy in Colon and Rectal Surgery* a useful distillation of the best of the "old" and the "new" strategies and techniques in colorectal surgery.

*Carol E.H. Scott-Conner, MD, PhD*

# Contents

# Contributors

*Susan M. Cera, MD*
Department of Colorectal Surgery
Chief of Endoscopy
Vice Chair Research and Education
Cleveland Clinic Florida
Weston, FL
USA

*Giovanna M. DaSilva, MD*
Research Fellow
Department of Colorectal Surgery
Cleveland Clinic Florida
Weston, FL
USA

*Amanda M. Metcalf, MD*
Department of Surgery
University of Iowa Carver College of Medicine
Iowa City, IA
USA

*Fabrizio Michelassi, MD*
Department of Surgery
The University of Chicago
The Pritzker School of Medicine
Chicago, IL
USA

*Dan Enger Ruiz, MD*
Department of General Surgery
Hospital Santa Helena
São Paulo
Brazil

*Danny M. Takanishi, MD*
Department of Surgery
The University of Chicago
The Pritzker School of Medicine
Chicago, IL
USA

*Steven D. Wexner, MD, FACS, FRCS, FRCS (Ed)*
Chairman
Department of Colorectal Surgery
Cleveland Clinic Florida
Weston, FL
USA

# Part I

## Large Intestine

# 1 Concepts in Surgery of the Large Intestine

Danny M. Takanishi
Fabrizio Michelassi

This chapter provides a comprehensive overview of essential concepts relating to the operative approach and strategy for colon and rectal surgery. Additional information is contained in the technical chapters that follow and the references at the end of the chapter.

## BENIGN CONDITIONS

### Diverticular Disease

*Diverticulosis* is defined by the presence of diverticula. Bleeding and septic complications are the major surgical concerns. Surgical management depends on the site of colonic involvement, the frequency of "attacks," elective or emergent basis, and the presence of synchronous lesions. Only 1% of patients with diverticulosis require surgery. The sigmoid and descending colon are most commonly involved, although generalized colonic involvement (pandiverticulosis) may occur.

*Diverticulitis*, the most common condition complicating diverticulosis, occurs in approximately 10–25% of patients [1,2]. Symptoms include pain and tenderness in the left lower quadrant, altered bowel habits, nausea, fever, and if the involved segment of colon is in contact with the bladder, urinary symptoms (frequency, dysuria, pneumaturia, fecaluria). A palpable mass may be noted in the lower abdomen or pelvis. Leukocytosis with a left shift is common. Computed tomography (CT) is the best confirmatory test. It provides additional information concerning transmural extension and abscess formation as well as the presence or absence of adjacent organ involvement [3]. Image-guided percutaneous drainage may obviate the need for emergent surgery if an abscess is detected. After resolution of the acute attack, endoscopic evaluation is valuable for assessing the extent of disease and ruling out synchronous pathology.

Initial therapy depends on clinical findings. Patients with mild tenderness and low grade fever may be cared for on an outpatient basis with oral antibiotics and a clear liquid diet. Patients with symptoms and signs severe enough to require hospitalization require intravenous broad-spectrum antibiotics, hydration, and bowel rest (and possibly nasogastric decompression). Most patients improve within 48–72 hours. Surgery is generally not indicated for the first such attack unless the course is complicated by perforation and free peritonitis or abscess formation. About 30–45% of patients have recurrent attacks and require surgical intervention [1,4].

The optimal treatment is resection of the primary disease with primary anastomosis. This can certainly be carried out after successful antibiotic treatment and gentle mechanical bowel preparation. Patients who fail antibiotic therapy should undergo a two-stage operation with segmental resection of the diseased segment of bowel, primary anastomosis, and a proximal loop ileostomy or colostomy. If an abscess has been encountered in the pelvis, an omental flap can be developed to fill the abscess cavity and separate it from the colorectal anastomosis. If the planned anastomosis seems to lie within the evacuated abscess cavity, it is wiser to perform a segmental resection with an end-colostomy and a Hartmann's rectal closure or mucous fistula. The gastrointestinal continuity can be reestablished at a later time. This approach is also preferred for cases of free perforation with generalized peritonitis.

There is little role for colonic diversion without resection. This temporizing approach is reserved primarily for the rare, high-risk individual with extensive co-morbidities, abscess formation, or localized peritonitis, who would not tolerate a major operative procedure. In this case a proximal diverting loop colostomy or loop ileostomy must be complemented by abscess drainage (operatively or percutaneously with radiographic guidance) to control sepsis. Staged resection and closure of the diverting stoma is performed at a later date.

Diverticulitis may occasionally present with signs of complete *obstruction*. In otherwise asymptomatic patients (absence of pain, tenderness, systemic signs of infection), resection of the affected segment with end-colostomy and Hartmann's closure of the rectosigmoid is generally performed. Another option is on-table colonic lavage with resection, primary anastomosis, and possibly a proximal loop diverting stoma. In the poorest-risk patient a diverting transverse loop colostomy is still an option as an initial step to a staged resection.

Patients with two or more documented episodes of diverticulitis or with a history of complications from diverticular disease (bleeding, high grade partial obstruction due to cicatricial narrowing, fistulas) are candidates for elective resection. Elective resection should be considered after the first episode of diverticulitis in young patients (less than 40 years old) and those who are immunosuppressed [1,2,4,5]. Although resection can be performed 1–3 weeks following the attack of acute diverticulitis, if all the signs of local inflammation have receded rapidly many surgeons prefer to delay the operation for 2–3 months, allowing complete patient recovery and resolution of the inflammatory reaction. Delaying definitive therapy beyond 3 months puts the patient at increased risk of recurrence with no additional technical advantage.

After standard mechanical and antibiotic bowel preparation resection is based on the gross extent of disease and should include all indurated and hypertrophied bowel. Generally the sigmoid colon is primarily involved, and resection can be limited to this region. The rectum does not need to be elevated from the presacral space. Unless the mesentery is so inflamed and edematous it becomes easier to divide it close to its base, it may be resected close to the bowel wall, a concept that holds true for all benign diseases with an inflammatory component. The anastomosis is done using bowel that is soft, pliable, and free of diverticula. The splenic flexure often requires mobilization to ensure a tension-free anastomosis.

Diverticulosis is one of the most common causes of massive *lower gastrointestinal bleeding*, especially in the elderly. In most patients the bleeding stops. If episodes recur or if there is any hemodynamic instability during the first episode, surgical intervention is mandatory. If the site can be localized, by endoscopic means or arteriography, segmental resection can be done. In an emergency situation with an unstable patient, a two-stage procedure is best, with primary resection and colostomy as the first step. If the bleeding site cannot be localized, an abdominal colectomy may be necessary after preoperative proctosigmoidoscopy has ruled out the presence of a bleeding site in the rectum and rectosigmoid. Whether a primary anastomosis is performed in the emergency setting or delayed for an elective procedure depends in part on the patient's hemodynamic and overall condition. If bleeding stops and the bleeding site had been identified, elective one-stage resection is carried out after bowel preparation.

*Colovesical fistulas* are the most common of all diverticular fistulas. Most are suspected on clinical presentation, with CT scanning probably the most sensitive test for confirming the clinical diagnosis. After appropriate bowel preparation, it is usually possible to perform one-stage, primary resection of the diseased sigmoid, with immediate anastomosis. The area of involvement in the bladder is generally small, and it may be excised and repaired by primary closure. If available, an omental interposition flap may be utilized. A Foley catheter is left in place for 7–10 days postoperatively to maintain bladder decompression.

Colonoscopy is the examination of choice for patients with chronic, occult blood loss and may also be useful for moderately severe lower gastrointestinal bleeding in the hemodynamically stable patient. If hemorrhage can be temporarily controlled, bowel preparation may be instituted and one-stage, segmental resection with primary anastomosis may be feasible.

For patients who are exsanguinating rapidly, volume resuscitation is paramount. Angiography is the test of choice and localizes the bleeding site in 75% of cases [6]. Selective infusion of vasopressin to stop or decrease the rate of hemorrhage followed by limited, segmental resection of the colon may be feasible. If brisk hemorrhage continues and angiography does not localize the source, subtotal colectomy should be performed after preoperative proctosigmoidoscopy has ruled out the rectum as the site of bleeding. Whether a primary anastomosis is performed in the emergency setting or delayed to an elective situation depends in part on the patient's hemodynamic and overall condition.

## Volvulus

Volvulus of the colon results from twisting of the mesentery, most commonly in the cecum and sigmoid. It is believed that the underlying predisposing factors include an elongated mesentery or a narrow base [7]. The resulting clinical presentation is one of bowel obstruction, which may progress rapidly to strangulation, gangrene, and perforation. The sigmoid is the site most frequently involved. Plain radiographs of the abdomen may demonstrate the dilated loop of colon in the right upper quadrant ("omega loop"), and barium enema demonstrates a "bird's beak" appearance of the barium terminating at the level of the torsion. If no peritoneal signs are present, perform rigid proctosigmoidoscopy to reduce and decompress the bowel. If the mucosa appears viable, a large red rubber tube can then be inserted through the rigid proctosigmoidoscope to stent the rectosigmoid junction and decompress the proximal colon. Subsequently, mechanical preparation can be instituted and elective one-stage sigmoid resection done, given the high recurrence rate if this approach is not taken [7]. If the volvulus cannot be reduced or if any evidence of impending gangrene is detected, emergent laparotomy is indicated. After operative reduction, the involved segment is resected as part of a planned two-stage procedure with an end-colostomy and mucous fistula or Hartmann's pouch. Alternatively in low-risk patients, intraoperative intestinal lavage can be performed and a primary colorectal anastomosis fashioned.

Cecal volvulus is the next most common colonic volvulus. It presents as small bowel obstruction. Plain radiographs of the abdomen may demonstrate features of a small bowel obstruction in association with a dilated cecum in the left upper quadrant. Emergency laparotomy is required. First reduce the volvulus and assess the viability of the bowel. If the bowel is viable, cecopexy is performed. A tube cecostomy can be added to increase the chances of a successful cecopexy. Simple reduction is inadequate and attended by a significant recurrence rate. Evidence of impending gangrene requires resection. Options include an end-ileostomy with mucous fistula. Primary anastomosis is safe in patients who are hemodynamically stable and in whom perforation or contamination has not occurred.

## Ischemic Colitis

Ischemic colitis is heterogeneous in terms of etiology, anatomic site of involvement, presentation, and degree of severity [8]. Although all areas of the colon can be involved, the splenic flexure and rectosigmoid (watershed areas) seem to be at particular risk [8,9]. Significant morbidity and mortality are in large part due to underlying conditions. A high index of suspicion is necessary for diagnosis. Many patients experience left flank and left lower quadrant pain, diarrhea, and blood per rectum. Colonoscopy is the diagnostic tool of choice. Plain radiographs of the abdomen and CT scans are useful primarily to exclude other causes of abdominal pain or the complications of perforation, pneumatosis, and portal vein air. Barium enema no longer has a role in the diagnosis and workup of this disease.

Initial treatment is supportive and consists of fluid resuscitation, bowel rest (possibly with nasogastric decompression), correction of anemia, and broad-spectrum antibiotics. Most attacks (80–90%) are self-limiting and heal with this approach. All require colonoscopy 6–8 weeks after the event. A small percentage (2%) of patients develop strictures [8,9]. Surgical resection is required if obstructive symptoms develop, or if cancer cannot be definitively excluded. After appropriate bowel preparation, an elective one-stage procedure is done, resecting the diseased segment of colon and performing the anastomosis in noninvolved, normal, viable bowel.

In a small group of cases ischemia progresses to necrosis and frank gangrene. These patients are quite toxic and ill, with evidence of sepsis, hemodynamic instability, and eventual shock. This mandates emergent laparotomy. The goals of surgery are (1) to assess the extent of ischemia by evaluating mesenteric flow (palpation, Doppler, intravenous fluorescein dye combined with a Wood's lamp) and by endoscopic evaluation of mucosal viability; and (2) to resect all nonviable, compromised bowel. Normal mucosa must be present at the margins of the resection. In general, an end-colostomy and a Hartmann's pouch or mucous fistula should be created (the latter has the unique advantage of allowing direct evaluation of the mucosa for evidence of ongoing ischemia); in the rare hemodynamically stable, low-risk patient, intraoperative cleansing of the proximal large bowel can be followed by a primary anastomosis. Another option is extension of the resection to include a subtotal colectomy with an ileorectal anastomosis. If the involvement is confined to the right colon, a primary anastomosis is feasible, provided there has been no major contamination and the patient is hemodynamically stable. If a primary anastomosis has been fashioned but there are doubts about intestinal viability, a planned second-look laparotomy is scheduled within 24 hours.

## Rectal Prolapse

Complete rectal prolapse (procidentia) presents with intussusception of the rectum into the anal canal [10], with the descent of all layers of the rectum through the anus. All patients should therefore undergo endoscopic evaluation to rule out a tumor etiology serving as the lead point and to assess for ulceration or other complications.

Surgical options all aim to correct the abnormal anatomy. Broadly categorized, techniques for repair are based on either an abdominal or a perineal approach. Factors considered during selection of a particular procedure include age, overall performance status, and the advantages or disadvantages of each technique [10,11].

*Abdominal approaches* include rectopexy alone, segmental resection alone, or a combination of the two. Rectopexy (e.g., the Ripstein procedure) (see Chapter 56) involves complete rectal mobilization to the pelvic floor with division of the lateral stalks. Suture rectopexy utilizes simple suturing of the rectum to the sacral fascia (posterior rectopexy) or the peritoneum, pelvic brim, or uterus (anterior rectopexy). Variations of this procedure diverge with the manner in which the rectum is suspended; nonreabsorbable sutures, Ivalon sponge (Wells' procedure), or Teflon/Marlex mesh (Ripstein procedure) have been well described [10,11]. Recurrence rates range from 2% to 16%, and complications include obstruction secondary to mesh wraps or sepsis related to the foreign body (e.g., full-thickness decubitus and pelvic abscesses). Segmental resection alone has also been successful, with recurrence rates comparable to those seen with the pexy procedures [11]. Associated complications are few, consisting primarily of anastomotic dehiscence. The lowest recurrence rates have been noted with the combination suture rectopexy and sigmoid resection.

*Perineal approaches* include simple encirclement of the anus and rectosigmoidectomy. The Thiersch procedure (see Chapter 63) has evolved over time but is rarely used owing to the high rates of recurrence and septic complications. Perineal rectosigmoidectomy involves resecting the prolapsed bowel starting 1–2 cm proximal to the dentate line. A primary anastomosis and a levatorplasty are then performed concomitantly. Recurrence rates vary significantly, from approximately 3% up to 60% in some series [12]. Theoretically, the reduction in rectal reservoir function could potentially result in urgency or incontinence.

It is generally accepted that transabdominal approaches are associated with lower rates of recurrence than the perineal approaches, which have higher recurrence rates but are safer options in high-risk or elderly patients [10,11]. What is still debatable and controversial is which procedures result in better functional outcomes. Unfortunately, too few randomized trials have compared the functional outcomes of the various techniques. Hence this important issue has not been addressed adequately.

## Familial Polyposis and Hereditary Colon Cancer Syndromes

*Familial adenomatous polyposis* (FAP) is the phenotypic result of a germline mutation of the adenomatous polyposis coli (*APC*) gene on chromosome 5q21 [13]. The disease is characterized by multiple adenomatous polyps in the large bowel that can be complicated by bleeding, obstruction (uncommon), a protein-losing enteropathy, and of considerable significance the development of adenocarcinomas. Extraintestinal manifestations are also common. The penetrance of this gene is high; this fact and the associated risk for carcinoma have provided the rationale to pursue a surgical approach as early as the late teenage years.

Current appropriate treatment requires total removal of the colorectal mucosa to avoid the later development of carcinoma, a complication that generally afflicts these patients by the age of 40, if not sooner. Although proctocolectomy with ileostomy removes the risk of colorectal cancer, it is obviously attended by loss of transanal defecation. This option, nowadays, is usually reserved for patients with advanced cancer of the rectum or anal incontinence. To avoid a permanent stoma, surgeons once performed subtotal colectomy with ileorectal anastomosis combined with electrocautery destruction of the remaining rectal polyps. Obviously, the remnant mucosa required close surveillance for the development of carcinoma. Review of the literature demonstrated a 30% incidence of rectal cancers after 20 years, so this procedure was indicated in only a small number of selected patients.

Today complete removal of colorectal cancer risk and maintenance of transanal defecation is achieved with a restorative proctocolectomy with ileal pouch/anal anastomosis [14]. The technique is described in Chapter 48. An alternative technique utilizing a stapled anastomosis (ileal pouch/distal rectal anastomosis) may yield slightly better functional results at the expense of risking recurrent polyposis in the retained mucosa, which presumably would render patients at higher risk for the development of dysplasia and adenocarcinoma. Currently, it is not possible to quantify the risk for the individual patient. Mutational analysis to pinpoint the specific locus of the gene mutation in the *FAP* gene in an individual patient may prove to be a method of selecting who can safely undergo an ileorectal anastomosis and who requires an ileal pouch/anal procedure or proctocolectomy because of a high risk for rectal cancer development in the retained rectum.

*Hereditary nonpolyposis colorectal cancer (HNPCC) syndrome* is the most common inherited disease predisposing to the development of colorectal cancer after FAP. This autosomal dominant syndrome is characterized by right-sided colon cancer usually by age 40–45 years, and increased incidence of synchronous and metachronous colorectal cancer, and an excess of extracolonic cancers, such as endometrial, ovarian, and upper gastrointestinal lesions. The predisposition to cancer in patients with HNPCC syndrome arises from germline mutations in mismatch repair (*MMR*) genes. A total abdominal colectomy is recommended as an alternative to lifetime endoscopic surveillance for selected *MMR* gene mutation carriers with colon adenomas. Prophylactic colectomy should be considered for patients whose colons are difficult to scope or for those in whom endoscopic polypectomy may be technically difficult.

## Inflammatory Bowel Disease

### *Crohn's Colitis*

Surgery is indicated for intractability (including individuals dependent on high doses of immunosuppressive agents and steroids), septic complications, chronic bleeding and anemia, stricture formation, fulminant colitis or toxic megacolon, and the development of dysplasia or adenocarcinoma [15]. Surgical treatment must be tailored to the anatomic extent of the macroscopic disease. If the colitis is limited to the right colon, a right hemicolectomy can suffice; if it extends past the splenic flexure, and the rectosigmoid is devoid of disease, an abdominal colectomy with ileosigmoid anastomosis is necessary. In the presence of pancolitis, a proctocolectomy with terminal ileostomy is the procedure of choice. A restorative proctocolectomy with ileal pouch/anal anastomosis is contraindicated in Crohn's disease because of the high risk of perineal and pelvic septic complications and the high Crohn's disease recurrence rate in the ileal pouch.

In case of fulminant colitis or toxic megacolon, many patients undergo total colectomy and end-ileostomy, with further surgery after a recovery period of 2–3 months. Completion proctectomy or an ileorectal anastomosis may be appropriate if the rectal stump is not diseased and there is good anal sphincter function without significant perineal disease [16]. In this acute emergency setting the colon is exquisitely friable. Exercise great care during operative manipulation to prevent rupture and peritoneal contamination. Do not attempt to separate the omentum from the transverse colon, as it may lead to inadvertent colonic perforation or may violate walled-off microabscesses.

Patients with extensive perineal disease complicated by acute and chronic sepsis should be treated by a staged approach with total colectomy and a short rectal pouch about 5 cm or less in length. Concomitant with this Hartmann coloproctectomy, fistulous tracts are opened and perirectal abscesses are drained. With subsequent resolution of perineal sepsis, intersphincteric resection of the rectal stump by a perineal approach can then be undertaken. This approach has significantly diminished the risk of perineal wound complications.

Although segmental colon resection is associated with a higher recurrence rate than proctocolectomy with ileostomy, it may avoid or delay a permanent stoma and facilitates retaining as much colon mucosa as possible. This is especially desirable in patients who have already suffered a sizable loss of small intestine. Thus sigmoid or left-sided colon disease is usually treated with a sigmoid or left colectomy; isolated rectal disease can be treated with abdominoperineal proctectomy with end-colostomy [17,18].

Anorectal complications of Crohn's disease must be approached based on their severity and extension and on the status of the rectal mucosa. If the rectum is not diseased, perianal abscesses can be drained, anorectal stenosis dilated, fistula in ano surgically treated, and rectovaginal fistula repaired with good expectation of complete healing. If the perineal disease is severe or the rectal mucosa is diseased (or both), a rectal ablative procedure is the only surgical procedure that can avoid the complications and return the patient to a satisfactory quality of life.

A genetically engineered monoclonal antibody, Infliximab, has been found to be efficacious in a randomized trial for treating fistulas in Crohn's disease patients. Long-term follow-up is necessary; but if these data are validated, this agent may prove to offer another option to the challenging and often complex management of perineal Crohn's fistulas.

### *Ulcerative Colitis*

Unlike Crohn's disease, which can affect any portion of the gastrointestinal tract, ulcerative colitis is limited to the colon and rectum. The surgical indications are similar for both diseases, however, and include medical intractability, fulminant colitis and toxic megacolon, stricture formation, hemorrhage, and the presence of dysplasia and carcinoma [15,19]. In the pediatric population, delayed growth and maturation may also be an indication, though less so than for Crohn's disease.

Proctocolectomy/end-ileostomy has the advantage of removing the entire target end-organ and curing the patient, usually with one surgical procedure. Although a major disadvantage is that the procedure results in a permanent stoma, it represents the best option for individuals with poor anal sphincter function, an advanced rectal carcinoma, and advanced age [15]. A variation on this theme is construction of a continent, or Kock, ileostomy. The benefit of this approach is that it allows patients an opportunity to maintain control over evacuation, but the technique is not without complications.

The ileal pouch/anal procedure is probably the most popular option in terms of patient preference. With experience in major centers accruing since the 1980s along with concomitant long-term patient follow-up, this operation has an excellent success rate and good functional results [20–26]. In the absence of dysplastic or malignant degeneration a complete mucosectomy is not mandatory, and the ileoanal anastomosis can be performed with a circular stapler 0.5–2.0 cm proximal to the dentate line. This modification makes the procedure easier, increases the chance of avoiding a temporary ileostomy (onestep restorative proctocolectomy with ileoanal pouch anastomosis), allows the procedure to be performed in obese patients, and maintains the lower rectal mucosa with its proprioceptive sensation indispensable for distinguishing flatus from liquid and solid stool.

Total abdominal colectomy and ileorectal anastomosis has been used in the past. Because of the retained rectum, ongoing surveillance for the early detection of dysplasia or carcinoma is mandatory [27–31]. This approach therefore is limited to patients with rectal sparing (which is unusual given that the disease has a tendency to manifest in the rectum first), elderly patients, and patients whose ulcerative colitis is complicated by a stage IV colon cancer.

Subtotal colectomy/end-ileostomy is the favored approach in patients with fulminant colitis intractable to medical therapy, toxic megacolon, or acute bleeding. In most cases, the subjects are severely ill individuals, many of whom are debilitated, on high-dose steroids, or highly catabolic with systemic manifestations of hemodynamic instability or sepsis. This procedure removes the diseased colon, allowing resolution of the systemic manifestations and quiescence of the associated rectal involvement. After a period of recovery, patients remain candidates for a completion proctectomy with the creation of an ileal pouch/anal procedure. From an operative standpoint this staged approach has the added advantage of allowing associated pelvic inflammation to subside. Pelvic dissection in the acute setting causes potentially more blood loss and greater risk of injury to the pelvic autonomic nerves or rectum during dissection, further compounding the risk of pelvic septic complications [32].

### *Indeterminate Colitis*

In approximately 5–10% of patients with inflammatory colitis the diagnosis of Crohn's or ulcerative colitis is still equivocal even after a thorough endoscopic and histopathologic evaluation. In patients with medically intractable disease requiring surgery, in both the emergent setting and the elective setting, the preferred approach is generally subtotal colectomy with end-ileostomy and closure of the rectal stump [33]. This approach allows for the possibility of a completion restorative proctectomy and ileal pouch/anal procedure if the histologic evaluation of the specimen demonstrates ulcerative colitis, while avoiding the unfortunate situation of performing an ileal pouch/anal procedure in an individual later diagnosed as having Crohn's disease [34].

## Polyps

The *hyperplastic polyp* is the most common type of polyp. It tends to be diminutive, is often multiple, harbors no malignant potential, and is easily removed endoscopically by simple biopsy in most cases. *Adenomatous polyps* and *villous adenomas* are premalignant lesions, based on observations of their natural history and an improved understanding of the molecular events in the adenoma–carcinoma sequence of colorectal cancer [35]. The risk of invasive cancer increases with polyp size, morphology (sessile), and histology (degree of villous component) [35–37]. Most polyps are initially excised endoscopically. Lesions less than 2 cm are amenable to endoscopic polypectomy; larger lesions may require partial snare excision or multiple piecemeal excisions. If histopathologic examination of the specimen excludes the presence of carcinoma, endoscopic removal is all that is needed. If the polyp cannot be removed endoscopically or is extremely large (and malignancy cannot be excluded), the patient must undergo operative polypectomy or segmental colon resection [35]. In these cases it is useful to inject the site with India ink at endoscopy to facilitate intraoperative identification.

Subsequent management is guided by the presence of invasive cancer and the likelihood of lymph node metastasis. Haggit et al. developed a prognostic schema that may be used to identify patients adequately treated by endoscopic excision alone [37,38]. Endoscopic removal of a polyp found to have malignant degeneration is considered sufficient if the following conditions have been met.

1. Endoscopic removal has provided an adequate margin of resection.
2. The lesion is well to moderately differentiated.
3. There is no lymphovascular invasion.
4. There is no evidence of invasion of the submucosa of the colonic wall.

All patients treated in this fashion require follow-up colonoscopy in 3–6 months to assess for local recurrence. If the polyp shows malignant degeneration, the margins of excision are less than 2 mm, and there is invasion of the submucosa, a poor histologic grade, or lymphatic/vascular invasion, the patient stands at increased risk for lymph node involvement or local recurrence by the carcinoma. In these instances, segmental colectomy is generally selected.

Cyclooxygenase-2 (COX-2) inhibitors may modify the management of colonic polyps in the future. Accumulating data suggest that this class may diminish the risk of developing adenomas and carcinomas [39]. Investigations are currently underway to elucidate the role these compounds play in colorectal carcinogenesis. This holds the promise of a potentially effective strategy in the nonoperative management of premalignant tumors of the colon and rectum.

## MALIGNANT CONDITIONS

### Colorectal Cancer

#### *Extent of Resection*

The surgical management of colorectal carcinoma is based on two principles: rendering patients disease-free when feasible and palliating any symptoms attributable to the malignancy. The concept of the "extent of resection" for curative intent has undergone considerable evolution as better understanding of the magnitude of lymphadenectomy and proximal, distal, and radial margins has accrued. In the case of colon cancers, resection is generally based on the vascular anatomy to ensure removal of the entire lymph node drainage basin [39]. This complete mesenteric excision frequently is associated with proximal and distal margins longer than 5–6 cm, which are more than adequate to minimize anastomotic and locoregional recurrences. The radial margin, not a frequent issue in colon cancers, becomes a consideration when the tumor invades adjacent organs. In this case, en bloc resection of the involved adjacent organs or viscera is required, provided distant disease is not present to preclude curative resection.

In the case of rectal cancer, including distal and radial margins is equally important to prevent locoregional recurrences, but it is rendered more challenging by the desire to save the anal sphincter complex and by the anatomic constraints of the pelvis. Optimal initial treatment is important, as local recurrences are often not salvageable for cure, and up to 25% of patients dying from rectal cancers have disease limited strictly to the pelvis. In addition, pelvic recurrences are quite symptomatic, with bleeding, tenesmus, anal sphincter dysfunction and incontinence, pelvic sepsis, bowel and urinary obstruction, and severe perineal pain secondary to bone and nerve plexus involvement [39]. Neoadjuvant or adjuvant radiation therapy (with or without chemotherapy) forms a major part of the multimodality approach to treating rectal carcinomas to enhance locoregional control.

Contemporary studies have not demonstrated any survival benefit of "high" lymphovascular ligation of a major vessel compared to a "low" ligation closer to the cancer [39]. Extended pelvic lymphadenectomy or high ligation of the inferior mesenteric artery for surgical management of rectal cancer has conferred no survival benefit, and current practice emphasizes ligation of the inferior mesenteric artery distal to the origin of the left colic artery [39]. The role of the sentinel node biopsy is being evaluated.

The surgical approach to a rectal cancer also depends on its distance from the anal verge. For cancers proximal to 5–7 cm from the anal verge, adequate oncologic clearance and gastrointestinal continuity restoration may be achieved with a low anterior resection using modern anastomotic techniques [40]. For coloanal anastomosis at the level of the dentate line, a colonic J-pouch reservoir may be added (see Intestinal Pouch Reservoirs, below).

#### *Colorectal Cancer with Synchronous Pathology*

Synchronous lesions are relatively common in colorectal carcinoma; hence there is a need to study the entire colon preoperatively or intraoperatively, generally by total colonoscopy. In a series of 228 patients with colorectal cancer evaluated at the University of Chicago, 45.6% had synchronous lesions and 11.0% required a surgical resection more extensive than what would have been dictated by the primary tumor [41]. Eleven patients (4.9%) had synchronous adenocarcinoma, in agreement with already reported data.

#### *Synchronous Benign or Premalignant Conditions*

In the case of coexisting *diverticular disease*, oncologic considerations and the location of significantly diseased bowel guide the extent of resection. The anastomosis must be constructed in a region of healthy tissue without diverticula or muscular hypertrophy.

*Synchronous polyps* outside the planned resection field should be addressed. If the colon cancer and the synchronous polyp(s) are present within the same segment of colon, a standard resection is performed. If the involved areas are noncontiguous, attempt preoperative endoscopic resection. If the polyp is confirmed to be benign but too large for endoscopic resection, colostomy with operative polypectomy combined with segmental colon resection may be a feasible option. If the polyp is located on the mesenteric side or is too large for surgical resection through a colostomy or if it harbors a malignancy, an extended colon resection is often necessary to remove both the polyp and the cancer and to avoid two anastomotic suture lines.

In the setting of *ulcerative colitis*, the principles of resection are based on the need to remove the target organ and the primary tumor concomitantly. With ulcerative colitis this often requires a restorative proctocolectomy with construction of an endileostomy or ileal pouch/anal procedure. A proctocolectomy will ileostomy may be necessary for rectal cancers. A subtotal colectomy with ileorectal anastomosis may be an alternative in the presence of a metastatic colon cancer.

The goals of management for *familial polyposis* are analogous to that for ulcerative colitis. Optimal management generally involves a restorative proctocolectomy to remove all involved diseased large bowel at risk for the development of metachronous carcinomas and avoid a permanent stoma. Proctocolectomy with ileostomy may be necessary in the presence of a rectal cancer.

A total abdominal colectomy is recommended for *MMR gene mutation carriers* with a colon carcinoma. Postmenopausal women should be advised to consider a prophylactic hysterectomy and bilateral salpingo-oophorectomy.

## Synchronous Cancer

The reported incidence of synchronous cancers varies between 1.5% and 10.7% [41]. The approach is to treat each cancer conceptually as a separate lesion. If the two are within a contiguous portion of colon, a standard primary resection is done; if they involve two noncontiguous regions, an extended resection is done so only one anastomosis must be created. It may necessitate subtotal colectomy.

## Preoperative Evaluation

*Total colonoscopy* with appropriate biopsy is the "gold standard" for diagnosis and confirmation of the presence of malignancies and synchronous pathology. Careful histologic evaluation is important for both cancer and benign conditions. Barium enema examination and the newer virtual reality imaging (still investigational) have limited roles because tissue sampling is not possible [39]. These studies are used primarily when total colonoscopy is not feasible.

*Precise measurement of location for carcinoma of the rectum* is generally done by digital rectal examination and rigid proctosigmoidoscopy. Each assesses the distance between the anal verge and the lower border of the tumor. Digital examination also allows assessment of the distance between the anorectal ring and the distal edge of the tumor. It is this distance that determines, in part, the surgical options available to an individual patient, most importantly the feasibility of sphincter preservation. Digital evaluation also provides an initial determination of tumor size, depth, location, and mobility. Finally, it assists in identifying those tumors potentially amenable to local excision techniques.

*Precise preoperative staging* assists in proper surgical planning and has become increasingly important as multimodality (including neoadjuvant) treatment gains widespread popularity. Standard staging studies include chest radiography or thoracic CT and CT of the abdomen and pelvis to determine if measurable pulmonary, hepatic, or peritoneal metastases are present and if adjacent organ involvement exists. Ultrasonography, in experienced hands, is equivalent to the CT scan as an imaging modality to detect liver metastases. Both have supplanted the use of liver chemistries for this goal [39]. Magnetic resonance imaging is not thought to offer additional advantage. Other staging studies (CT scans of the head or bone scans) are used only in symptomatic patients [39].

Digital examination and endorectal ultrasonography are more accurate than CT scans for determining the *local extent of rectal cancer* [39,42]. Endorectal ultrasonography is particularly useful for measuring the precise depth of invasion and the status of the perirectal lymph nodes.

Determination of the *carcinoembryonic antigen (CEA) level* has no value for preoperative staging of a colon or rectal carcinoma. It may be helpful as a baseline, however, for postoperative follow-up.

Finally, *patient age and overall performance status* (including co-morbid medical illnesses, nutritional status) are important issues when determining the timing and selection of the surgical procedure(s). Assessment of the general status is important when choosing the operative approach. High-risk, elderly patients with multiple co-morbidities are better served by less extensive resections, with attendant decreased anesthesia time, more rapid recovery, and less morbidity and mortality. Advanced age alone is not considered a contraindication to operative intervention in the emergent or the elective setting.

Patients who are debilitated, cachectic, or otherwise infirm may require nutritional support and restitution of metabolic and intravascular volume deficits before any planned procedure (if delay does not further compromise the patient's condition).

*Obesity* may preclude restoration of gastrointestinal continuity and maintenance of transanal defecation because of technical constraints. Patients must be informed of this possibility during preoperative treatment planning discussions. Stoma site selection also poses a significant challenge in this group of patients (see Intestinal Stomas, below).

### *Neoadjuvant Therapy for Rectal Adenocarcinoma*

Trials of preoperative (neoadjuvant) or postoperative radiation therapy for rectal adenocarcinoma have shown decreased local recurrence in the treated cohorts [43–53]. Perceived advantages of preoperative versus postoperative radiotherapy include optimal radiosensitivity of well oxygenated neoplastic cells still undisturbed by the surgical dissection and the possibility of decreasing the size of the perirectal infiltration allowing for a negative radial margin. In addition, preoperative radiotherapy avoids irradiation of the freshly fashioned anastomosis. The preoperative dose delivered and the duration of that delivery continue to be sources of considerable debate. A randomized trial from Lyon demonstrated that a longer interval to surgery (6–8 weeks compared to 2 weeks) resulted in significantly better tumor regression and downstaging with no differences appreciated in terms of local control, survival, or complication rate at a median follow-up of approximately 3 years [54]. Although most reports indicate that better local control is achievable with pre- or postoperative adjuvant therapy of advanced rectal cancers, most reports fail to demonstrate that neoadjuvant therapy translates into improved control and overall survival when compared to postoperative treatment [47,51,52].

## Squamous Carcinoma of the Anus

The *Nigro protocol* is used for squamous cell carcinoma of the anal region. This combined regimen of external beam radiation, 5-fluorouracil, and mitomycin C allows preservation of sphincter function and yields improved 5-year survival compared to that of historical controls who underwent abdominoperineal resection. Overall 5-year survival rates with modern modifications of this protocol exceed 80% [55,56]. For those with persistent or recur-rent disease, salvage abdominoperineal resection may result in more than 50% long-term survival [56].

## Surgical Approach and Strategy

### *Preoperative Preparation*

Although *mechanical bowel preparations* have been used for decades, currently no clinical trial data support this practice. A meta-analysis based on three clinical trials showed that patients who underwent mechanical bowel preparation had a higher rate of wound infections and anastomotic leaks. The prevailing concern regarding the potential risk of intraoperative peritoneal contamination and the facilitation of intraoperative colonic manipulation continues to favor use of mechanical bowel preparations. Polyethylene glycol (colonic lavage) solutions are most commonly used. A clear liquid diet for 1–2 days prior to the operative procedure is another component of the traditional bowel preparation.

The concept of *antimicrobial prophylaxis* has been studied extensively for years. Debate centers on the optimum route of administration, what constitutes the best antibiotic, and the value of combination regimens of oral and parenteral agents. The most common regimens include preoperative oral neomycin and erythromycin only, parenterally administered second-generation cephalosporins only, and a combination of the two. Oral antibiotics should be given within 24 hours of the procedure. The timing of parenteral agents is guided by the goal of adequate tissue levels at operation. This generally means dosing one-half hour before the skin incision.

The extent or need for *postoperative parenteral antibiotic administration* is also unknown. From the standpoint of prophylaxis there appears to be no benefit beyond two or three doses postoperatively or for a period beyond 24 hours.

Patients who have been on *steroids* as part of their medical regimen for inflammatory bowel disease or collagen-vascular disorders require preoperative pharmacologic doses in preparation for the metabolic stress of general anesthesia and a major operative procedure. Supplementation is done to prevent precipitation of adrenal insufficiency during the perioperative period. A "rapid taper" schedule is followed over the subsequent days until the patient is at the preoperative oral dose equivalent. A sample regimen is hydrocortisone intravenously 100mg q8h on the day of surgery, followed by 75mg q8h for the next 24 hours, then 50mg q8h for 24 hours, then 50mg q12h by postoperative day 3.

### *Laparotomy Versus Laparoscopy*

*Open laparotomy* is the traditional approach and is emphasized in the chapters that follow. The procedure begins with thorough evaluation of the extent of disease and assessment for associated diseases before planned resection. This includes evaluation of adjacent organ involvement and regional lymph node involvement and determination of the presence or absence of distant (usually hepatic) disease. All four quadrants of the abdomen are examined, including the entire small bowel, along with careful exploration of the pelvis and gynecologic organs and all peritoneal surfaces.

Innovations in *minimally invasive surgery* have been extended to colorectal surgery, and many "open" procedures have been adapted to this approach [57–68]. Comparative studies continue to accrue, substantiating earlier hypotheses of safety and feasibility. Accurate comparative assessments of diminished postoperative pain and ileus, shorter hospital stay, shortened postoperative convalescence compared to that after open procedures, and cost differences continue to be areas of some controversy. Preliminary analyses of data demonstrate that an equivalent resection may be accomplished [39,57,58,61,62,64,65]. Laparoscopy is also useful for staging and abdominal exploration prior to laparotomy for recurrent or metastatic disease. By detecting peritoneal implants, laparoscopy may spare patients the morbidity of an unnecessary laparotomy in this setting [39]. Port-site metastases in patients who have undergone the procedure with a "curative" resection remain a concern. Trials are currently in progress to determine the exact incidence of this phenomenon and to elucidate its etiology.

## *Alternatives to Formal Resection of Rectal Cancer*

***Simple transanal excision*** is the most common local approach to rectal polyps and cancers. With the patient in lithotomy or jack-knife position, an anal retractor is placed for exposure and a headlight utilized to visualize the anorectal canal. The tumor is excised with electrocautery obtaining a full-thickness biopsy (deep margin is perirectal fat) with a 1 cm margin around the tumor. The defect may be left open or closed with absorbable sutures. Complications are rare, and there is no postoperative pain. This approach is used [36,39] in tumors that are

Well to moderately dif3ferentiated

Small (<3 cm)

Nonulcerated

Involve less than one-fourth the circumference of the rectum

Exophytic

Mobile

Tis or T1 lesions (as determined by endorectal ultrasonography)

Demonstrating no evidence of lymphovascular invasion

Without palpable perirectal lymphadenopathy

Within 10 cm of anal verge.

Positive margins or unfavorable histopathologic characteristics require surgical resection. Data from clinical trials show that *adjuvant radiation* reduces recurrence rates significantly after transanal excision in well selected patients, in contrast to surgery alone [39]. These data must be interpreted with caution because many of these studies are small with short follow-up; and so far there has been no evidence that this combination of treatment has any effect on overall survival. Along this line of thought, T2 lesions have been subjected to chemoradiation as adjuvant treatment, particularly because of the higher likelihood of regional node involvement with increasing depth of invasion [39]. This modality has been associated with low morbidity (less than 10%) and no operative mortality. Yet with the maturation of some clinical studies, the recurrence rates for locally resected T2 lesions approximate 15–25% even after postoperative chemotherapy, suggesting that formal resection is still the treatment of choice for these tumors.

*Transanal endoscopic microsurgery* offers a transanal approach to lesions located in the proximal rectum and rectosigmoid. Essentially, a large-bore proctoscope allows resection of the tumor with specially constructed graspers, scissors, needle-holders, and cautery while viewing the procedure on a video screen. Full-thickness excision with primary closure is achieved. This approach is utilized primarily for adenomas and Tis and T1 cancers. Local recurrence rates appear comparable to those seen with open surgical approaches, with less morbidity and shorter hospitalization [69–73].

*Electrocoagulation* and *laser fulguration* represent other transanal ablative techniques. These techniques are limited in that full-thickness resections and wide margins usually cannot be obtained [74]. Hence they should be restricted to patients whose medical condition and general status precludes major surgery and those who already have identifiable distant metastasis.

The *posterior approach* may be useful for resecting benign rectal polyps that would otherwise be difficult to reach through the anal route because of size, location, or distance from the anal verge. This approach is ideal for polyps located 7–13 cm from the anal verge, especially if located on the anterior or lateral rectal wall.

*Endocavitary irradiation (papillon technique)* is based on use of a low-voltage generator to irradiate a rectal carcinoma through a proctoscope. This has the benefit of a more limited extent of radiation injury compared to external beam irradiation, and adjacent organs are therefore spared injury. This factor is exploited using large doses (up to 15,000 cGy) directed to the tumor bed, often combined with an iridium 192 implant [75,76]. It is done as an outpatient procedure for cure or palliation. The morbidity is minimal, except that many patients require local anesthesia or sedation owing to the large proctoscope utilized, and some develop varying degrees of incontinence due to sphincter injury. Again, a major disadvantage of this procedure and similar "ablation" techniques is the absence of an intact specimen to allow comprehensive histologic examination, which may influence the decision for additional therapy. For this reason, when a local approach is chosen the choice is usually between a transanal approach (with or without endoscopic microsurgery) or a posterior approach.

## Specific Interoperative Considerations During Operations for Colorectal Cancer

Many techniques, such as the Turnbull "no touch" technique were previously advocated in an attempt to minimize locoregional and distant failure [77]. As our understanding of cancer biology has improved based on observational, natural history studies and the advent of molecular biology and cancer genetics, it has become increasingly clear that to a great extent it is the biology of the specific tumor that governs disease-free survival. However, analysis of data involving patterns of recurrence has allowed formulation of a few principles that may affect the disease-free interval and ultimately survival.

The most significant surgeon-controlled factor that diminishes the risk of local recurrence is an operative conduct aimed at obtaining *negative proximal, distal, and radial resection margins*. This may necessitate the use of intraoperative frozen section control and en bloc resection if there is adjacent organ involvement. Suture line recurrence constitutes a form of local failure, and strategies to prevent this occurrence are similar to those expounded to prevent local recurrences in general.

*Minimize manipulation of the tumor* and, in particular, avoid breaching the colonic wall with significant spillage of tumor cells into the peritoneal cavity. It is not clear exactly what tumor inoculum size is necessary for implantation and propagation to occur, as host factors play an important role. If the involved segment of large bowel is adherent to an adjacent organ or structure, perform an en bloc resection rather than attempting to dissect the tumor free in patients where the resection has curative intent.

The surgical principles governing control of locoregional recurrence pertain to prevention of distant failure as well. There is a growing body of literature that substantiates the theory that inadequate local control, by virtue of persistent disease, increases the propensity for distant disease [39].

## Strategies for Complex Situations

Patients who are *septic* because of abscess or perforation require fluid resuscitation and broad-spectrum parenteral antibiotics. Initial antibiotic coverage should include agents effective against Enterobacteriaceae and obligate anaerobes such as *Bacteroides* species and *Clostridium*. Bowel rest is also an important component of management, as many patients have an associated ileus depending on the degree of the septic insult.

In instances of *colonic perforation*, whether due to benign or malignant disease, an emergent resection to control the septic process is imperative. Constructing an anastomosis in the presence of peritoneal contamination, especially if generalized, is attended by a significant risk of anastomotic leakage. Consequently, the most common and safest option is represented by a segmental colon resection with a proximal end-stoma and closure of the distal colon or construction of a mucous fistula. Alternatively, if the perforation is localized and walled off, resection with primary anastomosis and proximal diverting loop ileostomy is often possible. This approach has the advantage of not requiring a formal laparotomy to reconstitute gastrointestinal continuity at a later time. If a good-risk, healthy patient is found to have a localized cecal perforation, an ileocolonic anastomosis following right colectomy may be done, provided the two intestinal segments to be anastomosed are free of inflammation. The anastomosis should be placed in the upper abdomen, away from the abscess cavity. Omentum may be used to wrap the anastomosis as an added precaution. If contamination and inflammation are not well localized or if the patient has significant co-morbidity, hemodynamic instability, or pulmonary insufficiency, primary anastomosis is hazardous and should not be attempted. For more extensive colonic involvement, as may be the case with fulminant colitis with perforation, or in the setting with a cecal perforation resulting from a distal left colonic carcinoma obstruction, a subtotal colectomy with end-ileostomy and mucous fistula or Hartmann's pouch may be the best option.

The approach to management of *abscesses* is analogous to that for a localized perforation, with a few additional principles. First, any undrained inflammatory exudate and pus must be evacuated. Second, depending on the degree of necrosis and the age of the abscess, débridement may be required to remove all devitalized tissue. Drain placement may be necessary for the perioperative period, depending on the degree of residual contamination. Finally, an omental flap may be useful to fill the drained abscess cavity and separate it from the abdominal cavity.

*Fistulas* can usually be managed by one-stage, primary resection of the diseased segment of colon, with primary anastomosis after bowel preparation. If there is an associated abscess with substantial contamination and sepsis, the procedure may require staging. The abscess cavity may have to be drained, débrided, and filled with an omental flap. Reconstruction of the gastrointestinal continuity may have to be delayed in favor of a proximal stoma and distal Hartmann pouch/mucous fistula. Alternatively, a primary anastomosis with proximal diverting loop ileostomy may be undertaken.

In patients with *large bowel obstruction* the standard approach has been a stage resection with creation of an ostomy and later reconstruction of the gastrointestinal tract. This is due, in large part, to an inability to prepare the obstructed colon adequately combined with concern of fashioning an anastomosis using dilated, edematous bowel. Three techniques warrant discussion, as they are useful adjuncts in the management of this condition. For the first two techniques, intestinal decompression and lavage, data attest to the safety, efficacy, cost-effectiveness, and improved quality of life that has resulted from their implementation [78–84]. For the third technique, use of metallic stents, data are sparse but nevertheless promising.

*Intestinal decompression* involves creating a colotomy proximal to the site of obstruction and within the confines of the intestinal segment to be resected to decompress the proximal bowel with a large-bore catheter or suction device [79–81]. This generally takes 10–15 minutes. A theoretic benefit is decreased colonic distension, which facilitates abdominal closure and improves colonic perfusion and tone. The technique appears to be safe and efficacious.

*On-table intestinal lavage* (intraoperative antegrade irrigation) has gained favor as a method to cleanse the colon mechanically at surgery and to facilitate one-stage colonic resection and primary anastomosis. Key elements to the successful outcome of this approach are the absence of significant peritoneal contamination, no intraoperative hemodynamic instability, and a patient with an otherwise excellent performance status with minimal co-morbid disease [82–84]. The most common method involves mobilizing the obstructed colon and distal intestinal transection; draining the proximal intestinal end into a large bucket via a plastic conduit (the authors prefer an ultrasonographic/endoscopic plastic sleeve); placing a large Foley catheter into the cecum (often via the stump of the removed appendix) and securing it in place with a purse-string suture; and lavaging the colon with saline until the effluent is clear [79,82]. This technique is more cumbersome than intestinal decompression and requires a longer time to complete (approximately 30–45 minutes). Currently, no prospective randomized trial has compared the outcome of intestinal decompression alone to decompression plus on-table colonic lavage prior to primary colon anastomosis. One retrospective analysis demonstrated no additional benefit with the addition of lavage [82].

*Metallic stents or endoprostheses* have been used for benign strictures and malignant obstruction [85–89]. Data from small, single-institution series show excellent results, probably attributable in part to careful patient selection. The procedures have been easily adapted to endoscopic or fluoroscopic deployment, are well tolerated, can be performed on an outpatient basis with minimal sedation, and provide palliation (to avoid colostomy in a terminally ill patient) or allow mechanical bowel preparation in anticipation of a single-stage resection and anastomosis.

## Primary Anastomosis versus Staged Procedures

Patients presenting with *malignant large bowel obstruction* generally undergo a staged resection and creation of a temporary ostomy with later takedown of the ostomy to restore gut continuity. Although options for on-table decompression and cleansing exist, as previously described, many of these patients are elderly and have associated medical illnesses that preclude prolonged anesthesia.

An attempt to construct an anastomosis in the presence of *generalized peritoneal contamination* is associated with a significant risk of anastomotic leakage. Hemodynamic instability, pulmonary and renal insufficiency, and even frank shock argue for a short but definitive operation that does not further compromise the tenuous physiologic status of these patients. Therefore the prevailing standard of care dictates that in the presence of generalized peritonitis or septic shock (or both) a primary anastomosis is contraindicated. Occasionally, in the presence of walled-off perforations or localized abscesses a primary anastomosis can be fashioned as detailed above.

*Hemodynamic instability* predisposes a patient to systemic perioperative morbidity and mortality as a result of impaired end-organ perfusion and oxygen delivery (e.g., risk of cardiac ischemic events or cerebrovascular accident) and to local complications related to anastomotic integrity and dehiscence. Additionally, the clinical manifestation of hemodynamic instability itself is a harbinger of an underlying disease process that generally defines an already poor-risk patient population. Thus if colonic resection is required, a staged approach is often a better option than fashioning a primary anastomosis.

Patients who are *severely malnourished* lack physiologic reserves for wound healing and the immune response to potential infectious agents. A staged approach (rather than primary anastomosis) allows an adequate interval for restitution of the patient to an anabolic phase and positive nitrogen balance.

Patients with medically intractable *indeterminate colitis* should undergo subtotal colectomy with end-ileostomy and closure of the rectal stump. This approach spares patients a permanent ileostomy and allows the possibility of a restorative proctectomy and ileal pouch/anal procedure if histopathologic examination of the specimen demonstrates ulcerative colitis, while avoiding performing an ileal pouch/anal procedure in an individual later diagnosed as having Crohn's disease.

## Technical Factors for Safe Anastomosis

A properly constructed anastomosis is attended by a dehiscence rate of less than 2%. Reported data reveal that the radiographic leak rate is actually much higher than the appreciated clinically detected rate, particularly for rectal cancer, though the clinical significance of this finding is not clear. To obtain these excellent results, proper patient selection (as described above) and attention to the following technical details is of utmost importance.

The cut edge of the mesentery of each intestinal segment should have *demonstrable pulsatile arterial blood flow*. The bowel wall should be pink, soft, and pliable; and the transected edge should demonstrate bleeding or mild oozing of bright red blood, confirming an intact blood supply. Intramural hematomas at the site of the anastomosis or a hematoma in the adjacent mesentery may impair blood flow and should be avoided by handling and manipulating the bowel and mesentery gently during mobilization, resection, and construction of the anastomosis.

*Accurate seromuscular apposition* must be achieved. Submucosa must be included in each suture, as this layer contributes to anastomotic strength, a function of its connective tissue component. Great care should be exercised to be certain there are no blood clots or pericolonic fat (mesentery or appendices epiploicae) interposed between the two ends of the bowel at the anastomosis. This often requires that a 1 cm cuff of bowel be completely cleared of fat, mesentery, and epiploic appendices. Most anastomotic leaks appear to occur on the mesenteric side of the bowel, presumably related to inadequate clearing of supporting, investing fatty tissue of the mesentery. If a hand-sewn technique is elected, good inversion of all layers of the bowel should be achieved without compromising luminal patency. Sutures should be tied to obtain tissue approximation, avoiding excessive force and strangulation necrosis of the bowel wall, which would result in anastomotic dehiscence.

The *mesenteric defect* should be closed with absorbable or nonabsorbable, interrupted or continuous suture technique to prevent an internal hernia. The exception to this rule is represented by the mesenteric defect obtained after a distal rectosigmoid or low anterior resection. The risk of internal herniation after these resections and anastomoses is sufficiently low that attempts to close these mesenteric defect are usually not pursued.

The anastomosis must be constructed *without tension*. Adequate mobilization may require division of peritoneal attachments and ligaments, such as those that suspend the splenic flexure.

*Avoid contamination* during intestinal mobilization and resection or at the time of the construction of the anastomosis. This requires proper technique during the mobilization phase, use of noncrushing bowel clamps on both ends of the bowel during bowel resection and anastomotic construction, and simultaneous liberal use of laparotomy pads to partition off the anastomotic site from the rest of the peritoneal cavity. Irrigation of the peritoneal cavity prior to abdominal closure also dilutes bacterial counts and limits the degree of any contamination.

*Accumulation of blood (or serum)* in the vicinity of an anastomosis not only may compromise the blood supply to the anastomosis but may provide a nidus for infection. Subsequent localized sepsis may predispose to abscess formation and anastomotic dehiscence. Treatment begins with prevention. Principles of meticulous hemostasis and asepsis require ardent adherence. Transient, early postoperative closed suction drainage of the presacral space may be a useful adjunct for resections carried distal to the peritoneal reflection to prevent accumulation of blood and tissue fluid.

Closure of the pelvic peritoneum may result in considerable *perianastomotic deadspace*. This may result in the collection of tissue exudate, which invites infection. The pelvic peritoneum is thus best left open to allow the small bowel to descend into the pelvis and fill the deadspace. Other options include creating an omental pedicle flap or a rectus muscle flap and bringing it down into the pelvis, effectively obliterating any deadspace [90].

*Distal obstruction causes anastomotic failure.* All efforts are made to ensure that there is no coexisting distal obstruction prior to construction of any bowel anastomosis. Preoperative radiographic contrast studies and pre- or intraoperative endoscopic studies provide useful information in this regard.

### Other Factors Affecting Anastomotic Healing

*Preoperative radiation therapy* was believed by many to be the Achilles heel of the neoadjuvant approach to treatment of rectal cancers. Although irradiation impairs healing, in the setting of rectal cancer the anastomotic complication rates of preoperative irradiation have compared favorably to those seen with adjuvant approaches.

Prolonged administration of *high-dose steroids* impairs wound healing. This class of drugs results in muscle- and protein-wasting, a condition that predisposes to negative nitrogen balance and a catabolic state. After prolonged steroid administration there is weakening of the cellular desmosomic plaques and inhibition of fibroblast activity, which account for the slower anastomotic healing noted in humans (confirmed in animal models by measuring bursting pressures of colonic anastomoses as the endpoint) [91–95]. To complicate matters, immune function, a necessary component of wound healing and important for minimizing infectious complications, is suppressed.

*Carcinoma at the anastomotic margin* contributes to anastomotic leakage and "suture-line" recurrence. This situation is rarely encountered today, as the principles of negative proximal and distal margins are well appreciated, and the use of intraoperative frozen section control of resection margins (if close or in doubt) is standard practice.

### Technical Considerations and Adjuncts

After constructing an ileal pouch/anal anastomosis without a diverting ileostomy, it is advisable to *drain the pouch* for 5–7 days by way of a transanal catheter. This allows drainage of secretions, blood and fecal material, avoids overdistension of the pouch, and minimizes suture-line dehiscences. The same concept can be used after closing a rectal stump during an emergency colectomy, especially if the closure has been challenging and the rectum appears tense with blood and secretions.

*Biodegradable intraluminal tubes* have proved feasible adjuncts for construction of anastomoses in the setting of septic processes and colonic obstruction in both animal models and humans [96,97]. Many materials have been used for this purpose, with the most popular being latex condoms. Results in small prospective series have demonstrated that the use of these devices is safe and technically uncomplicated. The risk of dehiscence and other complications in the setting of unprepared colon and even in instances of prior radiotherapy have been minimal. The technique generally involves using a sterile ring of a latex condom, which is sutured to the mucosa and submucosa of the proximal end of the bowel used for the anastomosis, followed by creation of the bowel anastomosis itself. The "tube" essentially intraluminally bridges or "bypasses" the anastomosis, which presumably allows better healing to occur by minimizing contact with stool.

The use of an *omental flap* can be desirable as it has many advantages in selected circumstances. Indeed, the omentum appears to be a major source of leukocytes and macrophages during intraabdominal septic processes, has angiogenic properties, has the ability to fill deadspaces and abscess cavities, and partitions off inflamed organs or an anastomosis to prevent generalized peritonitis or dehiscences. Furthermore, it can be used to exclude the small bowel from the pelvis when adjuvant therapy is likely during postoperative treatment of a rectal cancer [90].

There are differing opinions regarding the efficacy of *wrapping colorectal anastomoses with omentum*. Many surgeons traditionally have wrapped omentum (if enough is available to make it feasible) around colorectal anastomoses with the intent of reducing the risk or consequence of anastomotic leaks. A prospective, randomized French trial reported in 1999 demonstrated absolutely no benefit to this approach for colon or rectal anastomoses [90]. Omental wrapping of colorectal anastomoses does not appear to provide any additional benefit over the use of meticulous principles of surgical technique for anastomotic construction.

If *disparity exists between two ends of bowel*, there are a number of options that may be employed to construct an anastomosis. One maneuver is called the Cheatle slit, described in Figure 43-10, which involves creating a longitudinal incision along the antimesenteric border of the smaller limb of bowel to be anastomosed. Subtotal colectomy and low anterior resection are attended by a significant discrepancy between the two limbs of bowel. Use of a Cheatle slit in these circumstances to create an endto-end-anastomosis is often difficult owing to the large disparity of the size of the two intestinal lumens and the location of the anastomosis deep in the pelvis. A side-to-end anastomosis (ileoproctostomy or coloproctostomy) is usually an easier alternative. Furthermore, the end of the rectum can be invaginated into the side of the ileum or colon for additional protection against leakage without risking stenosis due to the relatively large anastomosis that can be achieved by this method. Alternatively, a side-to-side functional end-stapled anastomosis can be fashioned by initially stapling the two intestinal ends side by side with a linear stapler; the common lumen can then be closed by firing a second linear stapler across.

## INTESTINAL POUCH RESERVOIRS

Creation of intestinal pouch reservoirs is an integral component of restorative proctocolectomy for ulcerative colitis and familial polyposis. The pouches are of varied configurations, each with its own proponents, but the purpose served is identical, all with demonstrated excellent functional outcomes [98].

The *J-pouch* is a double-loop reservoir that has become the most common pouch because it is simple and easy to construct. It may be the best option for a narrow pelvis in an obese individual because it is less bulky than other configurations. It also may be the best option when performing a stapled anastomosis because of the ease at passage of the stapling device. The J-pouch offers minimal difficulty with evacuation and emptying; and in general, the functional results are good when the pouch is at least 15 cm in length. A brief comment regarding *colonic* J-pouches is in order. Similar to small bowel J-pouches, a 6- to 8-cm colonic pouch appears to improve the functional results after a proctectomy with coloanal anastomoses for treatment of rectal cancer. Stool frequency and urgency appear to be reduced compared to straight coloanal anastomoses [99–101]. This advantage is most apparent during the first 1–2 years of construction, after which equivalent functional outcomes tend to occur. Some studies advocating this approach have demonstrated a tendency toward a reduced incidence of anastomotic complications with the colonic J-pouch procedure, an observation that needs to be substantiated by larger studies.

*H-pouch* (also called the lateral H-pouch) is a double-loop reservoir designed to enhance the efficiency of pouch evacuation by placing the two segments of ileum in an isoperistaltic configuration [98]. The functional results are good if strict attention is paid to creating a short spout and a pouch length less than 12 cm. Two loops, placed in a slightly staggered alignment with respect to each other, may be an alternative to a J-pouch for patients with a short mesentery, rendering it difficult for the reservoir to reach the anus. As with the S-pouch, this configuration may pose difficulty with passage of stapling devices to create a stapled anastomosis. Additionally, like the S- and W-pouches, this type has the disadvantage of being more difficult to construct.

The *S-pouch* has a distal spout. This triple-loop configuration is helpful if there is technical difficulty with the pouch reaching the anus. It is more time-consuming to construct, as would be expected, and patients may experience difficulty with pouch evacuation, particularly if the outlet is longer than 2 cm [98].

The *W-pouch* is a quadruple-loop pouch with some important advantages over other pouches. In patients with partial loss of the terminal ileum this construction allows maintenance of pouch reservoir capacity (largest capacity of all types) [98]. Patients who fail other configurations in terms of functional results of high stool frequency and nocturnal incontinence may benefit from conversion to a large-capacity W-pouch, which results in decreased stool frequency. A disadvantage of this pouch is that its construction is difficult and time-consuming.

## INTESTINAL STOMAS

Intestinal stomas can be broadly categorized as temporary or permanent. The goal governing construction of a stoma is to allow the patient to return to an active life style. This is facilitated by appropriate stoma placement and protrusion to avoid local complications, especially those related to skin breakdown and appliance malfunction. The appropriate stoma site must be selected preoperatively for all elective procedures and for most emergent ones. Adequate mesenteric mobilization is necessary for stoma protrusion. End-ileostomies should protrude more than end-colostomies (1.0–1.5 cm vs. 0.5–1.0 cm) in view of the more liquid effluent. Protrusion helps bowel contents from seeping between the wafer of the appliance and the peristomal skin; it also prevents peristomal skin irritation and breakdown. Additional precautions include placement of sutures in the dermis during stomal maturation to prevent potential hypertropic scarring and intestinal cell implantation in the epidermis, which may render proper adherence of appliances difficult [102,103]. A snug fascial opening prevents postoperative herniation.

Preoperative site selection is important, as improper siting may result in poor fit of the appliance, with leakage and skin breakdown. Ideally, the site is chosen and marked preoperatively by the surgeon in consultation with an enterostomal therapist [104]. The location should be flat and away from skin creases and the costal or iliac margins; it should be in an area of normal, healthy-appearing skin that is visible to the patient. Have the patient sit, stand, and bend to select the best site. In general, the optimal location is approximately one-third the distance from the umbilicus to the anterior superior iliac spine. Place the stoma higher in obese individuals so they can see it.

One of the issues with temporary stomas is the *timing of closure* with restoration of gastrointestinal continuity. The underlying problem necessitating creation of the stoma should have been addressed and rectified. There should obviously be no distal obstruction. Anal sphincter mechanisms must be intact and function normally to ensure continence. Traditional teaching dictated that the surgeon wait 60–90 days before attempting closure. The purpose was to allow adequate time for overall recovery of the general physiologic status and adequate anastomotic healing if the temporary ostomy was created for the purpose of "protecting" an anastomosis. This time interval is more empiric than scientific, and no randomized, controlled trials have been conducted that have specifically identified the optimal timing for stomal closure. Certainly there are retrospective data that support ostomy closure prior to this interval without prohibitive complications [102,105,106].

*Loop ileostomies* are temporary stomas often created in the setting of sphincter-preservation procedures for rectal cancer, ulcerative colitis, and familial polyposis. These stomas require careful attention to detail during construction because the relatively high-volume effluent is highly irritating to the skin. In general, a site in the ileum is selected as distal as possible to maintain maximal absorptive surface area of the terminal ileum (the bowel distal to this site becomes effectively defunctionalized). If the loop ileostomy is performed in conjunction with a colorectal or coloanal anastomosis, the loop ileostomy should be placed 8–10 cm proximal to the ileocecal valve to facilitate subsequent closure. The mesentery is not fixed to the parietal peritoneum, thereby facilitating ease of takedown at a later time. A variation of this technique involves complete transection of the intestinal lumen with closure of the distal segment without division of the mesentery; both ends are brought out through the same abdominal wall site.

*Cecostomy*, used frequently in the past, is rarely performed today. Situations in which the procedure should be considered include the following: (1) patients with cecal volvulus at high risk of recurrence in whom resection of the colon is not necessary; and (2) patients with "pseudoobstruction" of the colon (Ogilvie syndrome) in whom an exploratory laparotomy was performed for presumptive mechanical obstruction and none was found or in whom repeated colonoscopies failed to decompress the distended colon and the patient develops signs and findings of impending cecal perforation. The procedure may be indicated during performance of an appendectomy when the wall of the cecum is indurated and friable and resection of the cecum is not otherwise desirable. Finally, it may be useful in the presence of an impending perforation of the cecum secondary to a mechanical obstruction of the colon. When the cecal diameter is more than 10 cm (measured on abdominal radiographs), there is appropriate concern about cecal perforation. If tenderness accompanies this finding, cecal exploration is mandatory to rule out ischemic necrosis of the cecal wall secondary to increased intraluminal pressure. Attempting a decompressing transverse colostomy without cecal evaluation risks a catastrophic perforation in areas of serosal tears and ischemic necrosis.

A cecostomy can be fashioned as a *tube* or a *skin-sutured cecostomy*. A tube cecostomy is more easily and expeditiously performed; and after it is no longer needed, the resulting fistula usually closes spontaneously soon after withdrawing the tube. Conversely, it requires significant nursing care and frequent irrigation and often becomes obstructed by semisolid fecal material. A skin-sutured cecotomy is a better decompressing and cleansing stoma, requiring much less nursing care, although it requires formal surgical closure when it is no longer needed.

*Loop colostomies* are rarely used nowadays. Preference is usually given to the loop ileostomy because of its ease of construction and subsequent closure. The only remaining indication to use of the loop colostomy is probably the bed-ridden patient with an unresectable, obstructing left colon cancer.

The *Kock continent ileostomy* involves complementary construction of a pouch and a continent "nipple valve." This modification obviates the requirement for patients to wear an appliance to collect and contain ileal excretions. Evacuation involves intubation of the pouch by the patient a few times daily.

This operation is attended by many complications that require reoperation (in the range of 15–20% and up to 30% in some large series). As a result, the Kock ileostomy cannot be recommended for general use. This procedure may be considered in patients who are severely opposed to wearing a stomal appliance because of personal preference or peristomal complications and those who have previously undergone total proctocolectomy with a failed ileal pouch/anal procedure. This procedure is contraindicated in those with Crohn's disease and relatively contraindicated if a significant small bowel resection has previously been done, in those over 60 years of age, in obese patients, and in the presence of significant associated psychiatric illness. Furthermore, patients must be highly motivated and well informed about the procedure, its attendant complications, and the significant possibility of additional surgery to rectify complications.

## POSTOPERATIVE CARE

*Nasogastric intubation*, long a mainstay of the postoperative management of patients who undergo large bowel operations, was done on the premise that it served the purpose of gut decompression until bowel function returned. Disadvantages of routine nasogastric intubation include impairment of lower esophageal sphincter function predisposing to gastroesophageal reflux with consequent esophagitis, an increase in nasopharyngeal secretions and risk of developing paranasal sinusitis, and impairment of coughing and pulmonary toilet, which increases the risk of perioperative pulmonary morbidity. Numerous randomized trials have shown no benefit for nasogastric decompression, and this modality is therefore probably best limited to patients who require extensive intraoperative dissection because of adhesions, those who experience nausea, emesis, and abdominal distension during the perioperative period, and the cohort operated on because of intestinal obstruction or sepsis. In the elective setting, postoperative nasogastric decompression is not routinely necessary.

Similarly, the initiation of *postoperative feeding* has changed over the past two decades. Early practice was based, to an extent, on animal studies that illustrated that before the seventh postoperative day the intrinsic tensile strength of a wound was inadequate to withstand a disruptive force. Extrapolating to humans, many believed that it made sense to "rest" an anastomosis of the colon for 5–7 days following an operation. It was believed that any minor imperfection in the anastomosis had an opportunity to heal without resulting in leakage. Current standard practice calls for institution of oral feedings as soon as evidence of bowel function is present (usually normoactive bowel sounds in a nondistended patient who has or has not yet passed flatus or stool). Chronologically, this occurs between the third and fifth postoperative day. Surgical tradition has resulted in institution of clear liquids first, advancing to a general diet based on the patient's ability to "tolerate" the intake (absence of nausea, emesis, or cramping, with passing of flatus and stool). No randomized studies exist to substantiate the efficacy of commencing with a clear liquid diet and advancing it rather than instituting a general diet at the outset of the return of bowel function. Randomized trials have shown that early oral feeding (starting on the first postoperative day) after elective colorectal surgery is safe and generally well tolerated [107,108].

Colorectal surgery generally requires a *postoperative hospital stay* of 5–10 days. Patients were and still are traditionally discharged from the hospital when they are clinically stable and afebrile, able to tolerate an adequate oral intake to maintain hydration and nutritional repletion, have bowel function, and their pain is controlled through oral medications. Many factors hinder discharge: nausea, emesis, ileus, pain, fatigue, and the inability to care for drains, tubes, and ostomies competently. Laparoscopy has failed to reveal a consistent benefit for early discharge. A combination multimodality rehabilitation regimen with early oral nutrition, mobilization, and effective pain relief has reduced hospital stays for colorectal procedures to 2 days [109]. The success of this technique requires a motivated patient and an anesthesia team carefully integrated into the process at all steps. It requires use of epidural anesthesia with limited oral and parenteral narcotics (which contribute to bowel dysmotility) and limitation of crystalloid use intraoperatively to diminish bowel edema, and thus speed the return of function. In our experience this is a safe, efficacious regimen and has far-reaching consequences in costcontainment without sacrificing or compromising patient care.

### Management of Altered Sphincter Function

During convalescence, after restorative proctocolectomies for ulcerative colitis or familial polyposis and after sphincter-saving procedures for rectal cancers, attention is directed at careful evaluation of stool frequency, volume and consistency, urgency, degree of incontinence if present, constipation or difficulty with evacuation, development of anal stenosis, and occurrence of pouchitis. If incontinence occurs, it must be quantitated by recording the number of nocturnal and diurnal episodes, the need to wear a protective pad, and incontinence to flatus, liquid, or solid stools.

*Changes in diet* and administration of drugs to alter intestinal motility may ameliorate the frequency and consistency of bowel movements over time. Incontinence and stool frequency tend to disappear with time. Ileoanal or coloanal stenoses may have to be mechanically dilated under anesthesia to ease difficulty of evacuation. In the absence of a coloanal stenosis, suppositories or Fleet's enemas may be necessary to initiate a bowel movement.

### Urogenital Function

Low pelvic dissections for benign or malignant disease may be associated with complications such as urinary retention, dyspareunia, impotence (secondary to parasympathetic nerve damage), retrograde ejaculation (resulting from sympathetic nerve injury), and the development of rectourethral or rectovaginal fistulas. Preoperatively, a surgeon is well advised to pay careful attention to signs and symptoms of urogenital functional abnormalities.

Meticulous attention to detail during pelvic dissections, particularly for benign diseases that do not require extensive mesorectal resections, prevents the occurrence of some but not all of these complications. Some, such as urinary retention, though relatively frequent, are self-limiting; and resolution occurs with time. Others are more disabling and may severely affect the quality of life. Patients who are candidates for procedures attended by these risks require in-depth counseling to ensure an informed decision.

## CANCER SURVEILLANCE

Most colorectal cancer recurrences (80–85%) occur within the first 2 years of surgical resection for "curative intent" [39]. Up to two-thirds of patients whose lesions were resected for cure develop recurrent disease. Some of these patients may still be cured, particularly those with disease limited to the pelvis and those with isolated hepatic or pulmonary metastases. These patterns of failure have led surgeons to monitor patients closely during the first 2 years. If at 5 years patients are disease-free, the likelihood of recurrence decreases to 5% or less [39]. Many centers advocate patient evaluation every 3–4 months for the first 2–3 years, every 6 months for the remainder of the 5 years, then annually. Complete history and physical examination, stool for Hemoccult testing, hemoglobin and hematocrit levels assessing for anemia, liver function testing, carcinoembryonic antigen (CEA) assay, chest radiography, CT of the abdomen and pelvis, yearly endoscopy, transrectal ultrasonography (rectal cancer), radiolabeled-anti-CEA antibody imaging, and fluorodeoxyglucose positron emission tomography (if the plasma CEA level is rising) have been utilized. The most effective strategy for follow-up remains controversial. Many studies fail to demonstrate a statistically significant increase in survival based on early detection of recurrences, prior to the development of symptomatic disease [39].

## POUCH SURVEILLANCE

*Pouchitis* is the most common long-term morbidity associated with ileal pouch/anal anastomoses [110–113]. For unknown reasons, this condition occurs more frequently in patients who have had ulcerative colitis than in those with familial polyposis; and the incidence is even higher if pancolitis or extraintestinal manifestations were present. Among the many theories to explain this phenomenon are pouch outflow obstruction, stasis and bacterial overgrowth, abnormal mucus secretion, reduced levels of free fatty acids in the pouch, oxygen free radical injury secondary to ischemia, presence of antineutrophil cytoplasmic antibodies, and pouches that are created "too" large [110]. Clinically, patients present with low grade fever, fatigue and malaise, and frequent loose stools or frank diarrhea occasionally with passage of blood or associated with pelvic pain, cramps, and urgency, often with soiling and incontinence. The mucosa becomes inflamed with progression to ulceration in severe cases. In more than 50% of patients the first episode occurs within the first year of surgery, with the initial risk highest during the first 6 months after surgery [111,112].

Therapy often comprises a course of metronidazole or fluoroquinolone antibiotics. Daily dosing may be necessary for chronic pouchitis. If it fails, antiinflammatory agents are used (e.g., steroids or 5-aminosalicylic acid enemas). Approximately 10% of patients with pouchitis become intractable to medical therapy (chronic pouchitis). Follow-up in this cohort should include both endoscopic and histologic evaluation for the development of high-grade dysplasia. If this ensues, pouch removal is necessary because of the high risk of malignancy (particularly if villous atrophy is also noted). Conversion to an endileostomy with pouch removal may also be necessary because of the poor functional results associated with chronic pouchitis [114]. New biologic response-modifying modalities are currently under investigation and may prove to be promising alternatives for nonoperative management of this entity [115].

## REFERENCES

1. Roberts PL, Veidenheimer MC. Current management of diverticulitis. Adv Surg 1994;27:189.
2. Ferzoco LB, Raptopoulos V, Silen W. Acute diverticulitis. N Engl J Med 1998;338:1521.
3. Smith TR, Cho KC, Morehouse HT, et al. Comparison of computed tomography and contrast enema evaluation of diverticulitis. Dis Colon Rectum 1990; 33:1.
4. Schecter S, Mulvey J, Eisenstat TE. Management of uncomplicated acute diverticulitis: results of a survey. Dis Colon Rectum 1999;42:470.
5. Eusebio EB, Eisenberg MM. Natural history of diverticular disease of the colon in young patients. Am J Surg 1973;125:308.
6. Parker BM, Obeid FN, Sorensen VJ, et al. The management of massive lower gastrointestinal bleeding. Am Surg 1993;9:676.
7. Ballantyne GH, Brandner MD, Beart RW Jr, et al. Volvulus of the colon: incidence and mortality. Ann Surg 1985;202:83.
8. Bower TC, Ischemic colitis. Surg Clin North Am 1993;73:1037.
9. Gandhi SK, Hanson MM, Vernava AM, et al. Ischemic colitis. Dis Colon Rectum 1996;39:88.
10. Kim DS, Tsang CBS, Wong WD, et al. Complete rectal prolapse: evolution of management and results. Dis Colon Rectum 1999;42:460.
11. Madoff RD, Mellgren A. One hundred years of rectal prolapse surgery. Dis Colon Rectum 1999;42:441.
12. Altemeier WA, Culbertson WR, Schowengerdt C, et al. Nineteen years experience with the one-stage perineal repair of rectal prolapse. Ann Surg 1971;173: 993.
13. Kinzler KW, Nilbert MC, Su L-K, et al. Identification of FAP locus genes from chromosome 5q21. Science 1991;253:661.
14. Kartheuser AN, Parc R, Penna CP, et al. Ileal pouchanal anastomosis as the first choice operation in patients with familial adenomatous polyposis: a tenyear experience. Surgery 1996;119:615.
15. Michelassi F. Indications for surgical treatment in ulcerative colitis and Crohn's disease. In Michelassi F, Milsom JW (eds) Operative Strategies in Inflammatory Bowel Disease. New York, Springer-Verlag, 1999, pp 150–153.
16. Heppell J, Farkouh E, Dube S, et al. Toxic megacolon: an analysis of 70 cases. Dis Colon Rectum 1986;29: 789.
17. McLeod RS. Resection margins and recurrent Crohn's disease. Hepatogastroenterology 1990;37:63.
18. Heimann TM, Greenstein AJ, Lewis B, et al. Prediction of early symptomatic recurrence after intestinal resection in Crohn's disease. Ann Surg 1993;218:294.
19. Farouk R, Pemberton JH. Surgical options in ulcerative colitis. Surg Clin North Am 1997;77:85.
20. Milsom JW. Restorative proctocolectomy with ileoanal anastomosis. In Michelassi F, Milsom JW (eds) Operative Strategies in Inflammatory Bowel Disease. New York, Springer-Verlag, 1999, pp 173–183.
21. Gemlo BT, Wong WD, Rothenberger DA, et al. Ileal pouch-anal anastomosis: patterns of failure. Arch Surg 1992;127:784.
22. Fazio VW, Ziv Y, Church JM, et al. Ileal pouch-anal anastomoses complications and function in 1005 patients. Ann Surg 1995;222:120.
23. Miller R, Bartolo DC, Orrom WJ, et al. Improvement of anal sensation with preservation of the anal transition zone after ileoanal anastomosis for ulcerative colitis. Dis Colon Rectum 1990;33:414.
24. McIntyre PB, Pemberton JH, Beart RW, et al. Double-stapled vs. hand-sewn ileal pouch-anal anastomosis in patients with chronic ulcerative colitis. Dis Colon Rectum 1994;37:430.
25. Luukkonen P, Jarvinen HJ. Stapled vs. hand-sutured ileoanal anastomosis in restorative proctocolectomy: a prospective, randomized study. Arch Surg 1993; 128:437.
26. Gozzetti G, Poggioli G, Marchetti F, et al. Functional outcome in hand-sewn vs. stapled ileal pouch-anal anastomosis. Am J Surg 1994;168:325.
27. Khubchandani IT, Kontostolis SB. Outcome of ileorectal anastomosis in an inflammatory bowel disease surgery experience of three decades. Arch Surg 1994;129:866.
28. Longo WE, Oakley JR, Laverly IC, et al. Outcome of ileorectal anastomosis for Crohn's colitis. Dis Colon Rectum 1992;35:1066.
29. Ekbom A, Helmick C, Zack M, et al. Ulcerative colitis and colorectal cancer: a population-based study. N Engl J Med 1990;323:1228.
30. Pinczowski D, Ekbom A, Baron J, et al. Risk factors for colorectal cancer in patients with ulcerative colitis: a case-control study. Gastroenterology 1994; 107:117.
31. Taylor BA, Pemberton JH, Carpenter HA, et al. Dysplasia in chronic ulcerative colitis: implications for colonoscopic surveillance. Dis Colon Rectum 1992; 35:950.
32. Ziv Y, Fazio VW, Church JM, et al. Safety of urgent restorative proctocolectomy with ileal pouch-anal anastomosis for fulminant colitis. Dis Colon Rectum 1995;38:345.
33. Price AB. Overlap in the spectrum of nonspecific inflammatory bowel disease—"colitis indeterminate." J Clin Pathol 1978;31:567.

34. McIntyre PB, Pemberton JH, Wolff BG, et al. Indeterminate colitis: long-term outcome in patients after ileal pouch-anal anastomosis. Dis Colon Rectum 1995;38:51.
35. Stein BL, Coller JA. Management of malignant colorectal polyps. Surg Clin North Am 1993;73:47.
36. Cooper HS, Deppisch LM, Gourly WK, et al. Endoscopically removed malignant colorectal polyps: clinicopathologic correlations. Gastroenterology 1995; 108:1657.
37. Haggitt RC, Glotzbach RE, Soffer EE, et al. Prognostic factors in colorectal carcinomas arising in adenomas: implications for lesions removed by endoscopic polypectomy. Gastroenterology 1985;89:328.
38. Nivatvongs S, Rojanasakul A, Reiman HM, et al. The risk of lymph node metastases in colorectal polyps with invasive adenocarcinoma. Dis Colon Rectum 1991;34:323.
39. Laverly IC, Lopez-Kostner F, Pelley RJ, et al. Treatment of colon and rectal cancer. Surg Clin North Am 2000;80:535.
40. Hautefeuille P, Valleur P, Perniceni T. Functional and oncologic results after coloanal anastomosis for low rectal carcinoma. Ann Surg 1988;207:61.
41. Bat L, Neumann G, Shemesh E. The association of synchronous neoplasm with occluding colorectal cancer. Dis Colon Rectum 1985;28:149.
42. Kahn H, Alexander A, Rakinic J, et al. Preoperative staging of irradiated rectal cancers using digital rectal examination, computed tomography, endorectal ultrasound, and magnetic resonance imaging does not accurately predict T0,N0 pathology. Dis Colon Rectum 1997;40:140.
43. Fisher B, Wolmark N, Rockette H, et al. Postoperative adjuvant chemotherapy or radiation therapy for rectal cancer: results from the NSABP protocol R-01. J Natl Cancer Inst 1988;90:21.
44. Jessup JM, Bothe A, Stone MD, et al. Preservation of sphincter function in rectal carcinoma by a multimodality treatment approach. Surg Oncol Clin North Am 1992;1:137.
45. Papillon J, Gerard JP. Role of radiotherapy in anal preservation for cancer of the lower third of the rectum. Int J Radiat Oncol Biol Phys 1990;19:1219.
46. Minsky BD, Cohen AM, Enker WE, et al. Combined modality therapy of rectal cancer: decreased acute toxicity with the preoperative approach. J Clin Oncol 1992;10:1218.
47. Hyams DM, Mamounas EP, Petrelli N, et al. A clinical trial to evaluate the worth of preoperative multimodality therapy in patients with operable carcinoma of the rectum: a progress report of the national surgical breast and bowel project protocol r-03. Dis Colon Rectum 1997;40:131.
48. Bernini A, Deen KI, Madoff RD, et al. Preoperative adjuvant radiation with chemotherapy for rectal cancer: its impact on stage of disease and the role of endorectal ultrasound. Ann Surg Oncol 1996;3:131.
49. Shumate CR, Rich TA, Skibber JM, et al. Preoperative chemotherapy and radiation therapy for locally advanced primary and recurrent rectal carcinoma. A report of surgical morbidity. Cancer 1993;71:3690.
50. Minsky BD. Sphincter preservation in rectal cancer. Preoperative radiation therapy followed by low anterior resection with coloanal anastomosis. Semin Radiat Oncol 1998;8:30.
51. Mendenhall WM, Bland KI, Copeland EM III, et al. Does preoperative radiation therapy enhance the probability of local control and survival in high-risk distal rectal cancer? Ann Surg 1992;215:696.
52. Vauthey JN, Marsh RW, Zlotecki RA, et al. Recent advances in the treatment and outcome of locally advanced rectal cancer. Ann Surg 1999;229:745.
53. Wagman R, Minsky BD, Cohen AM, et al. Sphincter preservation in rectal cancer with preoperative radiation therapy and coloanal anastomosis: long term follow-up. Int J Radiat Oncol Biol Phys 1998;42:51.
54. Francois Y, Nemoz CJ, Baulieux J, et al. Influence of the interval between preoperative radiation therapy and surgery on downstaging and on the rate of sphincter-sparing surgery for rectal cancer: the Lyon R90–01 randomized trial. J Clin Oncol 1999;17: 2396.
55. Cho CC, Taylor CW III, Padmanabhan A, et al. Squamous cell carcinoma of the anal canal: management with combined chemoradiation therapy. Dis Colon Rectum 1991;34:675.
56. Nigro ND. The force of change in the management of squamous-cell cancer of the anal canal. Dis Colon Rectum 1991;34:482.
57. Franklin M, Rosenthal D, Abrego-Medina D, et al. Prospective comparison of open vs. laparoscopic colon surgery for carcinoma. Dis Colon Rectum 1996;39(suppl):35.
58. Milsom J, Bohm B, Hammermofer K, et al. A prospective, randomized trial comparing laparoscopic versus conventional techniques in colorectal cancer surgery: a preliminary report. J Am Coll Surg 1998; 187:46.
59. Philips EH, Franklin M, Caroll BJ, et al. Laparoscopic colectomy. Ann Surg 1992;216:703.
60. Puente I, Sosa JL, Sleeman D, et al. Laparoscopicassisted colorectal surgery. J Laparoendosc Surg 1994; 4:1.
61. Stage J, Schulze S, Moller P, et al. Prospective randomized study of laparoscopic versus open colonic resection for adenocarcinoma. Br J Surg 1997;84:391.
62. Talac R, Nelson H. Laparoscopic colon and rectal surgery. Surg Clin North Am 2000;9:1.
63. Eijsbouts QAJ, Heuff G, Sietses C, et al. Laparoscopic surgery in the treatment of colonic polyps. Br J Surg 1999;86:505.
64. Larach SW, Patankar SK, Ferrara A, et al. Complications of laparoscopic colorectal surgery: analysis and comparison of early vs. latter experience. Dis Colon Rectum 1997;40:592.

65. Kockerling F, Schneider C, Reymond MA, et al. Early results of a prospective multicenter study on 500 consecutive cases of laparoscopic colorectal surgery: laparoscopic colorectal surgery study group. Surg Endosc 1998;12:37.
66. Franklin ME Jr, Dorman JP, Jacobs M, et al. Is laparoscopic surgery applicable to complicated colonic diverticular disease? Surg Endosc 1997;11:1021.
67. Muckleroy SK, Ratzer ER, Fenoglio ME. Laparoscopic colon surgery for benign disease: a comparison to open surgery. J Soc Laparoendosc Surg 1999;3:33.
68. Sardinha TC, Wexner SD. Laparoscopy for inflammatory bowel disease: pros and cons. World J Surg 1998;22:370.
69. Heintz A, Morschel M, Jumginger T. Comparison of results after transanal endoscopic microsurgery and radical resection for T1 carcinoma of the rectum. Surg Endosc 1998;12:1145.
70. Saclarides TJ. Transanal endoscopic microsurgery: a single surgeon's experience. Arch Surg 1998;133: 595.
71. Winde G, Nottberg H, Keller R, et al. Surgical cure for early rectal carcinomas (T1): transanal endoscopic microsurgery vs. anterior resection. Dis Colon Rectum 1996;39:969.
72. Kreis ME, Jehle EC, Haug V, et al. Functional results after transanal endoscopic microsurgery. Dis Colon Rectum 1996;39:1116.
73. Smith LE, Ko ST, Saclarides T, et al. Transanal endoscopic microsurgery: initial registry results. Dis Colon Rectum 1996;39(suppl):79.
74. Salvati EP, Rubin RJ, Eisenstat TE, et al. Electrocoagulation of selected carcinoma of the rectum. Surg Gynecol Obstet 1988;166:393.
75. Papillon J. Intracavitary irradiation of early rectal cancer for cure: a series of 186 cases. Dis Colon Rectum 1994;37:88.
76. Papillon J. Surgical adjuvant therapy for rectal cancer: present options. Dis Colon Rectum 1994;37:144.
77. Turnbull RB, et al. Cancer of the colon: the influence of the no-touch isolation technique on survival rates. Ann Surg 1967;166:420.
78. Lau PW, Lo CY, Law WL. The role of one stage surgery in acute left-sided colonic obstruction. Am J Surg 1995;169:406.
79. MacKenzie S, Thomson SR, Baker LW. Management options in malignant obstruction of the left colon. Surg Gynecol Obstet 1992;174:337.
80. Naraynsingh V, Rampayl R, Maharaj D, et al. Prospective study of primary anastomosis without colonic lavage for patients with an obstructed left colon. Br J Surg 1999;86:1341.
81. Nyam DCNK, Seow Choen F, Leong AFPK, et al. Colonic decompression without on-table irrigation for obstructing left-sided colorectal tumours. Br J Surg 1996;83:786.
82. Forloni B, Reduzzi R, Paludetti A, et al. Intraoperative colonic lavage in emergency surgical treatment of left-sided colonic obstruction. Dis Colon Rectum 1998;41:23.
83. Kressner U, Autonsson J, Ejerblad S, et al. Intraoperative colonic lavage and primary anastomosis and alternative to Hartmann procedure in emergency surgery of the left colon. Eur J Surg 1994;160:287.
84. Murray JJ, Schoetz DJ, Coller JA, et al. Intraoperative colonic lavage and primary anastomosis in nonelective colon resection. Dis Colon Rectum 1991;34:527.
85. Rey JF, Romanczyk MG. Metal stents for palliation of rectal carcinoma: a preliminary report on 12 patients. Endoscopy 1995;27:501.
86. Saida Y, Sumiyama Y, Nagao J, et al. Stent endoprosthesis for obstructing colorectal cancers. Dis Colon Rectum 1996;39:552.
87. Mainar A, DeGregorio Ariza MA, Tejero E, et al. Acute colorectal obstruction: treatment with self-expandable metallic stent scheduled surgery: results of a multicenter study. Radiology 1999;210:65.
88. Binkert CA, Ledermann H, Jost R, et al. Acute colonic obstruction: clinical aspects and cost-effectiveness of preoperative palliative treatment with self-expanding metallic stents: a preliminary report. Radiology 1998; 206:199.
89. Akle CA. Endoprostheses for colonic strictures. Br J Surg 1998;85:310.
90. O'Leary DP. Use of the greater omentum in colorectal surgery. Dis Colon Rectum 1999;42:533.
91. Del Rio JV, Beck DE, Opelka FG. Chronic perioperative steroids and colonic anastomosis healing in rats. J Surg Res 1996;66:138.
92. Eubanks TR, Greenberg JJ, Dobrin PB, et al. The effects of different corticosteroids on the healing colonic anastomosis and cecum in a rat model. Am Surg 1997;63:266.
93. Furst MB, Stromber BV, Blatchford GJ, et al. Colonic anastomoses: bursting strength after corticosteroid treatment. Dis Colon Rectum 1994;37:12.
94. Ziv Y, Church JM, Fazio VW, et al. Effect of systemic steroids on ileal pouch-anal anastomosis in patients with ulcerative colitis. Dis Colon Rectum 1996;39: 504.
95. Cali RL, Ssmyrk TC, Blatchford GJ, et al. Effect of prostaglandin E1 and steroid on healing colonic anastomoses. Dis Colon Rectum 1993;36:1148.
96. Ruiz PL, Facciuto EM, Facciuto ME, et al. New intraluminal bypass tube for management of acutely obstructed left colon. Dis Colon Rectum 1995;38: 1108.
97. Yoon WH, Song IS, Chang ES. Intraluminal bypass technique using a condom for protection of coloanal anastomosis. Dis Colon Rectum 1994;37:1046.
98. Michelassi F, Takanishi D, McLeod RS, et al. Ileal reservoirs. In Michelassi F, Milsom JW (eds) Operative Strategies in Inflammatory Bowel Disease. New York, Springer-Verlag, 1999, pp 186–214.
99. Joo JS, Latulippe JF, Alabaz O, et al. Long-term functional evaluation of straight coloanal anastomosis and

colonic J-pouch: is the functional superiority of colonic J-pouch sustained? Dis Colon Rectum 1998; 41:740.

100. Dehni N, Tiret E, Singland JD, et al. Long-term functional outcome after low anterior resection: comparison of low colorectal anastomosis and colonic J-pouch-anal anastomosis. Dis Colon Rectum 1998;41: 817.
101. Read TE, Kodner IJ. Protectomy and coloanal anastomosis for rectal cancer. Arch Surg 1999;134:670.
102. Shellito PC. Complications of abdominal stoma surgery. Dis Colon Rectum 1998;41:1562.
103. Feinberg SM, McLeod RS, Cohen Z. Complications of loop ileostomy. Am J Surg 1987;153:102.
104. Bass EM, Del Pino A, Tan A, et al. Does preoperative stoma marking and education by the enterostomal therapist affect outcome? Dis Colon Rectum 1997; 40:440.
105. Parks SE, Hastings PR. Complications of colostomy closure. Am J Surg 1985;149:672.
106. Hull TL, Kobe I, Fazio VW. Comparison of handsewn with stapled loop ileostomy closures. Dis Colon Rectum 1996;39:1086.
107. Reissman P, Teoh TA, Cohen SM, et al. Is early oral feeding safe after elective colorectal surgery? A prospective randomized trial. Ann Surg 1995;222:73.
108. Nessim A, Wexner SD, Agachan F, et al. Is bowel confinement necessary after anorectal reconstructive surgery? A prospective randomized, surgeonblinded trial. Dis Colon Rectum 1999;42:16.
109. Kehlet H, Mogensen T. Hospital stay of 2 days after open sigmoidectomy with a multimodal rehabilitation programme. Br J Surg 1999;86:227.
110. Mignon M, Stettler C, Phillips SF. Pouchitis—a poorly understood entity. Dis Colon Rectum 1995;38:100.
111. Stahlberg D, Gullberg K, Liljeqvist L, et al. Pouchitis following pelvic pouch operation for ulcerative colitis: incidence, cumulative risk, and risk factors. Dis Colon Rectum 1996;39:1012.
112. Hurst RD, Molinari M, Chung TP, et al. Prospective study of the incidence, timing, and treatment of pouchitis in 104 consecutive patients after restorative proctocolectomy. Arch Surg 1996;131:497.
113. Nicholls RJ, Banerjee AK. Pouchitis: risk factors, etiology, and treatment. World J Surg 1998;22:347.
114. Keranen U, Luukkonen P, Jarvinen H. Functional results after restorative proctocolectomy complicated by pouchitis. Dis Colon Rectum 1997;40:764.
115. Sandborn WJ, McLeod R, Jewell DP. Medical therapy for induction and maintenance of remission in pouchitis: a systematic review. Inflamm Bowel Dis 1999; 5:33.

# 2 Right Colectomy for Cancer

## INDICATIONS

Malignancy of the ileocecal region, ascending colon, and transverse colon

## PREOPERATIVE PREPARATION

Colonoscopy to confirm the diagnosis and exclude other pathology

Computed tomography (CT) of abdomen

Mechanical and antibiotic bowel preparation

Perioperative antibiotics

## PITFALLS AND DANGER POINTS

Injury or inadvertent ligature of superior mesenteric vessels

Laceration of retroperitoneal duodenum

Trauma to right ureter

Avulsion of branch between inferior pancreaticoduodenal and middle colic veins

Failure of anastomosis

## OPERATIVE STRATEGY

The extent of the resection depends on the location of the tumor. For tumors of the cecum, the main trunk of the middle colic artery may be preserved **(Fig. 2–1)**. For tumors of the hepatic flexure or right transverse colon, it is necessary to ligate this vessel and resect additional colon **(Figs. 2–2, 2–3)**.

There are several anatomic advantages to the "no touch technique" described here, although the oncologic advantages are still debated. First, a dissection initiated at the origins of the middle colic and ileocolic vessels makes it possible to perform a more complete lymph node dissection in these two critical areas. Second, by devoting full attention to the lymphovascular pedicles early during the operation, before the anatomy has been distorted by traction *384 Right Colectomy for Cancer* or bleeding, the surgeon gains thorough knowledge of the anatomic variations that may occur in the vasculature of the colon. Finally, the surgeon becomes adept at performing the most dangerous step of this procedure—high ligation of the ileocolic vessels—without traumatizing the superior mesenteric artery and vein.

In most cases when the vascular pedicles are ligated close to their points of origin, it can be seen that the right colon is supplied by two vessels: the ileocolic trunk and the middle colic artery. The middle colic artery generally divides early in its course into right and left branches. The left branch forms a well developed marginal artery that connects with the left colic artery at the splenic flexure. When the proximal half of the transverse colon is removed, the left colic connection of this marginal artery supplies the remaining transverse colon. *Rarely*, a patient does not have good arterial flow from the divided marginal artery. In such a case the splenic flexure and sometimes the descending and sigmoid colon may have to be resected.

After the two major lymphovascular pedicles have been divided and ligated, the remainder of the mesentery to the right colon and the mesentery to the distal segment of the ileum should be divided. If occluding clamps are applied to the anticipated points of transection of the transverse colon and the ileum at this time, the entire specimen can be seen to be isolated from any vascular connection with the patient. This is all done before there is any manipulation of the tumor—hence the "no touch" technique. The specimen may now be removed by the traditional method of incising the peritoneum in the right paracolic gutter and elevating the right colon.

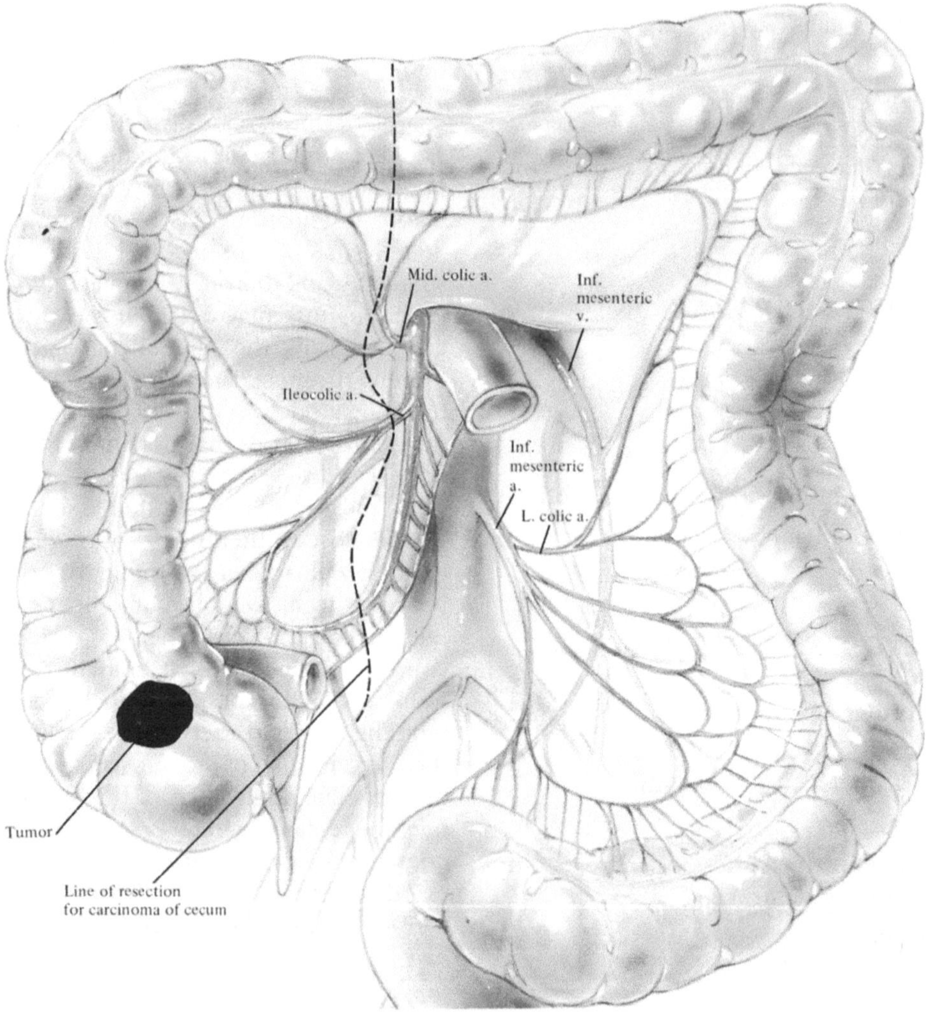
Mid. colic a.
Inf.
mesenteric
v.
Ileocolic a.
Inf.
mesenteric
a.
L. colic a.
Tumor
Line of resection
for carcinoma of cecum

Fig. 2–1

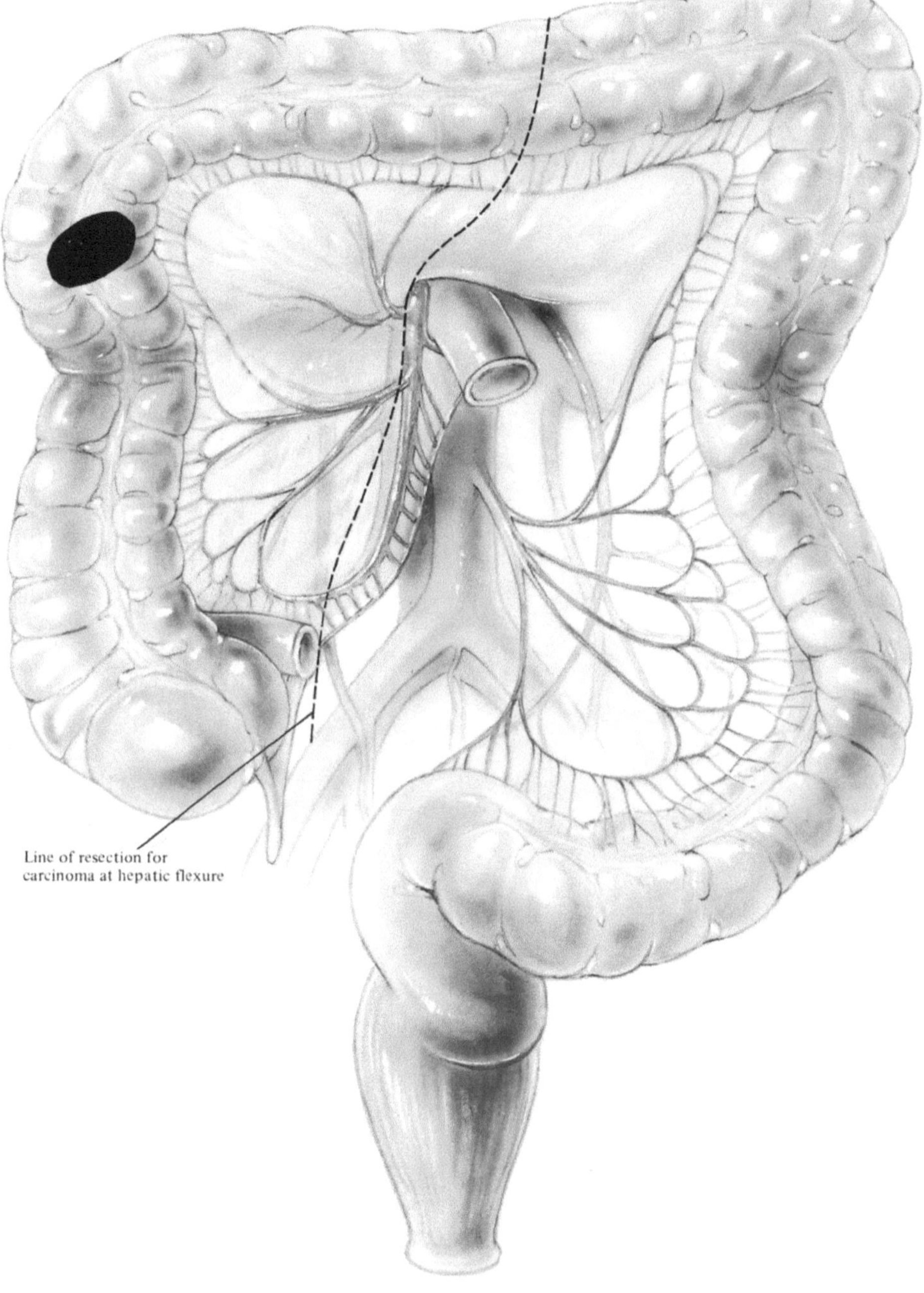


Fig. 2–2

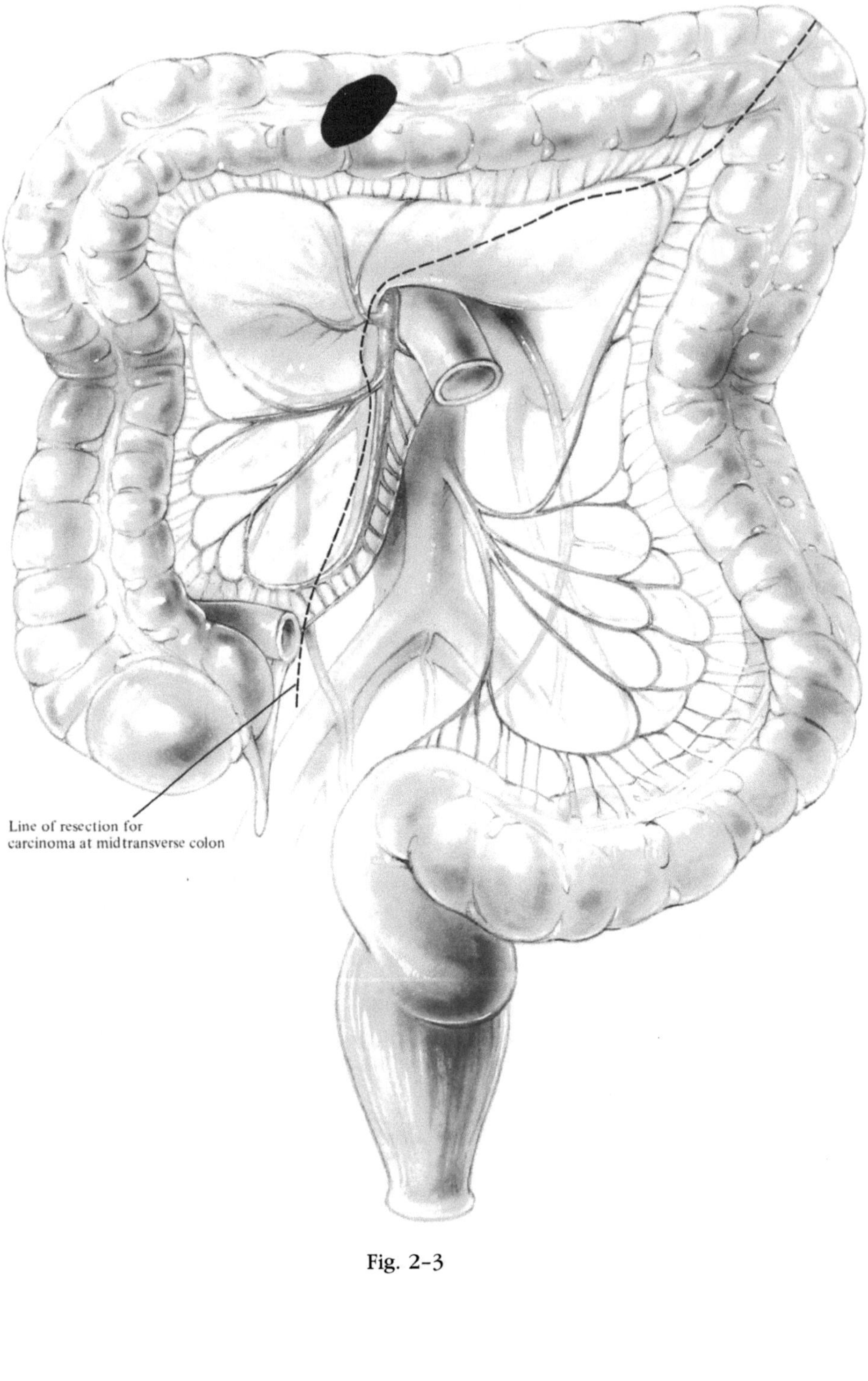


Fig. 2-3

# OPERATIVE TECHNIQUE (Right and Transverse Colectomy)

## Incision

Make a midline incision from the mid-epigastrium to a point about 8 cm below the umbilicus. Explore the abdomen for hepatic, pelvic, peritoneal, and nodal metastases. A solitary hepatic metastasis may well be resected at the same time the colectomy is performed. A moderate degree of hepatic metastasis is not a contraindication to removing a locally resectable colon carcinoma. Inspect the primary tumor but avoid manipulating it at this stage.

## Ligature of Colon Proximal and Distal to Tumor

Insert a blunt Mixter right-angle clamp through an avascular portion of the mesentery close to the colon, distal to the tumor, and draw a 3 mm umbilical tape through this puncture in the mesentery. Tie the umbilical tape firmly to occlude the lumen of the colon completely. Carry out an identical maneuver at a point on the terminal ileum, thereby completely occluding the lumen proximal and distal to the tumor.

## Omental Dissection

For a carcinoma located in the hepatic flexure, divide the adjacent omentum between serially applied Kelly hemostats just distal to the gastroepiploic arcade of the stomach **(Fig. 2–4)**. If the neoplasm is located in the cecum, there appears to be no merit in resecting the omentum. The omentum may be dissected (with scalpel and Metzenbaum scissors) off the right half of the transverse colon through the avascular plane, resecting only portions adhering to the cecal tumor. After this has been accomplished, with the transverse colon drawn in a caudal direction the middle colic vessels can be seen as they emerge from the lower border of the pancreas to cross over the retroperitoneal duodenum.

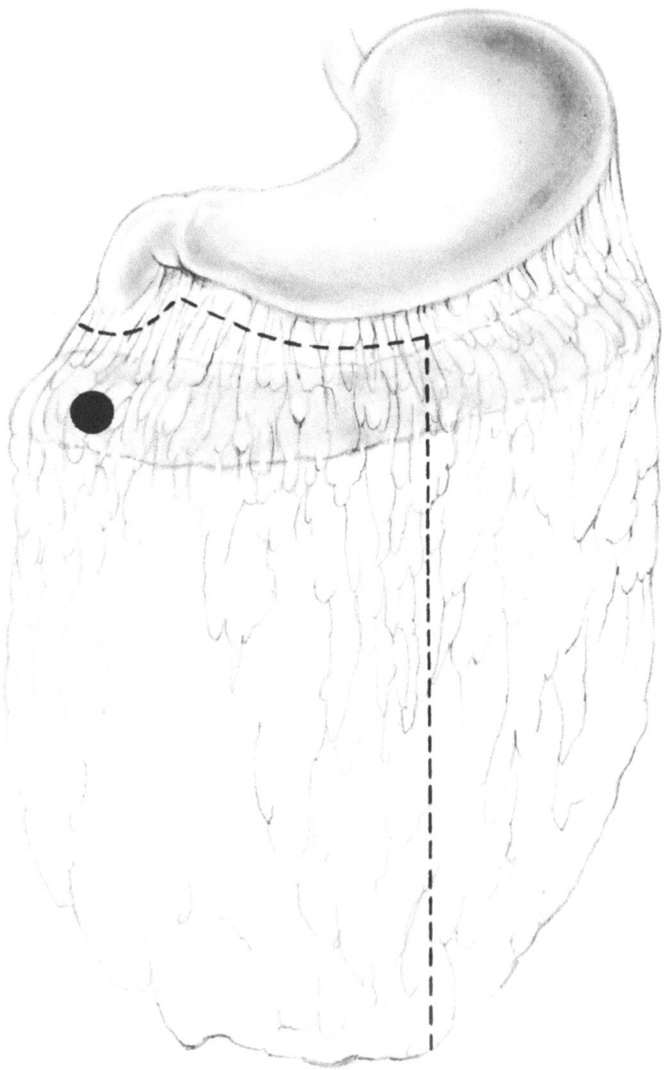

Fig. 2–4

## Division of Middle Colic Vessels

During operations for carcinoma of the cecum and the proximal 5–7 cm of the ascending colon, it is not necessary to divide the middle colic vessels before they branch (Fig. 2–1). The left branch of the middle colic vessel may be preserved and the right branch divided and ligated just beyond the bifurcation **(Fig. 2–5)**.

During operations for tumors near the hepatic flexure of the transverse colon, dissect the middle colic vessels up to the lower border of the pancreas (Figs. 2–2, 2–3, **2–6**). Be careful not to avulse a fairly large collateral branch that connects the inferior pancreaticoduodenal vein with the middle colic vein **(Fig. 2–7)**. If this is torn, considerable bleeding follows, as the proximal end of the pancreaticoduodenal vein retracts and is difficult to locate. Gentle dissection is necessary, as these structures are fragile. Place a Mixter clamp deep to the middle colic vessels at the appropriate point; then draw a 2-0 silk ligature around the vessels and ligate them. Sweep any surrounding lymph nodes down toward the specimen and place a second ligature 1.5 cm distal to the first. Divide the vessels 1 cm beyond the proximal ligature.

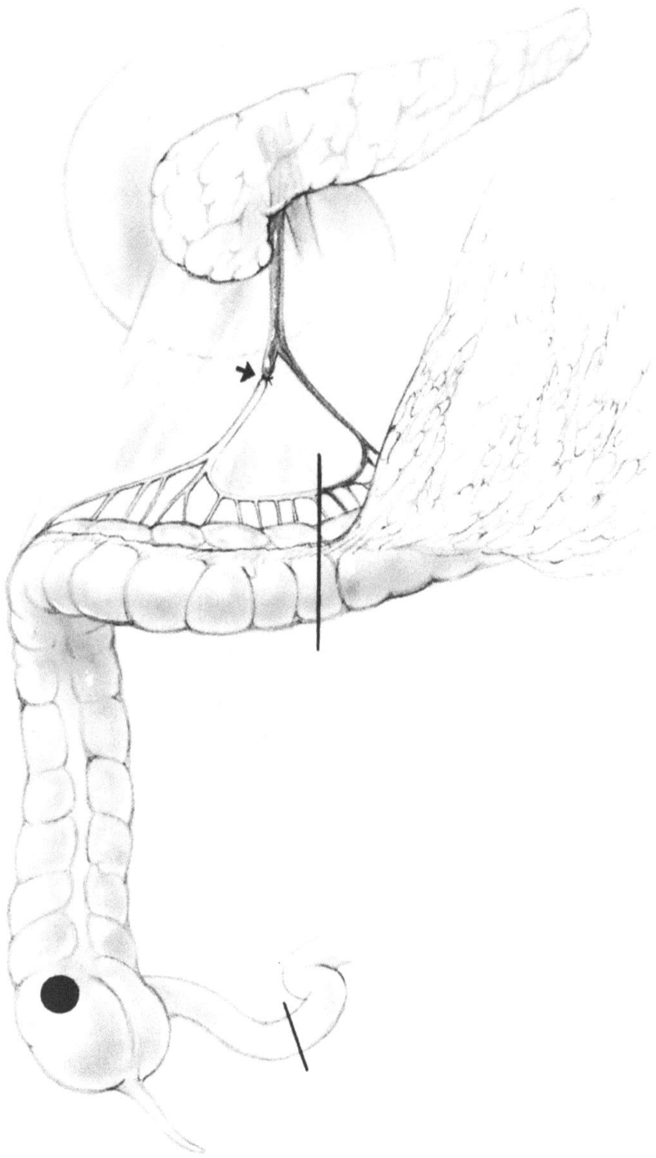

Fig. 2-5

Divide the mesocolon toward the point on the transverse colon already selected for division. Divide and ligate the marginal artery and clear the transverse colon of fat and areolar tissue in preparation for an anastomosis. Now apply an Allen clamp to the transverse colon, but to minimize bacterial contamination of the abdominal cavity do not transect the colon at this time.

## Division of Ileocolic Vessels

Retract the transverse colon in a cephalad direction. Pass the left index finger deep to the right mesocolon **(Fig. 2–8)**, inserting the finger through the incision already made in the transverse mesocolon. Gentle finger dissection should disclose, in front of the fingertip, a fairly large artery with vigorous pulsation; it is the ileocolic arterial trunk (Fig. 2–8). As the surgeon's index finger moves toward the patient's left, it palpates the adjacent superior mesenteric artery. After identifying these two major vessels, it is a simple matter to incise the peritoneum overlying the ileocolic artery with Metzenbaum scissors. By gentle dissection, remove areolar and lymphatic tissue from the circumference of the ileocolic artery and vein. After rechecking the location of the superior mesenteric vessels, pass a blunt Mixter right-angle clamp underneath the ileocolic artery and vein. Ligate the

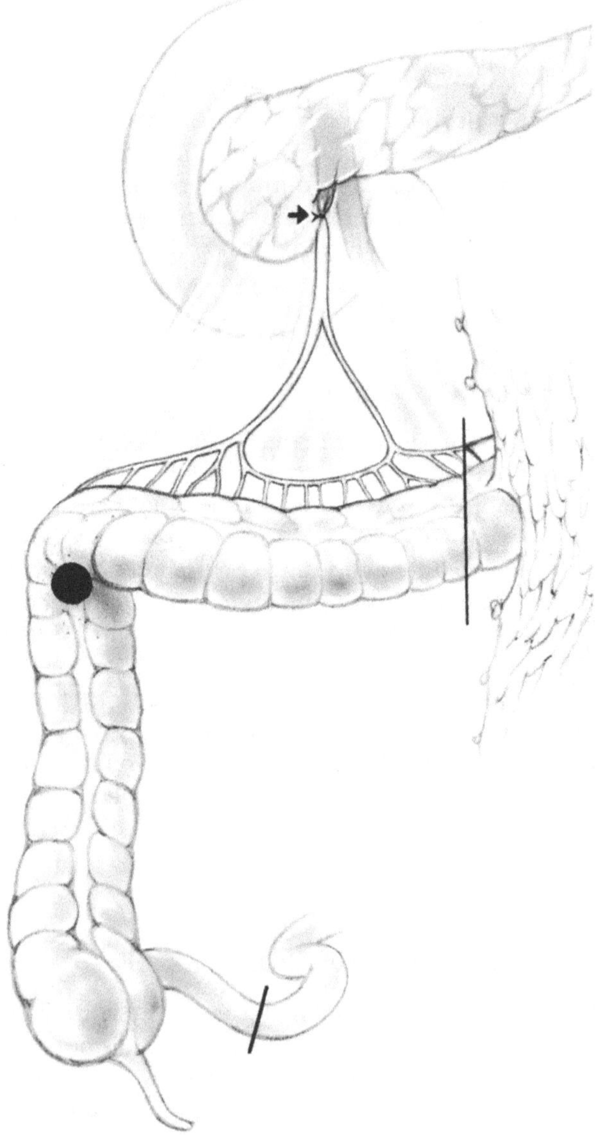

Fig. 2-6

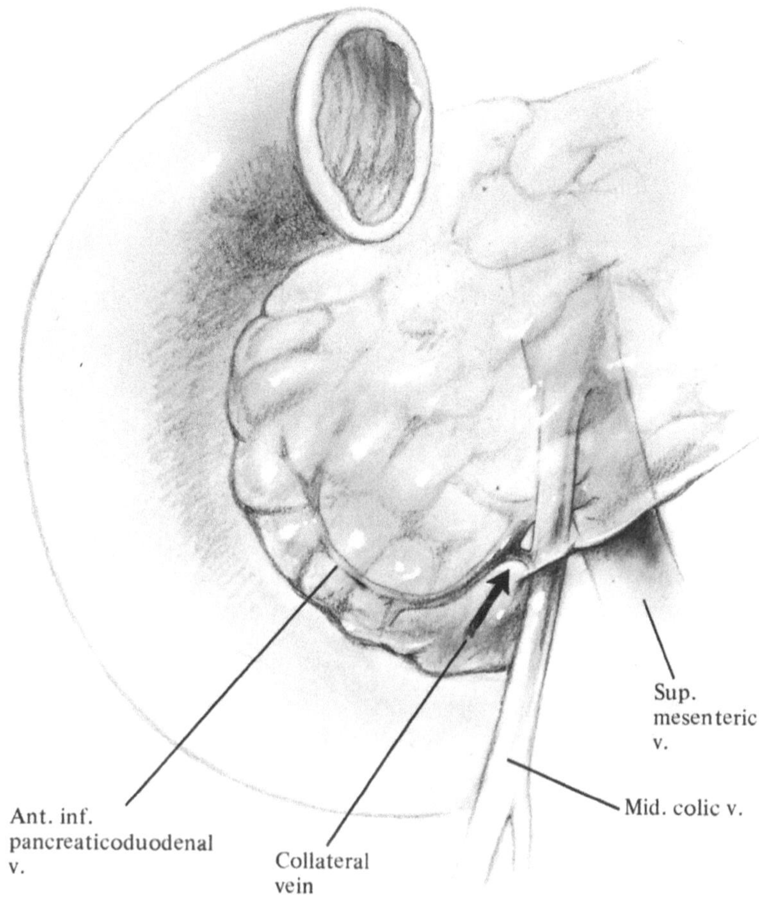


Fig. 2–7

vessels individually with 2-0 silk ligatures and divide them at a point about 1.5 cm distal to their junctions with the superior mesenteric vessels.

## Division of Ileal Mesentery

Pass the left index finger behind the remaining right mesocolon into an avascular area of 3–4 cm. This can be divided and leads to the mesentery of the terminal ileum. For neoplasms close to the ileocecal junction, include 10–15 cm of ileum in the specimen.

For tumors near the hepatic flexure, no more than 8–10 cm of ileum need be resected. In any case, divide the ileal mesentery between Crile hemostats applied serially until the wall of the ileum has been encountered. After ligating each of the hemostats with 3-0 or 2-0 PG, clear the areolar tissue from the circumference of the ileum in preparation for an anastomosis and apply an Allen clamp to this area. At this point the specimen has been isolated from any vascular connection with the host.

## Division of Right Paracolic Peritoneum

Retract the right colon in a medical direction and make an incision in the peritoneum of the paracolic gutter (Fig. 2–8). The left index finger may be inserted deep to this layer of peritoneum, which should then be transected over the index finger with Metzenbaum scissors or electrocautery. Continue this dissection until the hepatic flexure is free of lateral attachments. Rough dissection around the retroperitoneal duodenum may lacerate it inadvertently, so be aware of its location. Next, identify the right renocolic ligament and divide it by Metzenbaum dissection. When this is accomplished, the fascia of Gerota and the perirenal fat may be gently swept from the posterior aspect of the right mesocolon. Continue

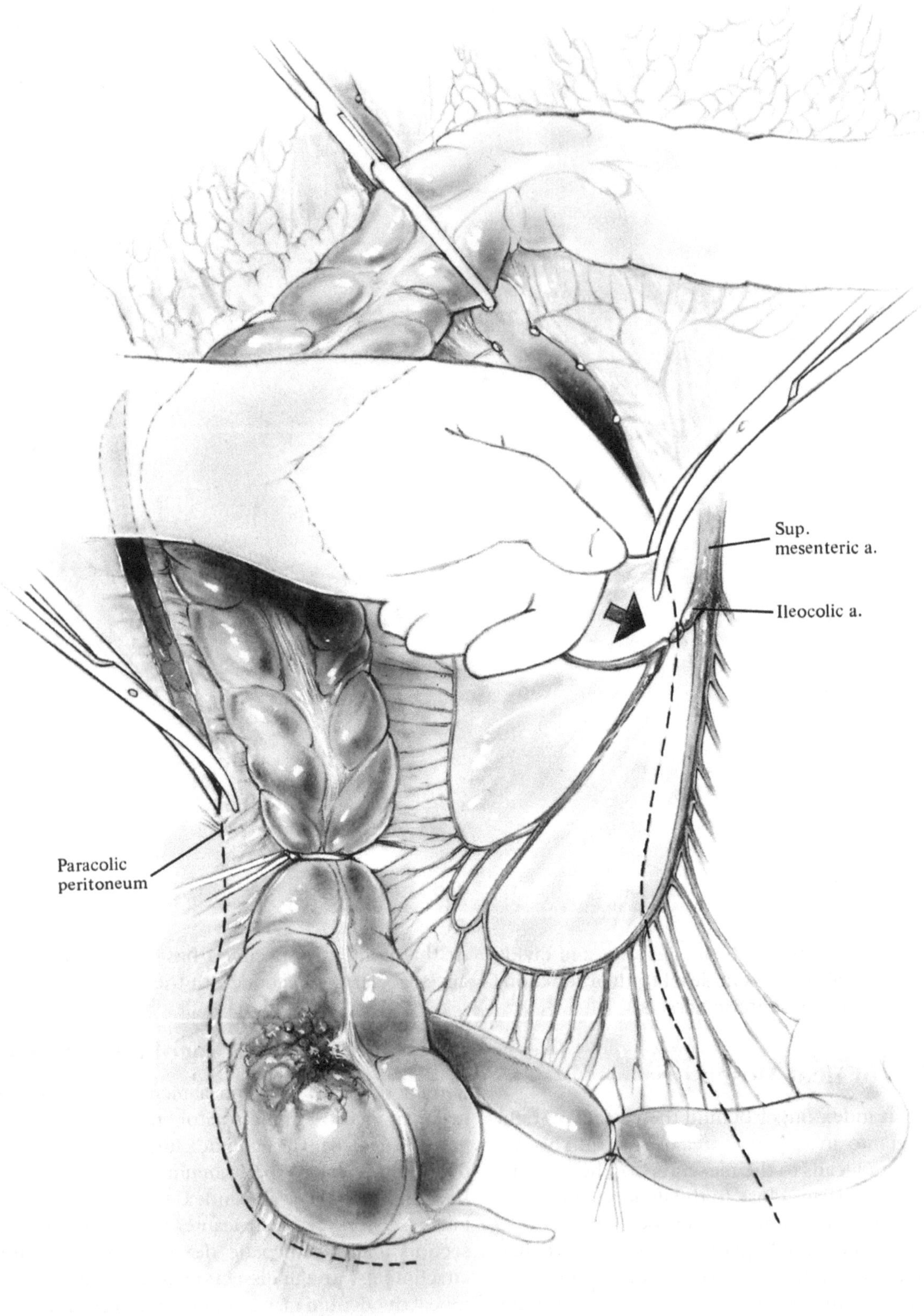


Fig. 2-8

this dissection caudally, eventually unroofing the ureter and gonadal vessel.

## Identification of Ureter

If the location of the ureter is not immediately evident, identify the right common iliac artery. The undisturbed ureter generally crosses the common iliac artery where it bifurcates into its internal and external branches. If the ureter is not in this location, elevate the lateral leaflet of the peritoneum, as the ureter may be adhering to the undersurface of this peritoneal flap. The ureter is often displaced by retraction of the peritoneal flap to which it adheres. If the ureter is not present on the lateral leaflet of peritoneum, similarly elevate and seek it on the medial leaflet of the peritoneum. Typical ureteral peristalsis should occur when the ureter is compressed with forceps.

The right colon remains attached to the peritoneum now only at the inferior and medial aspects of the cecum and ileum. There should be no difficulty dividing it.

## Division of Ileum and Colon

Protect the abdomen with large gauze pads and remove the specimen and the Allen clamps that had been applied to the ileum and transverse colon. If necessary, linen-shod Doyen noncrushing intestinal clamps may be applied to occlude the ileum and transverse colon at a point at least 10 cm from their cut edges in preparation for an open, two-layer end-to-end anastomosis **(Fig. 2–9)**.

Before the anastomosis is begun, the blood supply must be carefully evaluated. Generally there is no problem with the terminal ileum if no hematoma has been induced. Test the adequacy of the blood supply to the cut end of the colon by palpating the pulse in the marginal artery. For additional data about the blood supply, divide a small arterial branch near the cut end of the colon and observe the pulsatile arterial flow. If there is any question about the vigor of the blood supply, resect additional transverse colon.

## Ileocolic Two-Layer Sutured End-to-End Anastomosis

Align the cut ends of the ileum and transverse colon to face each other so their mesenteries are not twisted. Because the diameter of ileum is narrower than that of the colon, make a Cheatle slit with Metzenbaum scissors on the antimesenteric border of the ileum for a distance of 1–2 cm to help equalize these two diameters **(Fig. 2–10)**. Do not round off the corners of the slit.

Insert the first seromuscular layer of interrupted sutures using 4-0 silk on atraumatic needles. Initiate this layer by inserting the first Lembert suture at the antimesenteric border and the second at the mesenteric border to serve as guy sutures. Attach hemostats to each of these sutures. Drawing the two hemostats apart makes insertion of additional sutures by successive bisection more efficient **(Fig. 2–11)**. Now complete the anterior seromuscular layer of the anastomosis by inserting interrupted Lembert seromuscular sutures **(Fig. 2–12)**. After the entire anterior layer has been inserted and tied, cut the tails of all the sutures except the two guy sutures.

To provide exposure for the mucosal layer, invert the anterior aspect of the anastomosis by passing the hemostat containing the antimesenteric guy suture **(Fig. 2–13, A)** through the rent in the mesentery deep to the ileocolonic anastomosis. Then draw the mesenteric guy suture **(Fig. 2–13, B)** in the opposite direction and expose the mucosa for application of the first layer of mucosal sutures **(Fig. 2–14)**. Use 5-0 PG, double-armed, and begin the first suture at the midpoint **(Fig. 2–15A)**. Then pass the suture in a continuous fashion toward the patient's right to lock each stitch. Take relatively small bites (4 mm). When the right margin of the suture line is reached, tag the needle with a hemostat; with the second needle initiate the remainder of the mucosal approximation, going from the midpoint of the anastomosis toward the patient's left in a continuous locked fashion **(Fig. 2–15B)**. When this layer has been completed **(Fig. 2–15C)**, close the superficial mucosal layer of the anastomosis with continuous Connell or Cushing sutures beginning at each end of the anastomosis. Terminate the mucosal suture line in the midpoint of the superficial layer by tying the suture to its mate **(Fig. 2–16)**.

Accomplish the final seromuscular layer by inserting interrupted 4-0 silk Lembert sutures **(Fig. 2–17)**. Devote special attention to ensuring a secure closure at the mesenteric border. Then cut all the sutures and test the lumen with thumb and forefinger to gauge the width of the anastomotic stoma. It should admit the tip of the thumb.

Close the defect in the mesentery by continuous 2-0 PG sutures. Take care to avoid occluding important vessels running in the mesentery during the course of the continuous suture. If desired, a one-layer anastomosis can be constructed by the technique described above, simply by omitting the mucosal suture. If it is accomplished without error, the result is as successful as after the two-layer method.

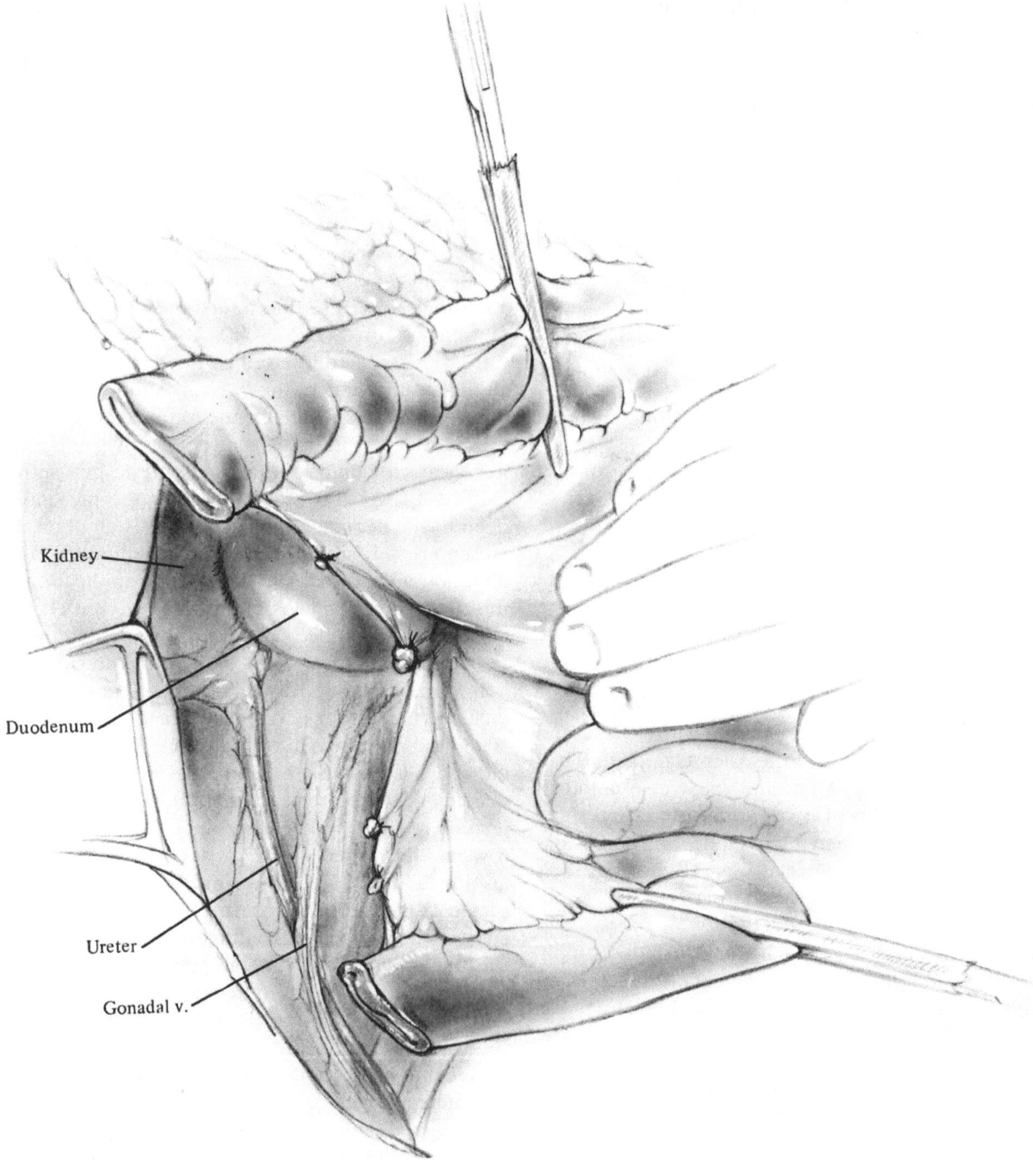


Fig. 2-9

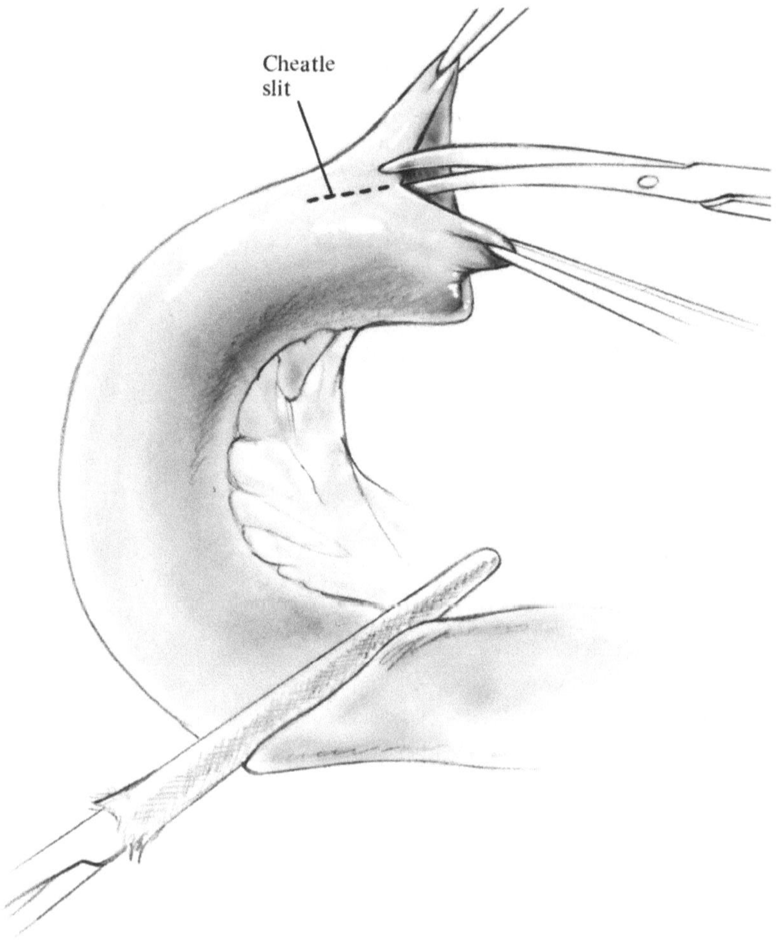


Fig. 2–10

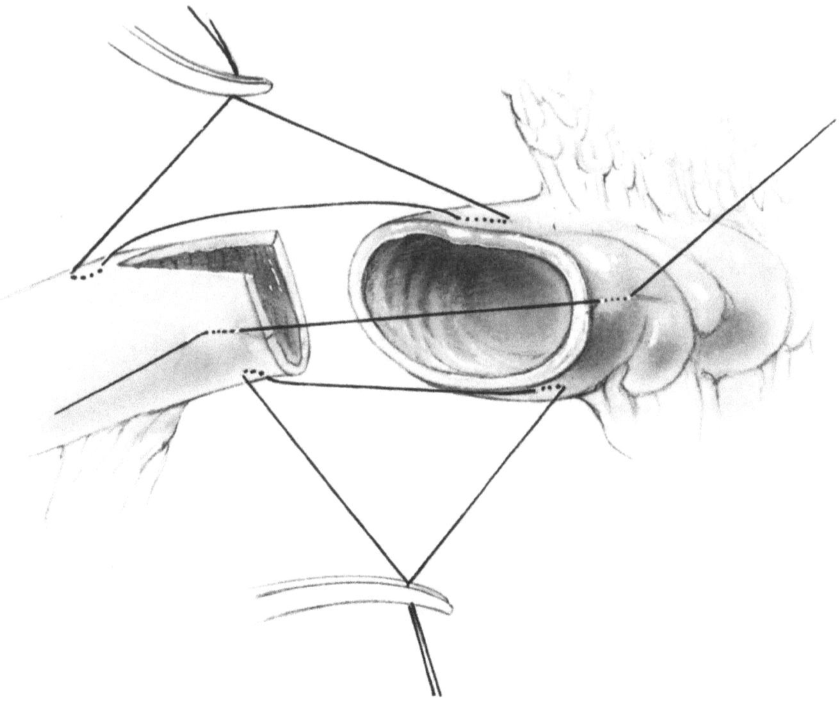

Fig. 2–11

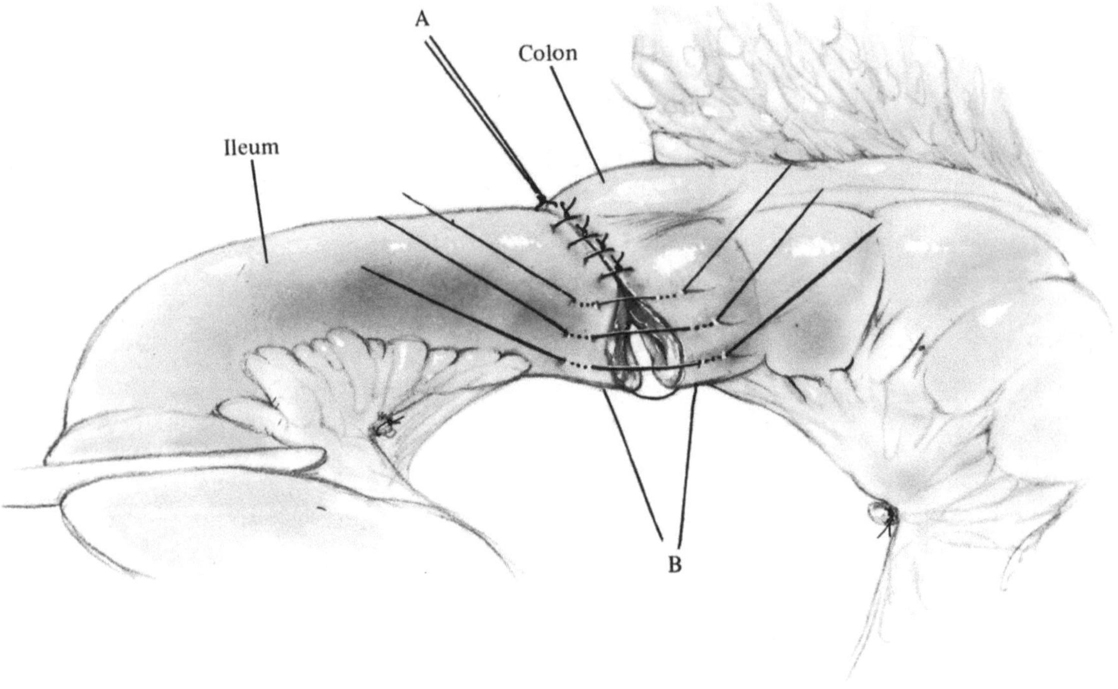


Fig. 2-12

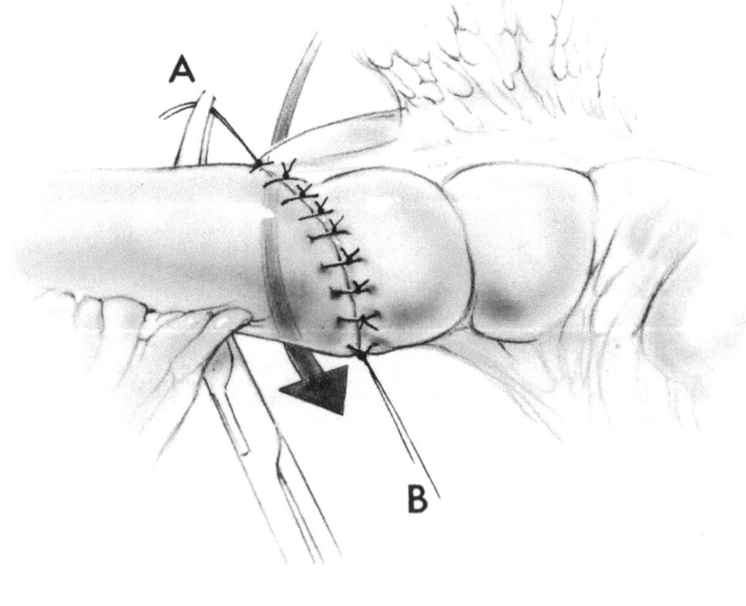


Fig. 2-13

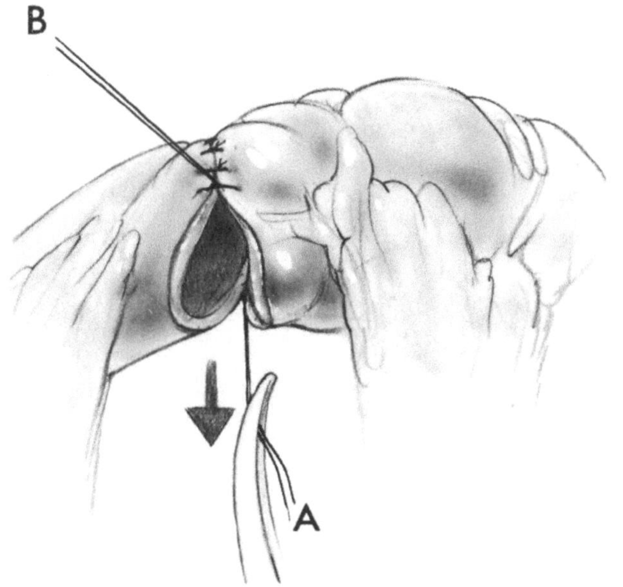


Fig. 2-14

## Anastomosis by Stapling, Functional End-to-End

To perform a stapled anastomosis, clear an area of mesentery and apply the 55/3.5 mm linear stapler transversely across the colon. Transect the colon flush with the stapler using a scalpel. Carry out the identical procedure at the selected site on the ileum. Alternatively, the bowel may be stapled and divided with the linear cutting stapler. Some oozing of blood should be evident despite the double row of staples. Control excessive bleeding by carefully applying electrocoagulation or chromic sutures. Align the ileum and colon side by side and with heavy scissors excise a triangular 8 mm wedge from the antimesenteric margins of both ileum and colon **(Fig. 2–18)**.

Insert one of the two forks of the cutting linear stapling instrument into the lumen of the ileum and the other into the colon, *hugging the antimesenteric border* of each **(Fig. 2–19)**. Neither segment of intestine should be stretched, as it may result in excessive thinning of the bowel, leaving inadequate substance for the staples to grasp. After ascertaining that both segments of the bowel are near the hub of the stapler, fire the device; this should result in a side-to-side anastomosis 4-5 cm long. Unlock and remove the device and inspect the staple line for bleeding and possible technical failure when closing the staples.

Now apply Allis clamps to the remaining defect in the anastomosis and close it by a final application of the 55/3.5 mm linear stapling instrument **(Fig. 2–20)**. Take care to include a portion of *each of the previously applied staples lines* in the final application of the stapler. However, when applying the Allis clamps, do not align points X and Y **(Fig. 2–21)** exactly opposite each other, as it would result in six staple lines meeting at one point. The alignment of these two points, as shown in **Figure 2–22**, produces the best results. Check the patency of the anastomosis by invaginating the colon through the anastomosis, which should admit the tips of two fingers. Then lightly touch the everted mucosa with the electrocautery instrument. During closure of the mesentery, cover the everted staple lines with adjoining mesentery or omentum if convenient.

We have modified Steichen's method of anastomosing ileum to colon, making it simpler by eliminating two applications of the stapler. With our technique the first step is to insert the cutting linear stapling device, one fork into the open end of ileum and the other fork into the open colon. Then fire the stapler, establishing a partial anastomosis between the antimesenteric borders of ileum and colon, as seen in Figure 2-21. Apply four or five Allis clamps to approximate the lips of the ileum and colon (in eversion) taking care that points X and Y are not in apposition. Then apply a 90/3.5 mm linear stapler underneath the Allis clamps and fire the staples. The end result is illustrated in **Figure 2–23**. In our experience this is the most efficient and reliable method for constructing an ileocolonic anastomosis.

## Wound Closure

The surgical team now changes gloves and discards all instruments used up to this point. Irrigate the operative field with saline. Cover the anastomosis with omentum if possible. Close the abdomen in routine fashion without drainage.

# POSTOPERATIVE CARE

Continue nasogastric suction for 1-3 days.

Delay oral intake of liquid and food until the fifth or sixth postoperative day.

If ileus persists, delay oral intake further and perform CT of the abdomen to exclude abscess, obstruction, or leak.

In the absence of preoperative intraabdominal sepsis, discontinue antibiotics after the operation.

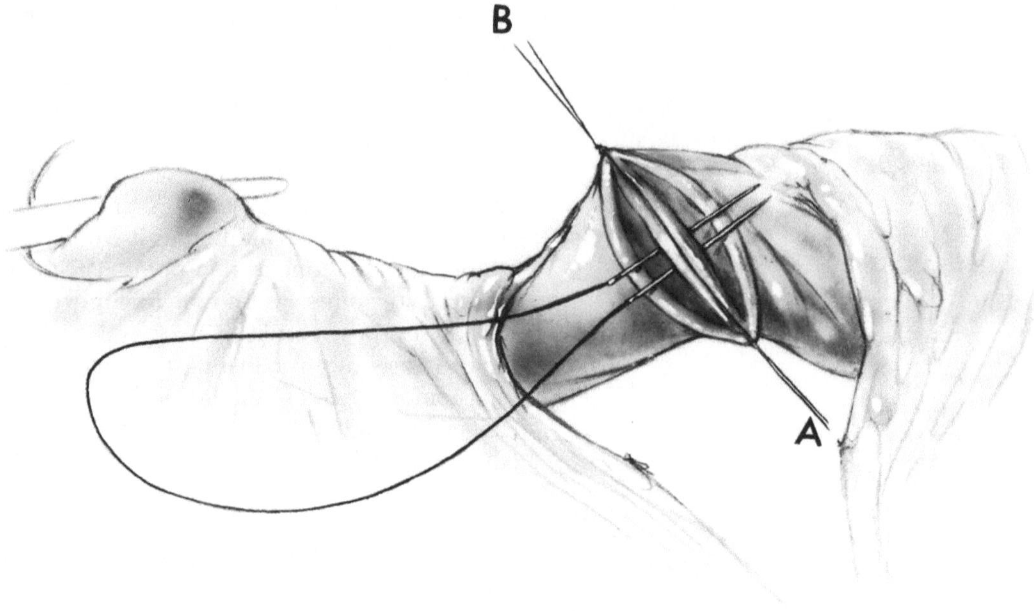


Fig. 2-15A

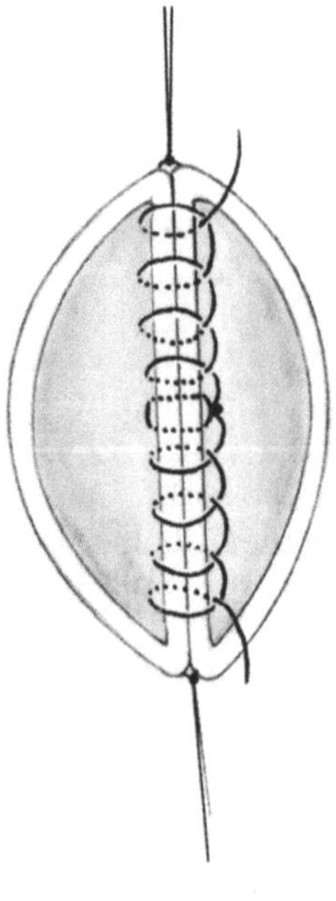

Fig. 2-15B

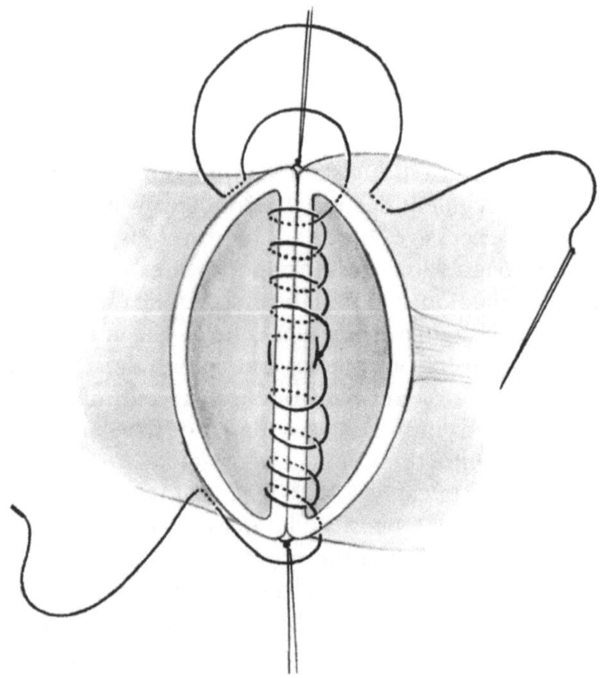

Fig. 2-15C

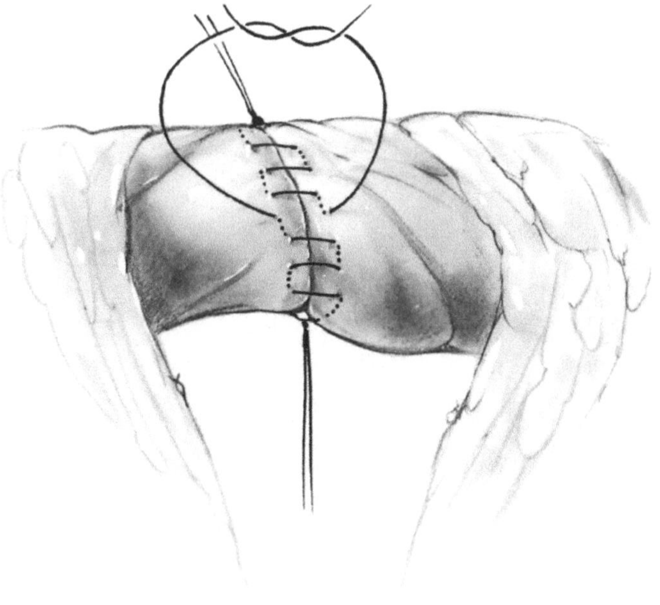

Fig. 2–16

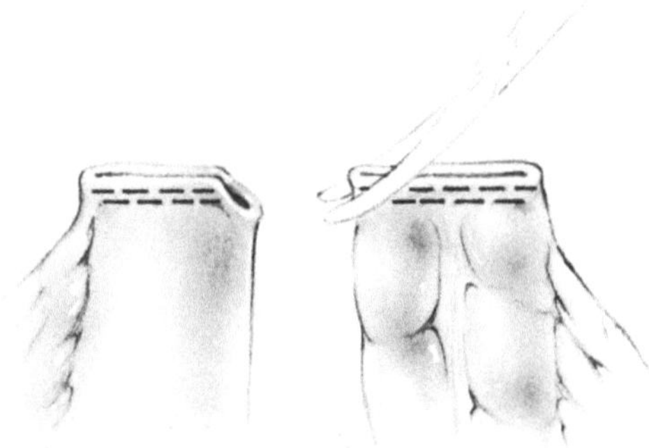

Fig. 2–18

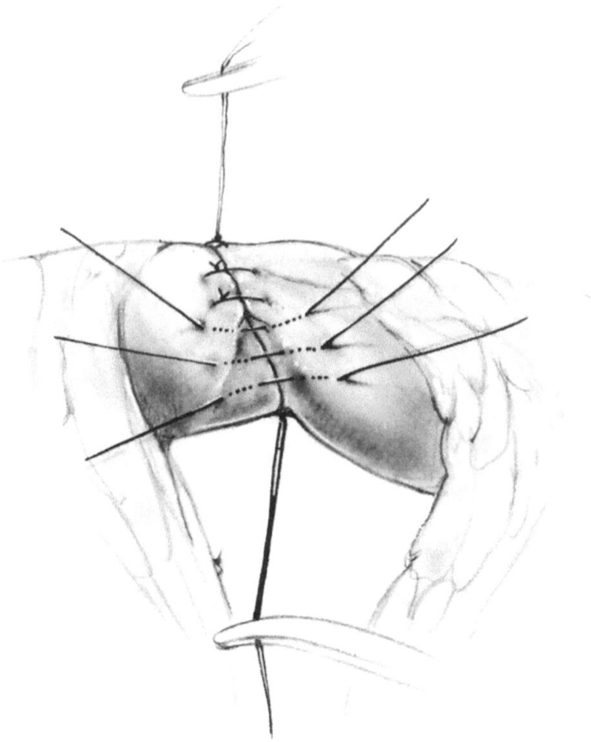

Fig. 2–17

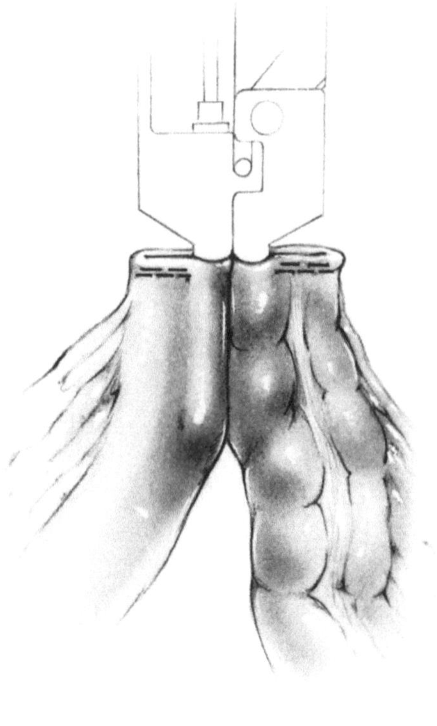

Fig. 2–19

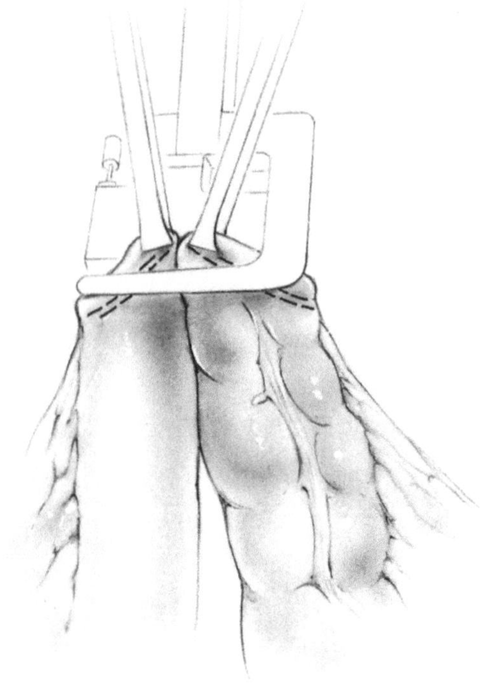

Fig. 2-20

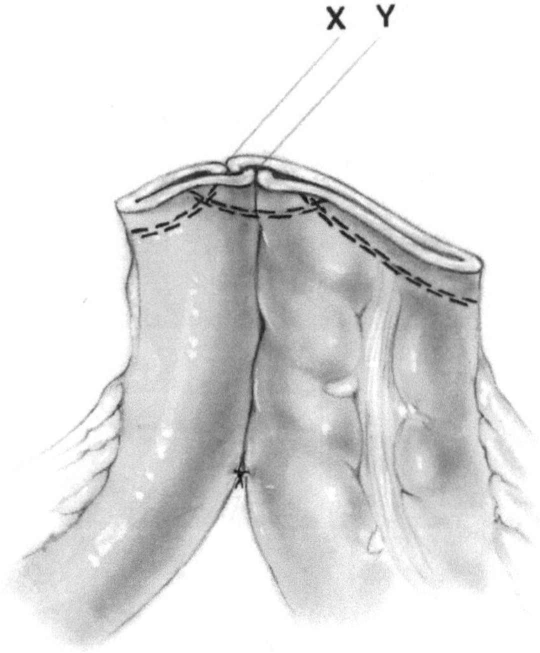


Fig. 2-22

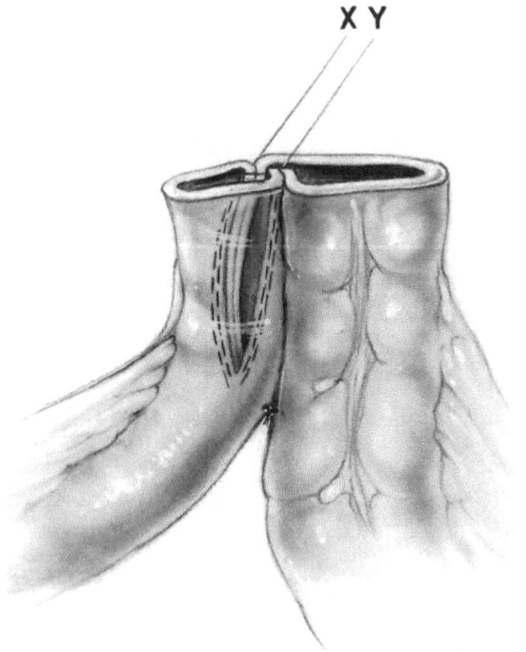


Fig. 2-21

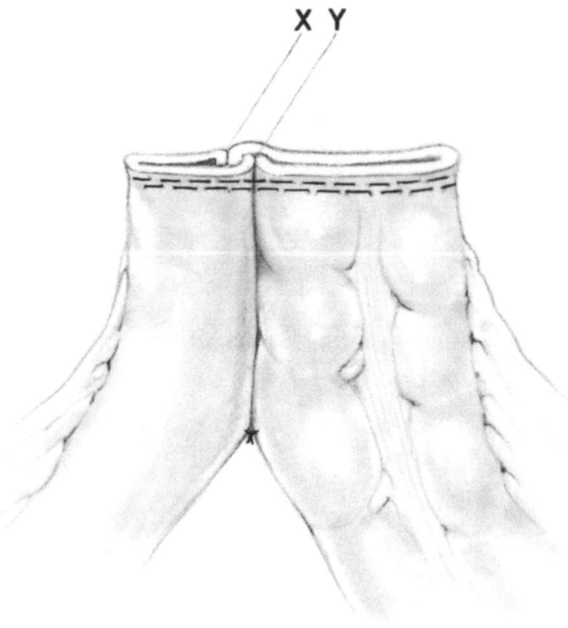


Fig. 2-23

## COMPLICATIONS

*Leakage* from an ileocolonic or colocolonic anastomosis may manifest as peritonitis, colocutaneous fistula, or localized intraperitoneal abscess. Localized or spreading peritonitis should be managed by prompt relaparotomy and exteriorization of both ends of the anastomosis.

*Sepsis* in the subhepatic, subphrenic, or pelvic areas is an occasional complication of anastomoses of the colon, even in the absence of leakage. CT of the abdomen generally provides the diagnosis, and percutaneous drainage is usually successful.

*Wound infection* requires prompt removal of all overlying skin sutures to permit wide drainage of the entire infected area.

## REFERENCES

Furstenberg S, Goldman S, Machado M, Jarhult J. Minilaparotomy approach to tumors of the right colon. Dis Colon Rectum 1998;41:997.

Heili MJ, Flowers SA, Fowler DL. Laparoscopic-assisted colectomy: a comparison of dissection techniques. J Soc Laparoendosc Surg 1999;3:27.

Leung KL, Meng WC, Lee JP, et al. Laparoscopic-assisted resection of right-sided colonic carcinoma: a casecontrol study. J Surg Oncol 1999;71:97.

Metcalf AM. Laparoscopic colectomy. Surg Clin North Am 2000;80:1321.

Schirmer BD. Laparoscopic colon resection. Surg Clin North Am 1996;76:571.

Young-Fadok TM, Nelson H. Laparoscopic right colectomy: five-step procedure. Dis Colon Rectum 2000; 2:267.

Young-Fadok TM, Radice E, Nelson H, Harmsen WS. Benefits of laparoscopic-assisted colectomy for colon polyps: a case-matched series. Mayo Clinic Proc 2000; 75:344.

# 3 Laparoscopic Right Hemicolectomy

Steven D. Wexner, MD
Susan M. Cera, MD

## INDICATIONS

Ileocolic Crohn's disease

Endoscopically irretrievable adenomatous polyps

Arteriovenous malformations

Cecal volvulus

Ischemia

Carcinoma

Right-sided diverticulitis

## PREOPERATIVE PREPARATION

Preoperatively, patients undergo an appropriate medical evaluation. Imaging studies including CT scan, barium studies, and colonoscopy are undertaken for preoperative planning to assess the location of disease, review any associated complications, and identify any synchronous lesions. Preoperative marking of polyps by endoscopic tattooing using India ink is necessary to ensure intraoperative identification of the lesion and to avoid the need for intraoperative colonoscopy. In patients with recurrent Crohn's disease or history of multiple laparotmoies, imaging studies are particularly important in providing "roadmaps" to define extent of previous resections, length of remaining bowel, and degree of previous mobilization of flexures. Preoperative mechanical and antibiotic bowel preparation consists of 45 cc sodium phosphate solution (Fleets phosphosoda; C.B. Fleet Co., Inc., Lynchburg, VA) PO at 4 pm and at 9 pm, each followed by 3–8 oz glasses of water, and 1 gm neomycin with 500 mg metronidazole at 7:00 and 11:00 pm. In addition, 2 gm of cefotetan are administered intravenously and 5000 units of heparin injected subcutaneously at the start of the operation.

## PITFALLS AND DANGER POINTS

Injury to liver, duodenum, or contents of the hepatoduodenal ligament

Hemorrhage from epigastric, mesenteric, iliac, or gonadal vessels

Inadvertent enterotomy or colotomy

Inadvertent retrorenal dissection

Anastomotic insufficiency or twist

## OPERATIVE STRATEGY

Elective laparoscopic right hemicolectomy is performed in a laparoscopic-assisted fashion with intracorporeal mobilization of the ileum, cecum, and hepatic flexure medially to the level of the duodenum and middle colic vessels. The bowel is then exteriorized through a small midline port incision extended to approximately 4 cm. Extracorporeal division of the mesentery is followed by resection of bowel and creation of a side-to-side functional end-to-end ileocolic anastomosis. The bowel is returned to the abdomen and re-insufflation allows final inspection of the intraperitoneal contents.

For patients with primary or recurrent Crohn's ileitis, significant inflammation and adhesions may be encountered. Dissection is initiated in areas free of inflammation to identify appropriate planes. Thorough inspection of the small bowel from the ileocecal valve to the jejunoduodenal junction using a two-instrument technique is essential to assess synchronous locations of disease which are addressed after maximal mobilization is accomplished laparoscopically. Resections, anastomoses, enterotomy repairs, and stricturoplasties are most easily performed extracorporeally through a limited incision, preferably midline to preserve future potential ostomy sites.

## OPERATIVE TECHNIQUE

### Room Setup and Trocar Placement

After the induction of general anesthesia, the patient is placed in the modified lithotomy position with the lower extremities in padded stirrups placed low for unimpeded movement of the instruments. Both arms are tucked at the patient's sides and extra care is taken to secure the patient to the bed because of the rotation and tilt required during surgery. A minimum of two monitors is needed and are placed one on each side of the patient at the head of the bed **(Fig. 3–1)**. Bilateral ureteral stents are placed by a urologist, followed by insertion of a urinary catheter and an orogastric tube. The patient's abdomen is shaved, prepped with povodine-iodine solution, and appropriately draped.

For port placement, the assistant stands to the right of the patient while the surgeon stays to the left. Three to four 10 mm trocars are employed for most procedures **(Fig. 3–2a and 3–2b)**. Initially, a 10 mm trocar is placed by the open Hasson technique in the supraumbilical position through which the camera is inserted. In the reoperative abdomen, the initial trocar can be placed in the left upper quadrant in a site remote from scars. The abdomen is insufflated to an intraabdominal pressure of 15 mm Hg. Two additional trocars are placed along the lateral edge of the left rectus muscle, 8-10 cm

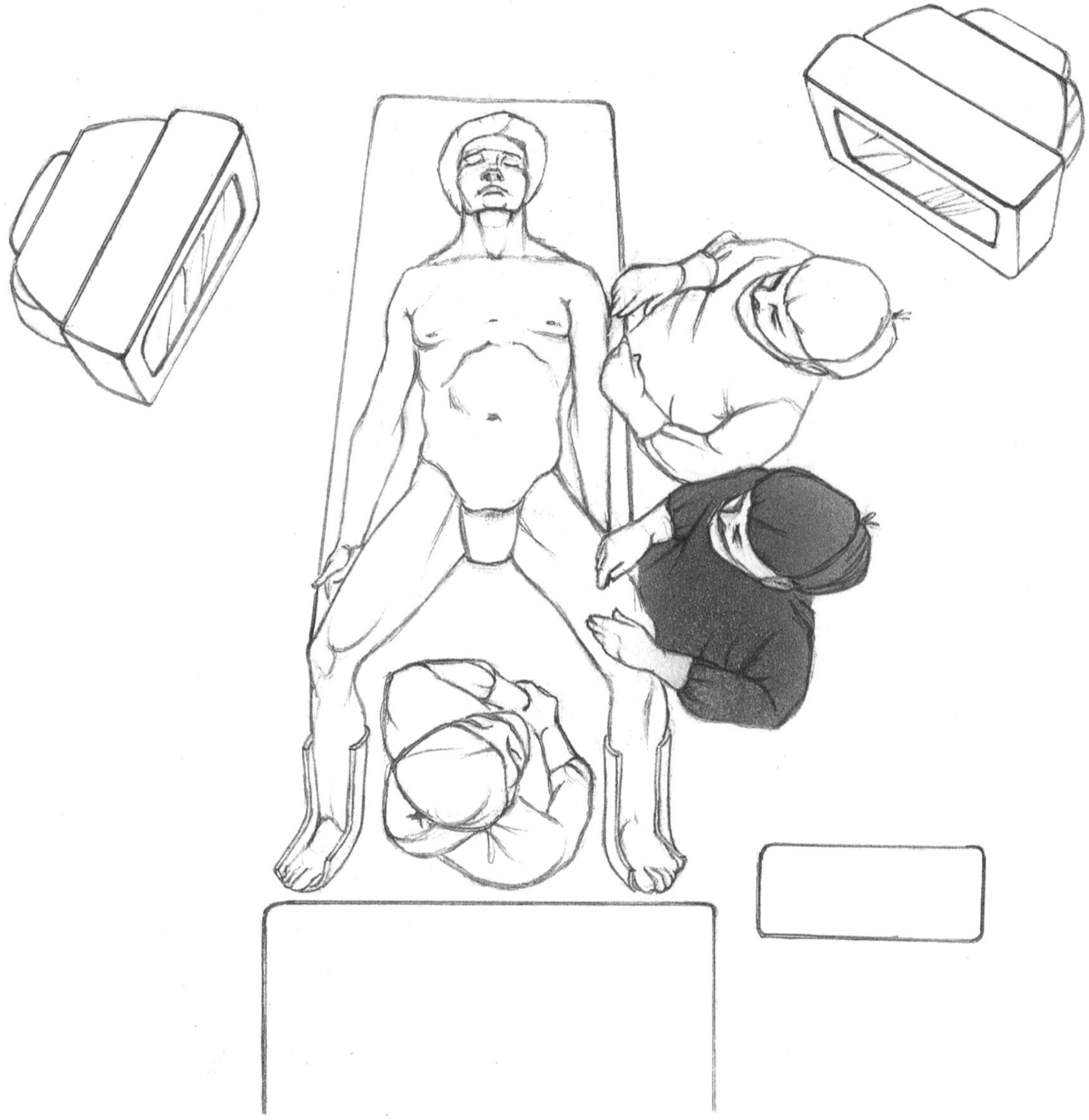

Fig. 3–1

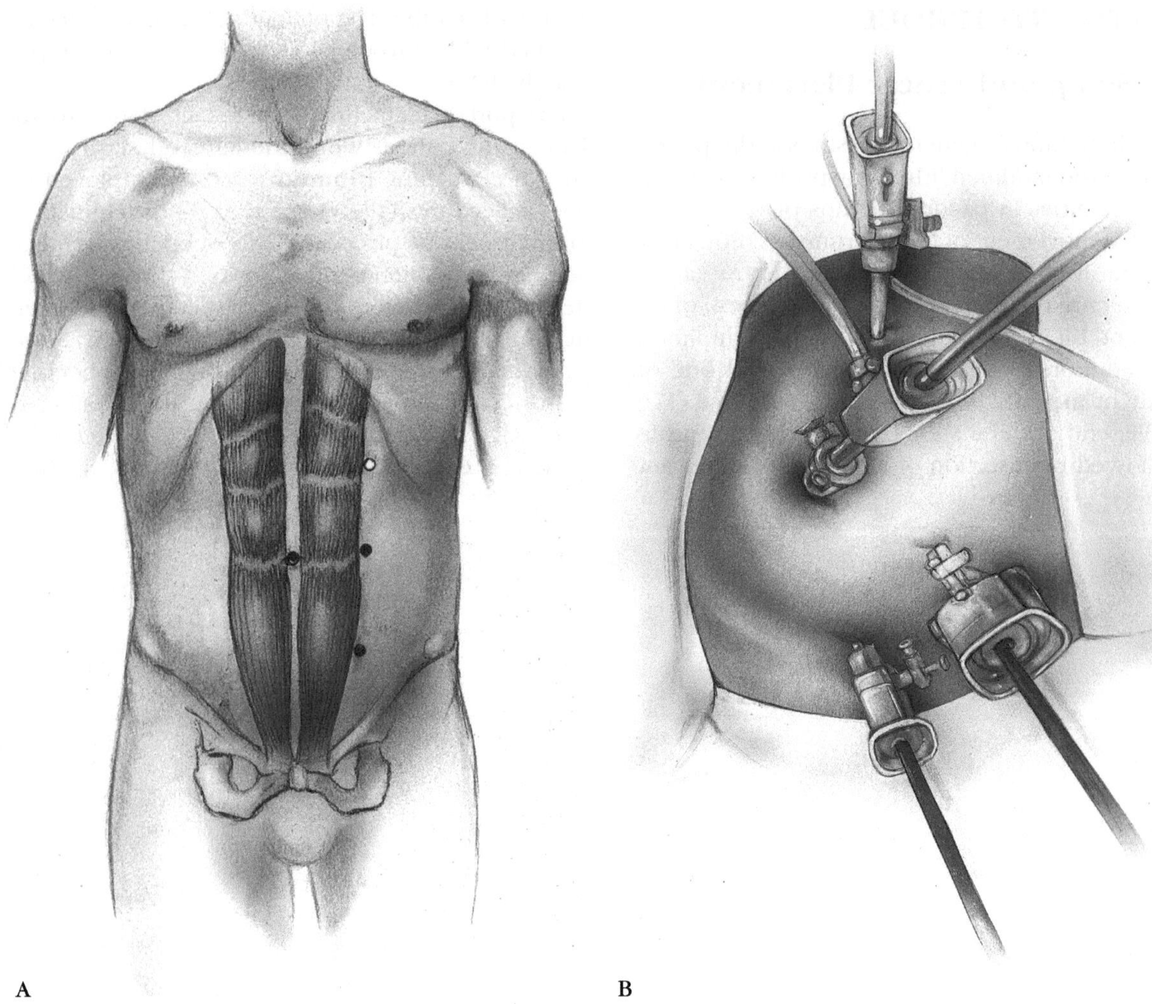


Fig. 3-2ab

apart, in the midabdomen and iliac fossa positions. This configuration allows adequate triangulation of the instruments to facilitate the dissection. All port placements should take into consideration the potential for future ostomy or drain sites. In obese patients or patients with extensive intraabdominal adhesions, an optional port can be placed in the left upper quadrant to assist in retraction during dissection of the hepatic flexure. Once all ports are placed, the assistant moves to the patient's left to direct the camera.

## Exploration

Exploration is undertaken to assess for adhesions and unexpected pathology and to define the extent of disease. In the cases of neoplasia, peritoneal surfaces and the liver are inspected for metastases. Extensive adhesions may require early conversion while large phlegmons or masses may require long incisions for removal obviating the need for a laparoscopic approach. Unexpected complications of inflammatory bowel disease mandates advanced laparoscopic skills and may necessitate conversion to laparotomy. Thorough inspection of the small bowel from the ileocecal valve to the jejunoduodenal junction using a two-instrument technique is essential to assess anatomy and identify pathology. Any synchronous "skip areas" of disease, such as inflammation or strictures, can be marked with sutures for subsequent resection or strictureplasty after the index resection has been accomplished through the midline incision.

## Mobilization of the Cecum

The operating table is tilted toward the patient's left side and Trendelenberg position is used to facilitate medial retraction of the right colon and prevent the small bowel from entering the field of dissection. The mesentery of the cecum is gently grasped and retracted medially using Babcock clamps placed through the left upper port. With the 10-mm ultrasonic shears placed through the left lower port, the peritoneum along the base of the terminal ileum mesentery and around the cecum is opened exposing the retroperitoneum **(Fig. 3–3a)**. Dissection is begun in an area free of inflammation and adhesions and proceeds in the avascular plane medially under the cecum to the level of the duodenum and superiorly to the hepatic flexure **(Fig. 3–3b)**. The lateral peritoneal attachments of the cecum are incised **(Fig. 3–4a)**. The ureter is identified in the retroperitoneum traversing the right iliac vessels in parallel with the gonadal vessels. Great care should be taken to identify the correct plane of dissection anterior to Gerota's fascia as more lateral dissection results in medial mobilization of the kidney with difficulty in subsequent mobilization of the hepatic flexure. Hemostasis of small vessels is important for visualization of the tissue planes during this portion of the procedure. Early identification of the duodenum is imperative in preventing injury and inadvertent electrocautery burns. For patients expected to have extensive intraabdominal adhesions and/or intraabdominal, pelvic, or retroperitoneal inflammation, ureteric catheters can be a valuable adjunct.

## Mobilization of the Hepatic Flexure

The surgeon often moves to a position between the patient's legs while working on the hepatic flexure and transverse colon. With the patient in steep

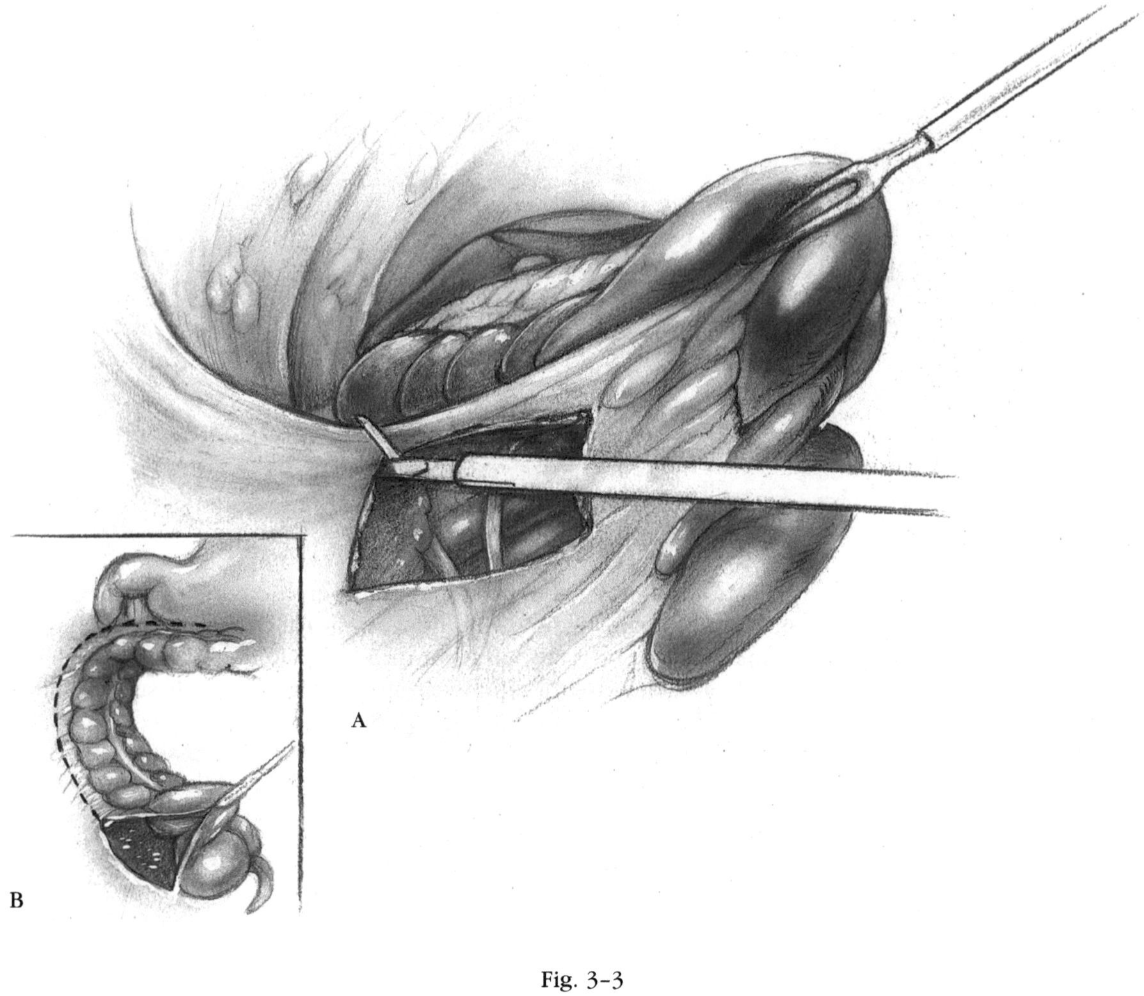


Fig. 3-3

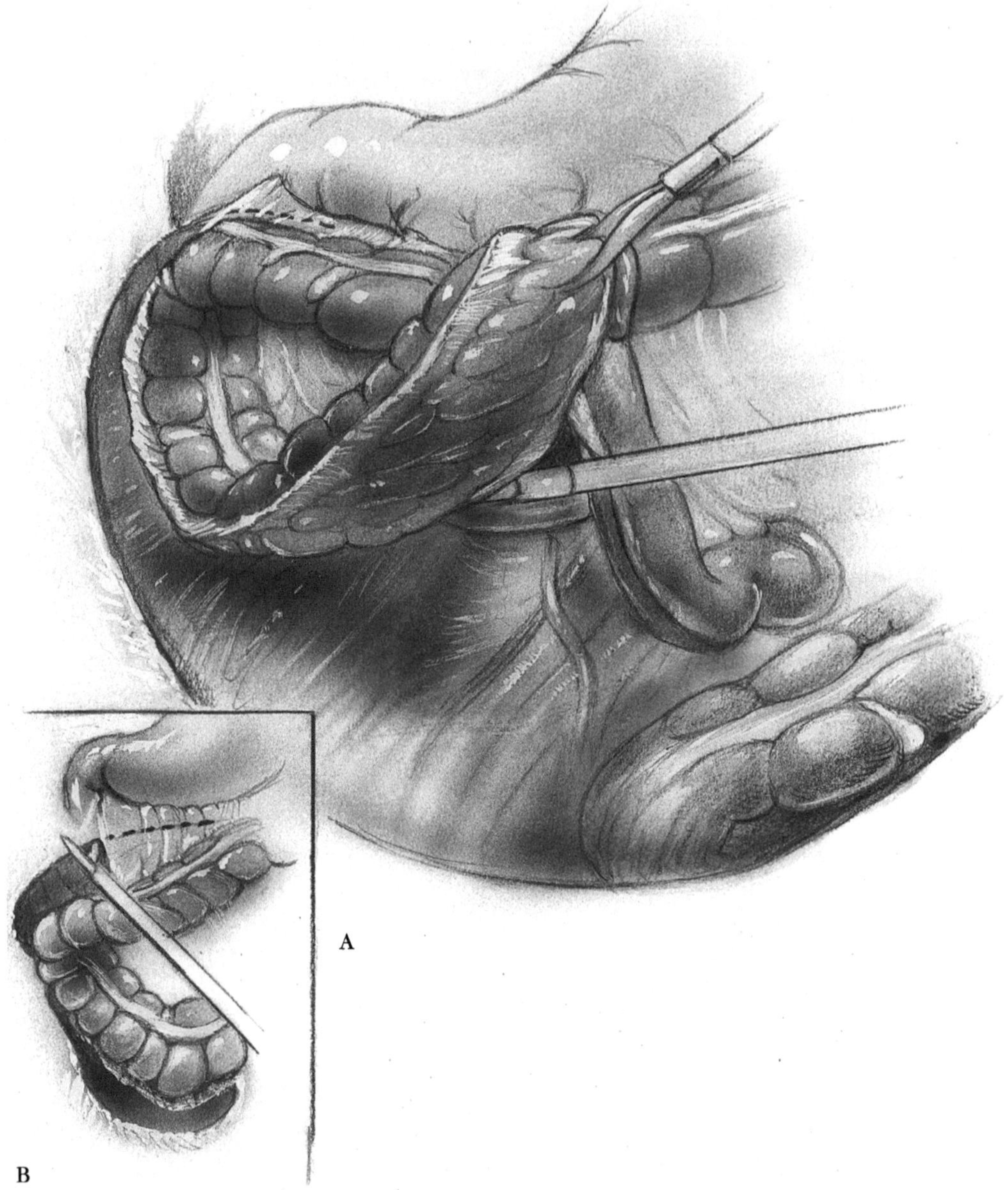

Fig. 3-4

reverse Trendelenberg position, dissection of the lateral attachments is continued around the hepatic flexure dividing the hepatocolic ligament **(Fig. 3–4b)**. With the transverse colon retracted caudad and the greater omentum retracted cephalad, the omentum is separated from the midtransverse colon to the hepatic flexure with the ultrasonic scalpel or scissors through the avascular omental-colic junction **(Fig. 3–5a and 3–5b)**. An optional fourth upper left-sided port may be placed to provide upward traction on the omentum and is particularly in the presence of significant obesity, inflammation, or adhesions (Fig 3-2a and 3-2b). It is generally best to mobilize the proximal transverse colon to the level of the middle colic vessels to ensure optimal length for mobilization into the midline. Upon completion of the mobilization, the right colon is suspended by its mesentery where the origins of the ileocolic, right colic, and middle colic arteries reside.

## Extracorporeal Resection and Anastomosis

Once appropriate mobilization has been achieved, the supraumbilical port site is extended to an approx-

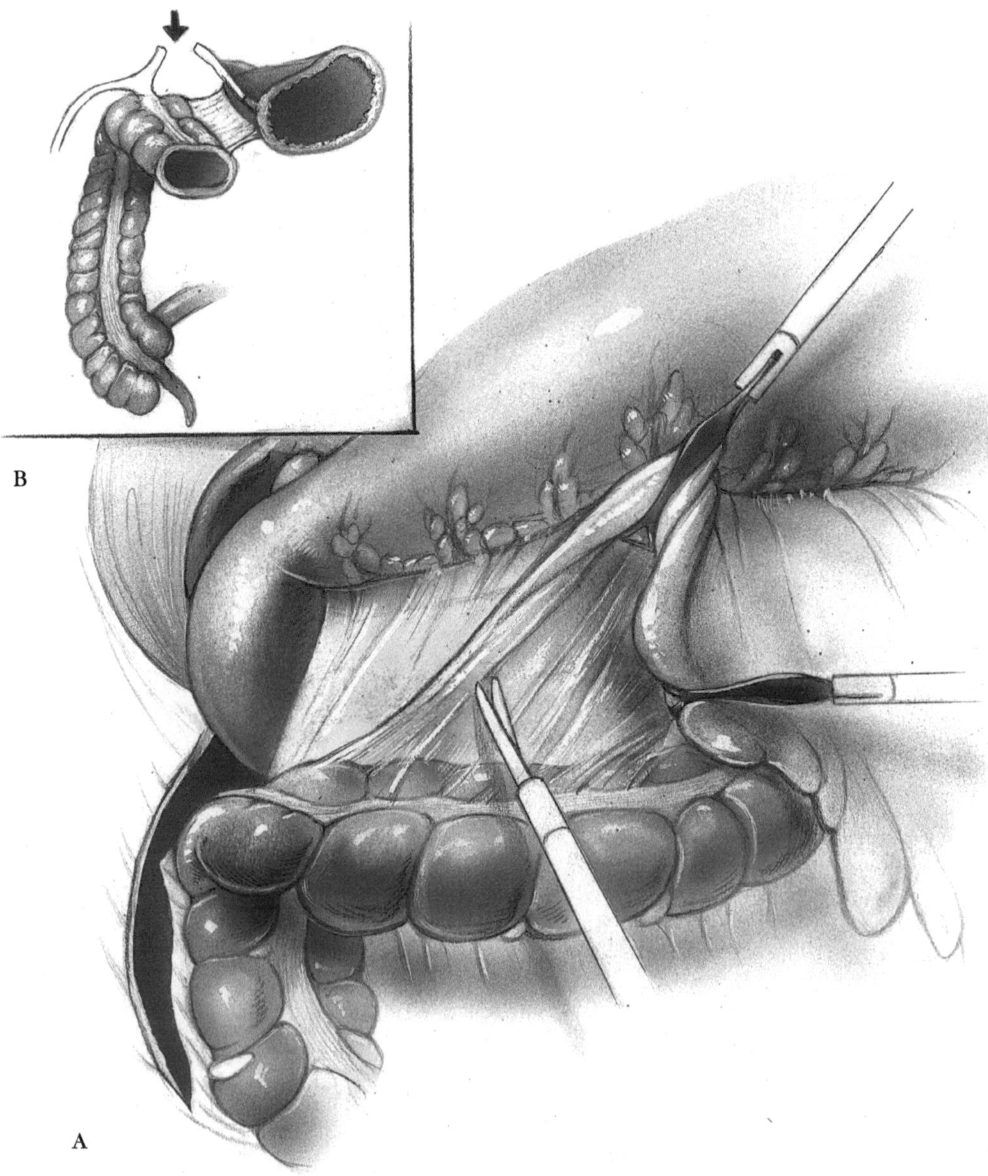


Fig. 3–5

imately 4 cm midline incision. A plastic, impervious wound drape is placed, the cecum is gently grasped, and the right colon is easily delivered through the wound **(Fig. 3–6)**. Points of transection on the ileum and colon are chosen and marked. The mesentery between these points is clamped, ligated, and divided prior to bowel resection to prevent twisting of the bowel and mesentery. Once the mesentery is divided, closure of the mesenteric defect with absorbable suture is begun but left untied. Linear cutting staplers are used to divide the ileum and transverse colon and, subsequently, to perform the side-to-side ileocolic anastomosis. The anastomosis should be tension-free, airtight, and well-vascularized. Closure of the mesenteric defect is then completed. Any synchronous lesions, strictures or phlegmons, can be addressed at this time. In patients with inflammatory bowel disease, it may be useful to inspect the entire length of the small bowel through this incision.

## Re-insufflation and Inspection

The fascia of the midline incision is closed with running absorbable sutures begun at each end but

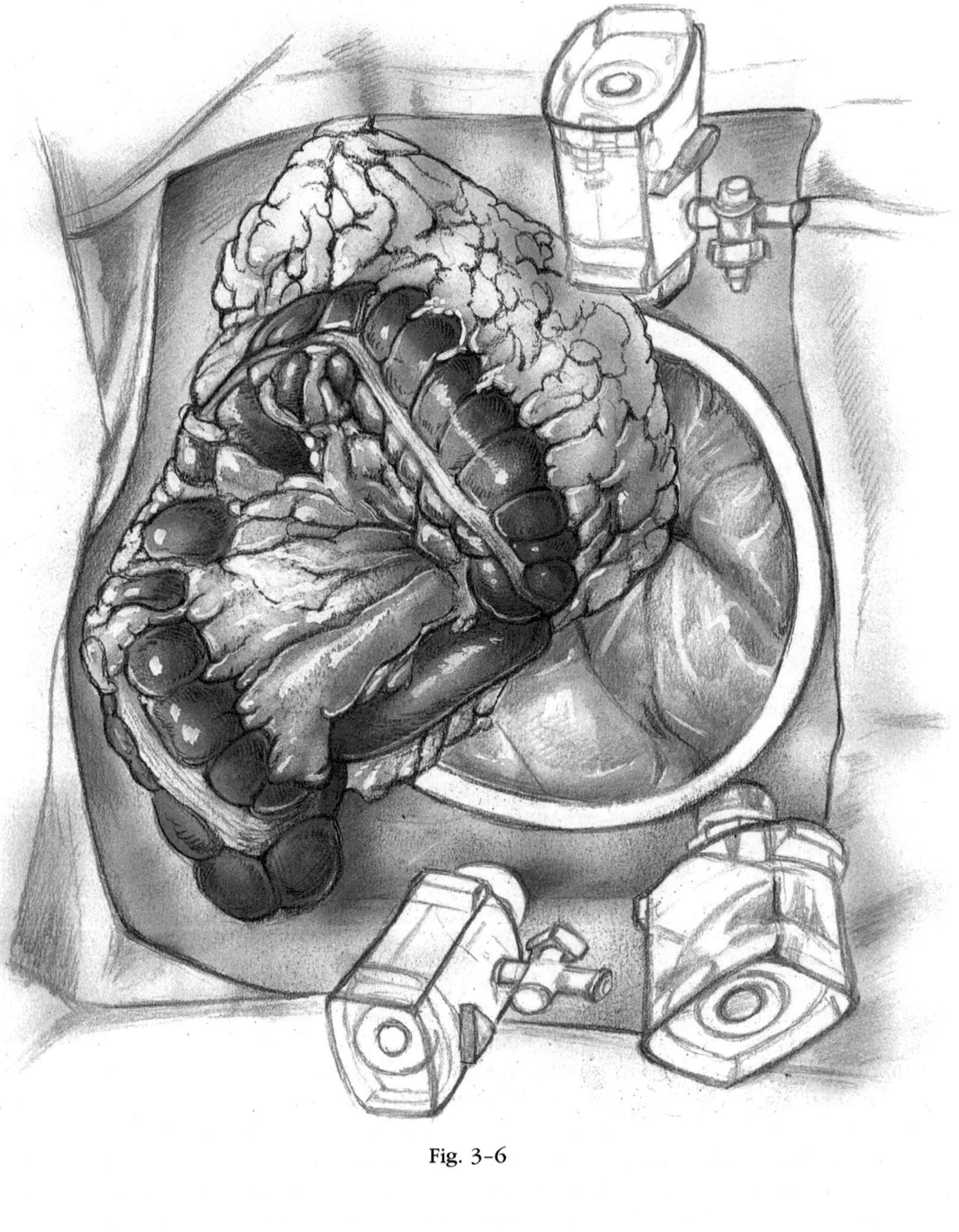

Fig. 3-6

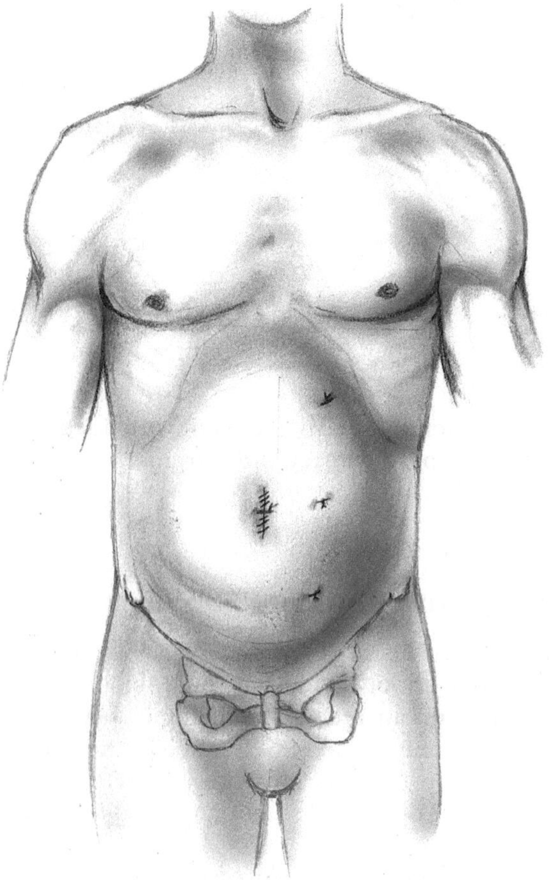

Fig. 3-7

left open in the midportion. The 10-mm cannula is reinserted and the abdomen reinsufflated. Inspection of the intraabdominal contents is undertaken to ensure no twisting of the mesentery and absence of hemorrhage in areas of pervious dissection. The ports are removed under direct vision and the midline fascia closed. The skin of the midline and port-site wounds are reapproximated with absorbable sutures and covered with adhesive strips and gauze dressings **(Fig. 3–7)**.

## POSTOPERATIVE CARE

Postoperatively, the patient is begun on clear liquids and a self-administered analgesic pump. On the first postoperative day, the bladder catheter is removed and pain is controlled with oral medication. The diet advanced with onset of bowel function and the patient discharged shortly thereafter.

## COMPLICATIONS

Anastomotic leak

Small bowel obstruction

Wound infection

Port site hernia

## REFERENCES

Wexner SD, Moscovitz ID. Laparoscopic colectomy in diverticular and Crohn's disease: minimal access surgery, Part 1. Surg Clin North Am 2000;80(4):1299–1319.

Miranda JA, Singh JJ. Laparoscopic right hemicolectomy. In MacFayden B, Wexner SDW (eds) Laparoscopic Surgery of the Abdomen. New York, Springer-Verlag, 2004, pp 359–363.

Cera C, Wexner SD. Diverticulitis. In Advanced Therapy of Minimally Invasive Surgery. New York, B.C. Decker (in press).

Wexner SD (Guest Ed). Laparoscopy for benign disease. Seminars in Laparoscopic Surgery. New York, Westminster Publications, 2003.

Wexner SD (Guest Ed). Laparoscopy for malignant disease. Seminars in Laparoscopic Surgery. New York, Westminster Publications, 2004.

# 4 Left Colectomy for Cancer

## INDICATIONS

Whereas malignancies of the proximal three-fourths of the transverse colon require excision of the right and transverse colon, cancers of the distal transverse colon, splenic flexure, descending colon, and sigmoid are treated by left hemicolectomy **(Figs. 4–1, 4–2)**.

## PREOPERATIVE PREPARATION

See Chapter 2.

## PITFALLS AND DANGER POINTS

Injury to spleen

Injury to ureter

Failure of anastomosis

## OPERATIVE STRATEGY

### Extent of Dissection

Lymph draining from malignancies of the left colon flows along the left colic or sigmoidal veins to the inferior mesenteric vessels. In the usual case, the inferior mesenteric artery should be divided at the aorta and the inferior mesenteric vein at the lower border of the pancreas.

Except for treating lesions situated in the distal sigmoid, the lower point of division of the colon is through the upper rectum, 2–3 cm above the promontory of the sacrum (Figs. 4–1, 4–2). Presacral elevation of the rectal stump need not be carried out, and the anastomosis should be intraperitoneal. The blood supply of a rectal stump of this length, arising from the inferior and middle hemorrhoidal arteries, is almost invariably of excellent quality. The blood supply of the proximal colonic segment, arising from the middle colic artery, generally is also excellent, provided care is exercised not to damage the marginal vessel at any point in its course.

### Liberation of Splenic Flexure

The splenic flexure of the colon may be completely liberated without dividing a single blood vessel if the surgeon can recognize anatomic planes accurately. The only blood vessels going to the colon are those arising from its mesentery. Bleeding during the course of this dissection arises from three sources.

1. Frequently, *downward traction on the colon and its attached omentum* avulses a patch of splenic capsule to which the omentum adheres. It is worthwhile to inspect the lower pole of the spleen at the *onset* of this dissection and to divide such areas of adhesion with Metzenbaum scissors under direct vision before applying traction.

2. Bleeding arises when the *surgeon does not recognize the plane* between the omentum and appendices epiploica attached to the distal transverse colon. The appendices may extend 1–3 cm cephalad to the transverse colon. When they are divided inadvertently, bleeding follows. Note that the character of the fat in the omentum is considerably different from that of the appendices. The former has the appearance of multiple small lobulations, each 4–6 mm in diameter, whereas the appendices epiploica contain fat that appears to have a completely smooth surface. If the proper plane between the omentum and appendices can be identified, the dissection is bloodless.

3. Bleeding can arise from the *use of blunt dissection* to divide the renocolic ligament. This ruptures a number of veins along the surface of Gerota's capsule, which overlies the kidney. Bleeding can be prevented by accurately identifying the renocolic ligament, delineating it carefully, and then dividing it with Metzenbaum scissors along the

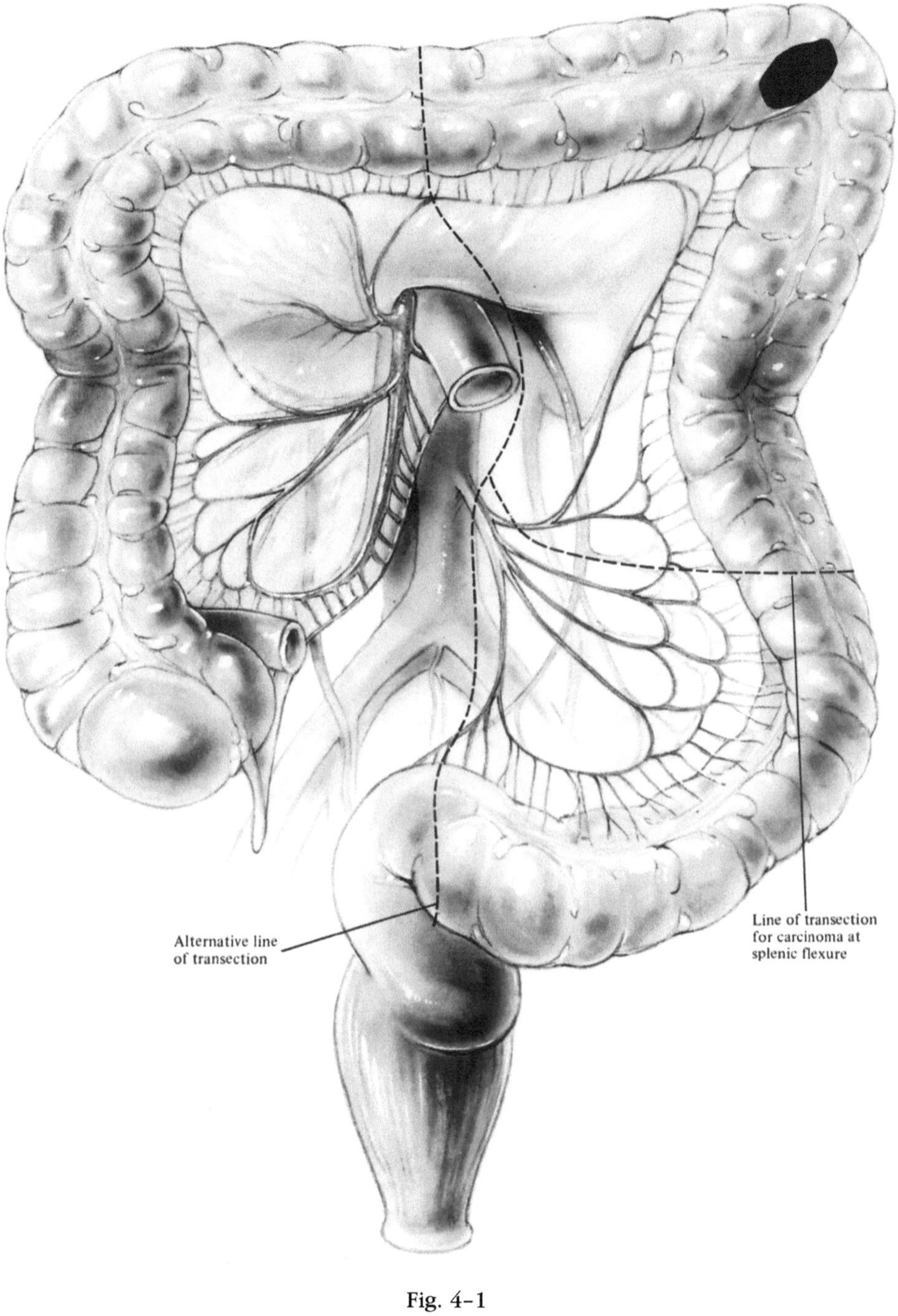
Alternative line
of transection
Line of transection
for carcinoma at
splenic flexure

Fig. 4–1

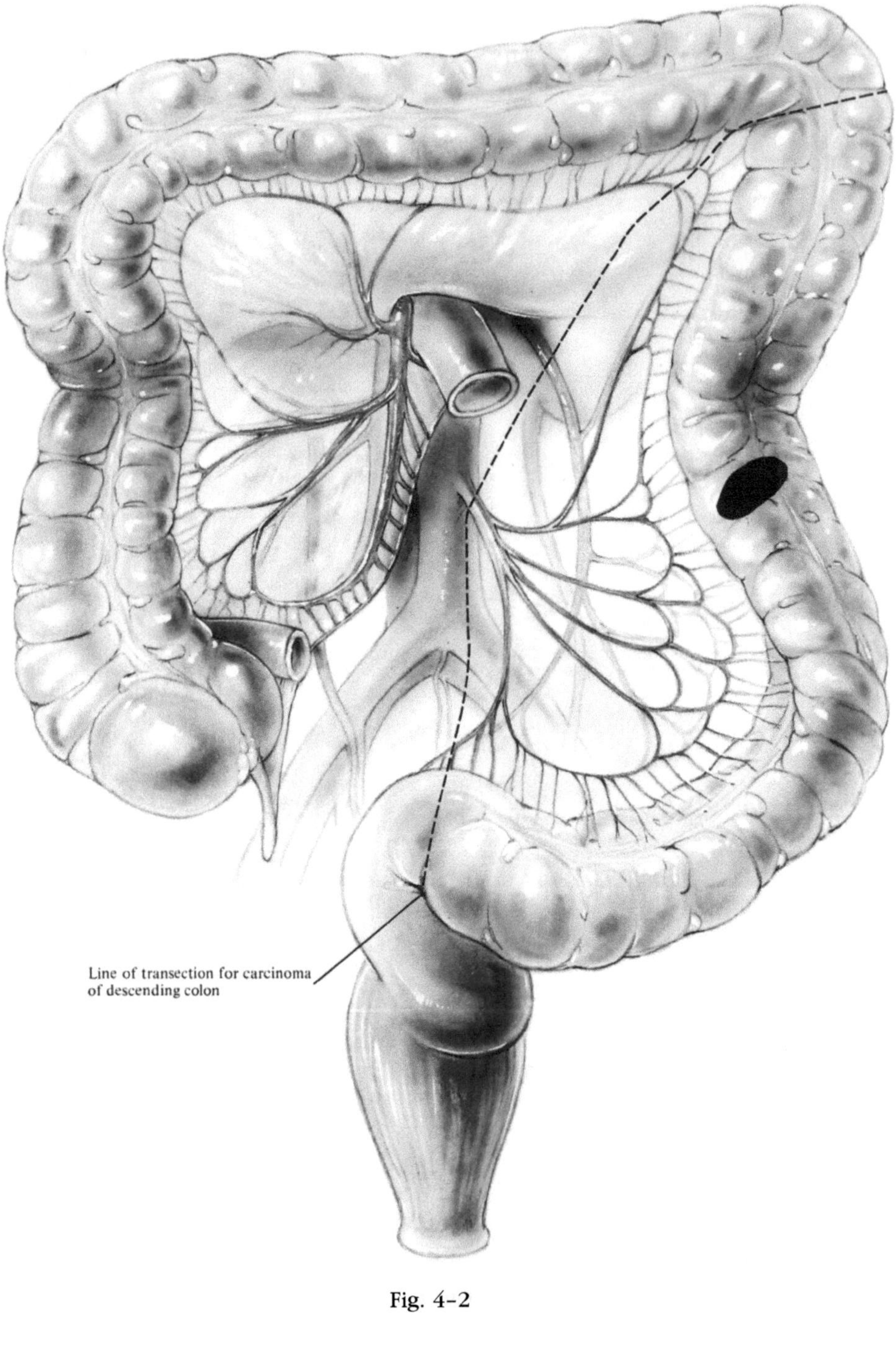


Fig. 4–2

medial margin of the renal capsule. Although the classic anatomy books do not generally describe a "renocolic ligament," it can be identified as a thin structure (see Figs. 4-4, 4-5) extending from the anterior surface of the renal capsule to the posterior surface of the mesocolon.

There are three essential steps to safe liberation of the splenic flexure. First, the obvious one is to incise the parietal peritoneum in the left paracolic gutter going cephalad to the splenic flexure. Second, dissect the left margin of the omentum from the distal transverse colon as well as from the left parietal peritoneum near the lower pole of the spleen (in patients who have this attachment). The third, least well understood step, is to identify and divide the renocolic ligament between the renal capsule and the posterior mesocolon. Then pass the index finger deep to this ligament in the region of the splenic flexure (see Fig. 4-5); this plane leads to the lienocolic ligament, which is also avascular and may be divided by Metzenbaum scissors provided this ligament is separated from underlying fatty tissue by finger dissection. The fatty tissue may contain an epiploic appendix with a blood vessel. After the lienocolic ligament has been divided, the index finger should lead to the next avascular "ligament," which extends from the pancreas to the transverse colon. This pancreaticocolic "ligament" comprises the upper portion of the transverse mesocolon. Dividing it frees the distal transverse colon and splenic flexure, except for the mesentery. For all practical purposes the renocolic, lienocolic, and pancreaticocolic "ligaments" comprise one continuous avascular membrane with multiple areas of attachment.

## No-Touch Technique

The no-touch technique is more difficult to apply to lesions of the left colon than to those on the right. In many cases it can be accomplished by liberating the sigmoid colon early in the procedure, identifying and ligating the inferior mesenteric vessels, and dividing the mesocolon—all before manipulating the tumor. Care must be taken to identify and protect the ureter.

In some cases the tumor's location or the obesity of the mesocolon make this approach more cumbersome for the surgeon, unlike the situation on the right side where the anatomy lends itself to adoption of the no-touch method as a routine procedure. Most surgeons content themselves with minimal manipulation of the tumor while they use the operative sequence of first liberating the left colon and then ligating the lymphovascular attachments.

## Technique of Anastomosis

Because the anastomosis is generally intraperitoneal and the rectal stump is largely covered by peritoneum, the leak rate in elective cases is less than 2%. Anastomosis may be done by the end-to-end technique or the Baker side-to-end method based on the preference of the surgeon.

If a stapling technique is desired, we prefer the functional end-to-end anastomosis (see Figs. 4-35 through 4-38). A circular stapling device (see Figs. 6-25 through 6-31) may also be used, but the internal diameter of the anastomosis resulting from this technique may be slightly narrow.

# OPERATIVE TECHNIQUE

## Incision and Exposure

Make a midline incision from a point about 4 cm below the xiphoid to the pubis **(Fig. 4–3a)** and open and explore the abdomen. Insert a Thompson retractor to elevate the left costal margin; it improves the exposure for the splenic flexure dissection. Exteriorize the small intestine and retract it to the patient's right. Apply umbilical tape ligatures to occlude the colon proximal and distal to the tumor.

## Liberation of Descending Colon and Sigmoid

Standing at the patient's left, make a long incision in the peritoneum of the left paracolic gutter between the descending colon and the white line of Toldt **(Fig. 4–3b)**. Use the left index finger to elevate this peritoneal layer and continue the incision upward with Metzenbaum scissors until the rightangle curve of the splenic flexure is reached. At this point the peritoneal incision must be moved close to the colon; otherwise the incision in the parietal peritoneum tends to continue upward and laterally toward the spleen. Similarly, with the index finger leading the way, use Metzenbaum scissors to complete the incision in a caudal direction, liberating the sigmoid colon from its lateral attachments down to the rectosigmoid region.

## Division of Renocolic Ligament

With the descending colon retracted toward the patient's right, a filmy attachment can be visualized covering the renal capsule and extending medially to attach to the posterior surface of the mesocolon

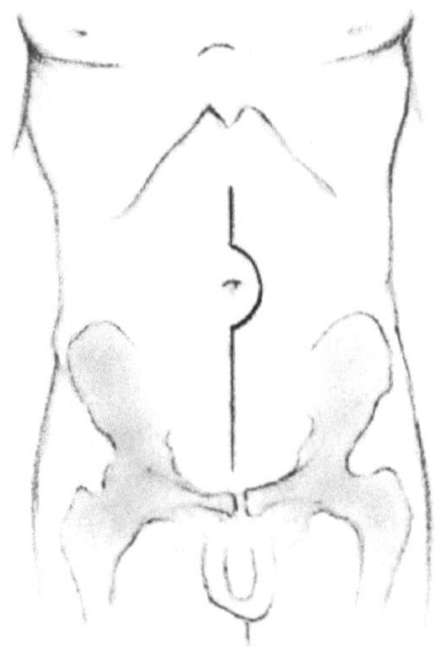

Fig. 4–3a

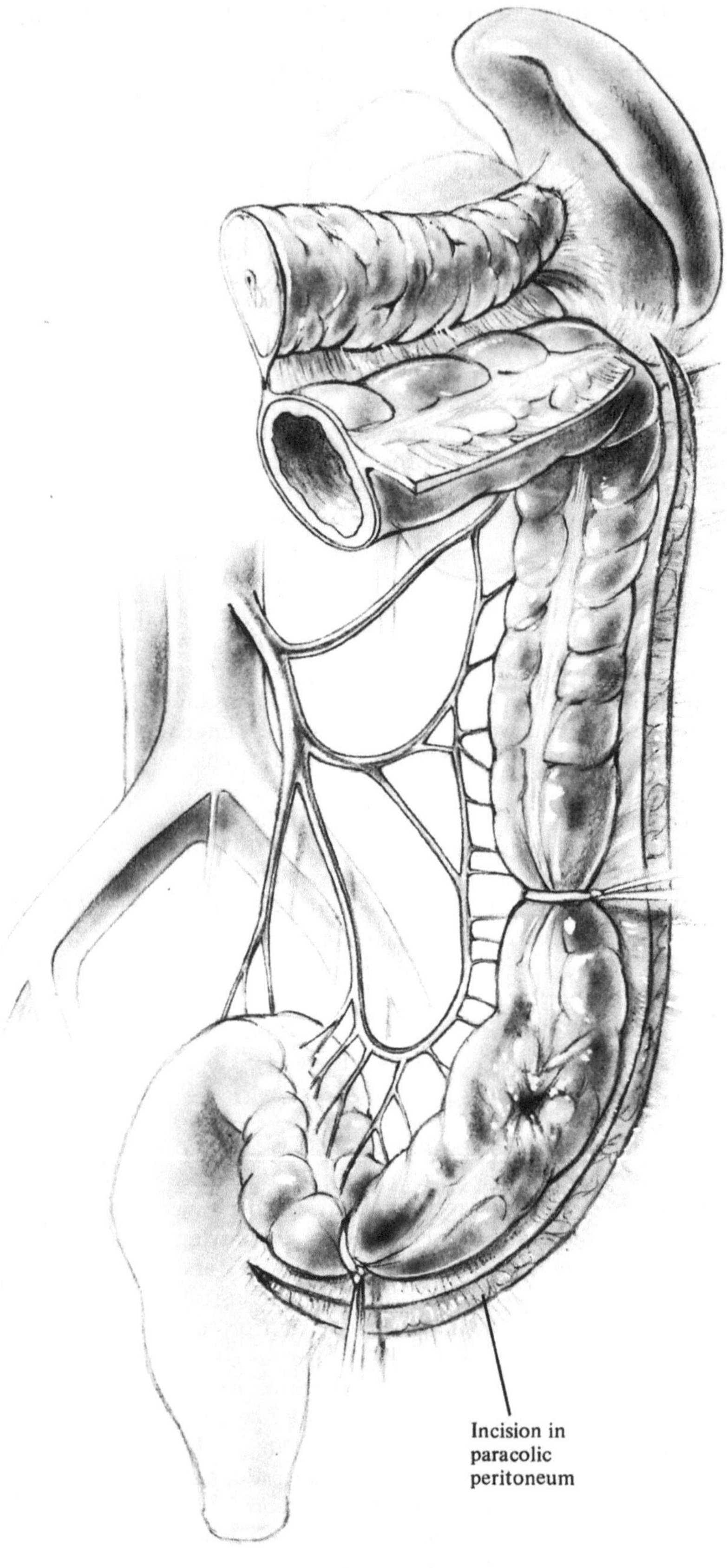


Fig. 4–3b

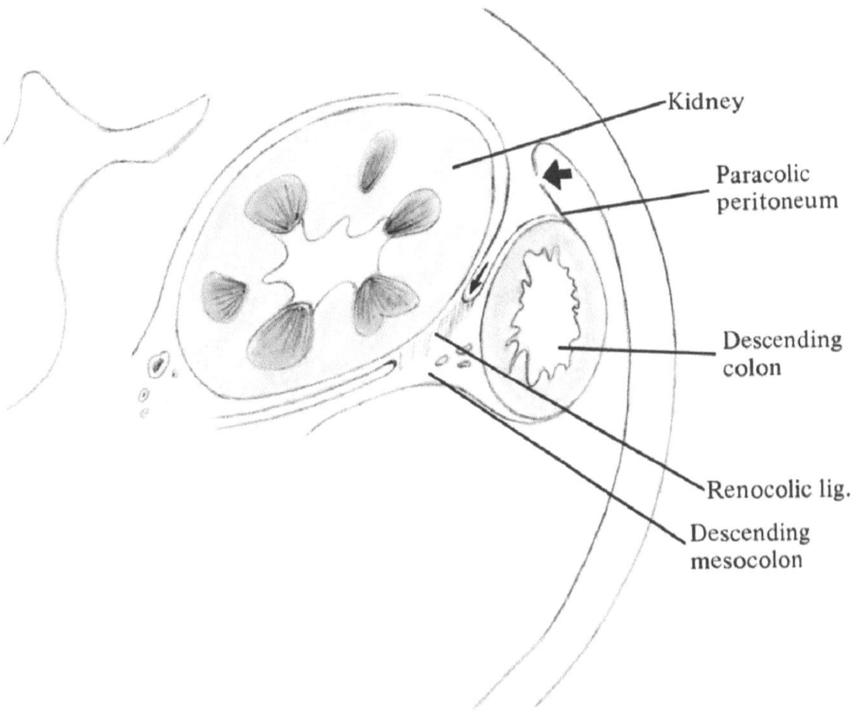


Fig. 4-4

**(Fig. 4–4)**. Most surgeons bluntly disrupt this renocolic attachment, which resembles a ligament, using a gauze pad in a sponge-holder; but this maneuver often tears small veins on the surface of the renal capsule and causes unnecessary bleeding. Instead, divide this structure with Metzenbaum scissors near the junction of the medial margin of the renal capsule and the adjacent mesocolon. Once the incision is initiated, delineate this fibrous structure by elevating it over an index finger **(Fig. 4–5)**. After the renocolic ligament has been divided, the upper ureter and gonadal vein lie exposed. Trace the ureter down to its entrance into the pelvis and encircle it with a Silastic loop tag for future identification.

## Splenic Flexure Dissection

The lower pole of the spleen can now be seen. Sharply divide any adhesions between the omentum and the capsule of the spleen to avoid inadvertent avulsion of the splenic capsule (due to traction on the omentum). If bleeding occurs because the splenic capsule has been torn, it can usually be controlled by applying a piece of topical hemostatic agent. Occasionally sutures on a fine atraumatic needle are helpful.

At this stage identify and divide the attachments between the omentum and the lateral aspect of the transverse colon. Remember to differentiate carefully between the fat of the appendices epiploica and the more lobulated fat of the omentum (see Operative Strategy, above). Free the omentum from the distal 10-12 cm of transverse colon **(Fig. 4–6)**. If the tumor is located in the distal transverse colon, leave the omentum attached to the tumor and divide the omentum just outside the gastroepiploic arcade.

Return now to the upper portion of the divided renocolic ligament. Insert the *right* index finger underneath the upper portion of this ligament and pinch it between the index finger and thumb; this maneuver localizes the lienocolic ligament **(Fig. 4–7)**. The ligament should be divided by the first assistant guided by the surgeon's right index finger. By inserting the index finger 5-6 cm farther medially, an avascular pancreaticocolic "ligament" **(Figs. 4-7, 4–8)** can be identified. It is an upper extension of the transverse mesocolon. After this structure has been divided, the distal transverse colon and splenic flexure become free of all posterior attachments. Control any bleeding in the area by sutureligature or electrocautery.

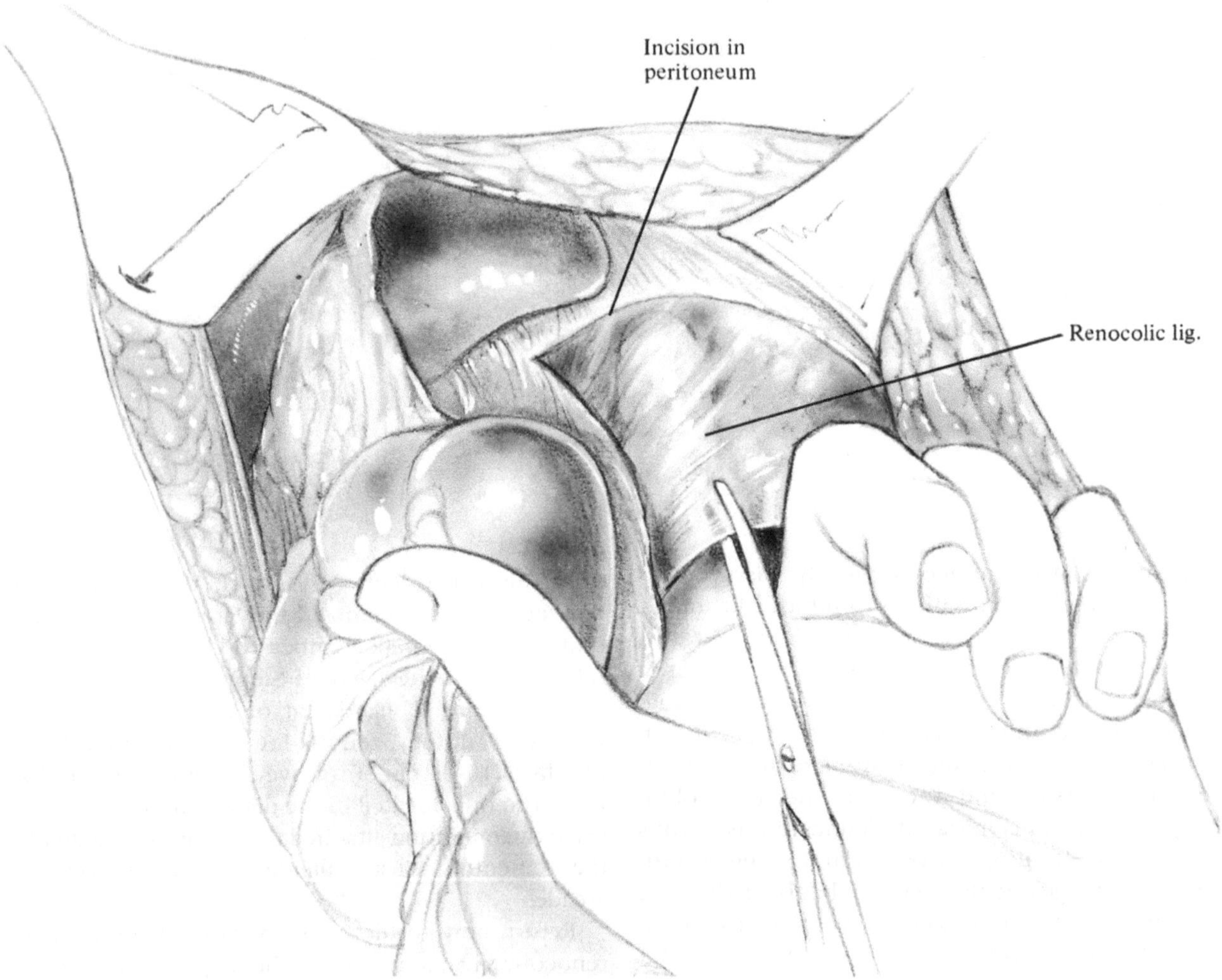


Fig. 4-5

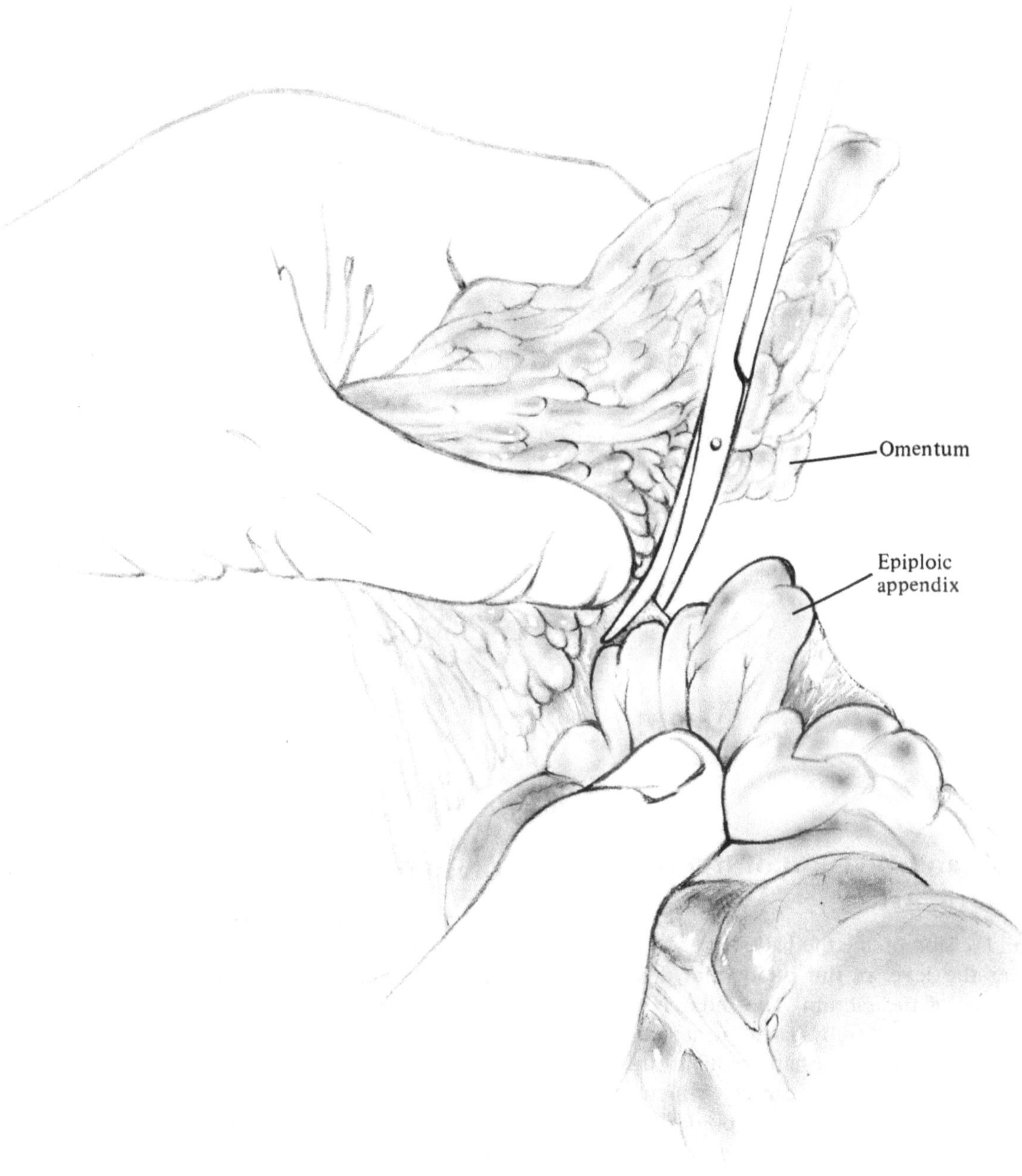


Fig. 4-6

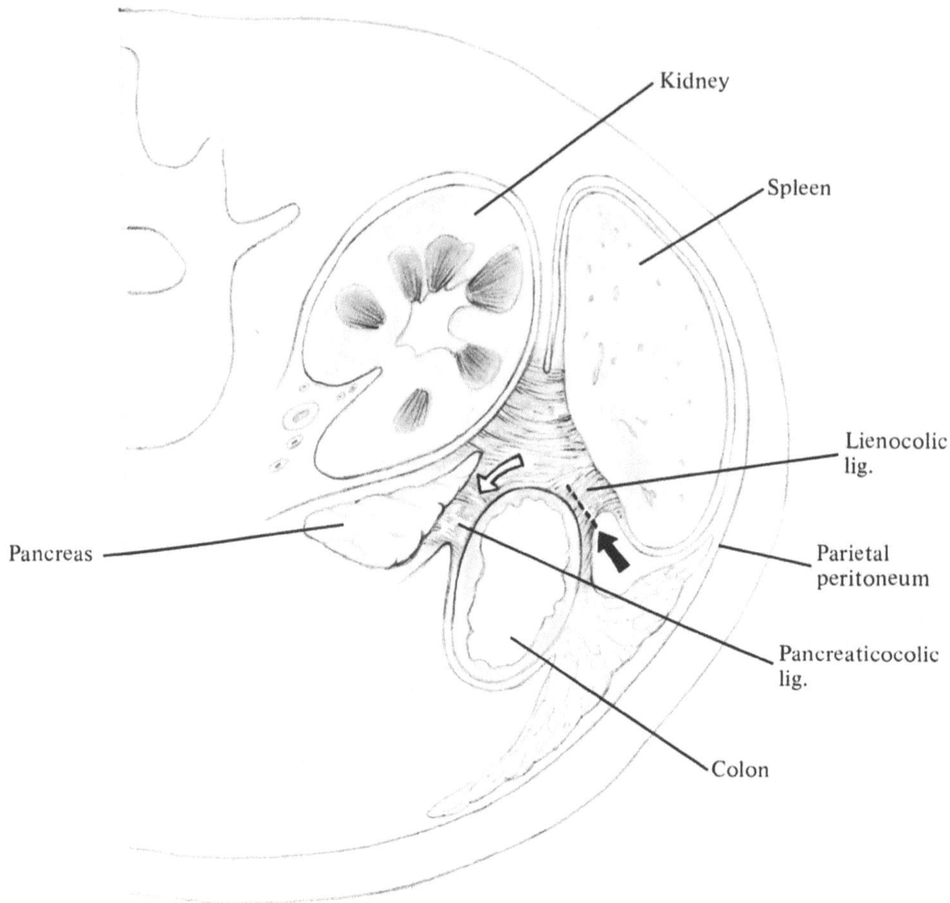


Fig. 4–7

## Ligation and Division of Inferior Mesenteric Artery

Make an incision on the medial aspect of the mesocolon from the level of the duodenum down to the promontory of the sacrum. The inferior mesenteric artery is easily identified by palpation at its origin from the aorta. Sweep the lymphatic tissue in this vicinity downward, skeletonizing the artery, which should be double-ligated with 2-0 silk at a point about 1.5 cm from the aorta **(Fig. 4–9)** and then divided. Sweep the preaortic areolar tissue and lymph nodes toward the specimen. It is not necessary to skeletonize the anterior wall of the aorta, as it could divide the preaortic sympathetic nerves, which would result in sexual dysfunction in male patients. If the preaortic dissection is carried out by gently sweeping the nodes laterally, the nerves are not divided inadvertently. Now divide the inferior mesenteric vein as it passes behind the duodenojejunal junction and pancreas.

## Division of Mesocolon

Depending on the location of the tumor, divide the mesocolon between clamps up to and including the marginal artery **(Fig. 4–10)**.

## Ligation and Division of Mesorectum

Separate the distally ligated pedicle of the inferior mesenteric artery and the divided mesocolon from the aorta and iliac vessels down to the promontory of the sacrum. Divide the vascular tissue around the rectum between pairs of hemostats sequentially until the wall of the upper rectum is visible. Then free the rectal stump of surrounding fat and areolar tissue at the point selected for the anastomosis. This point should be 2–3 cm above the promontory of the sacrum, where three-fourths of the rectum is covered anteriorly and laterally by peritoneum.

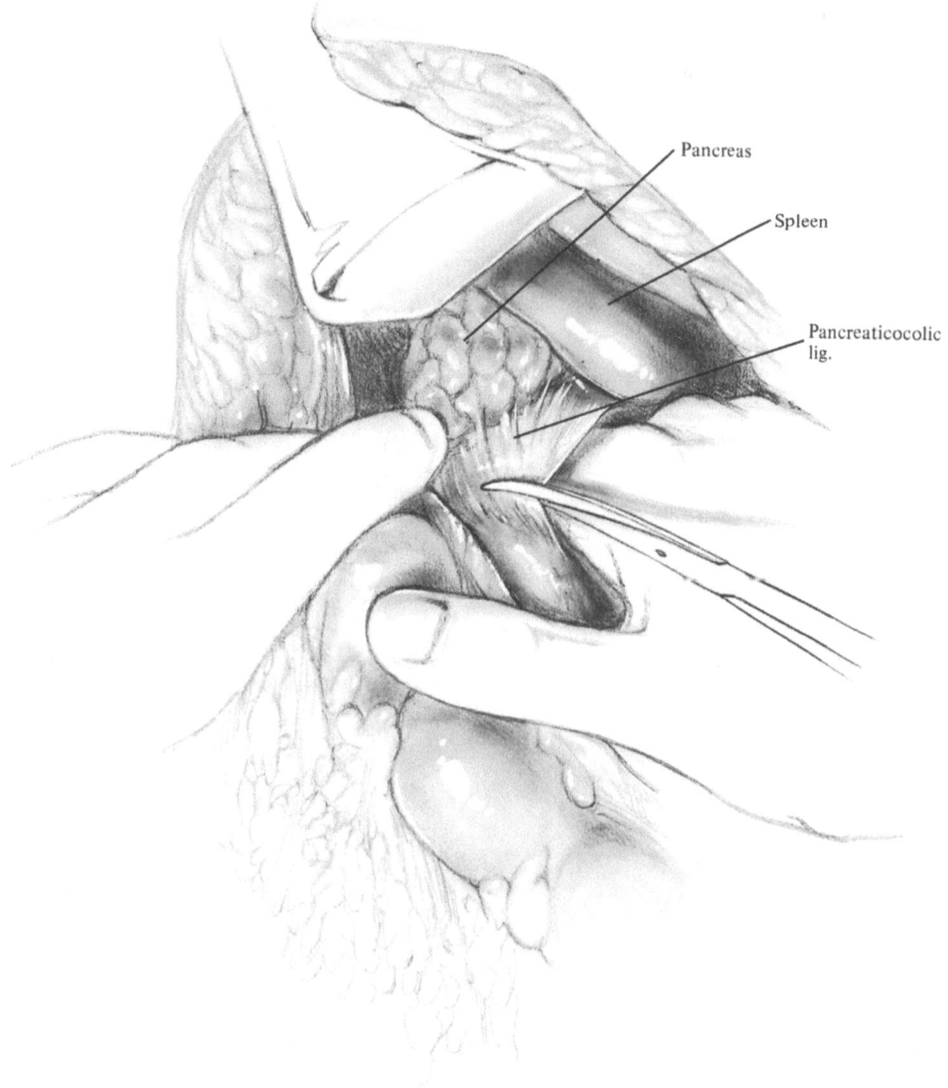


Fig. 4-8

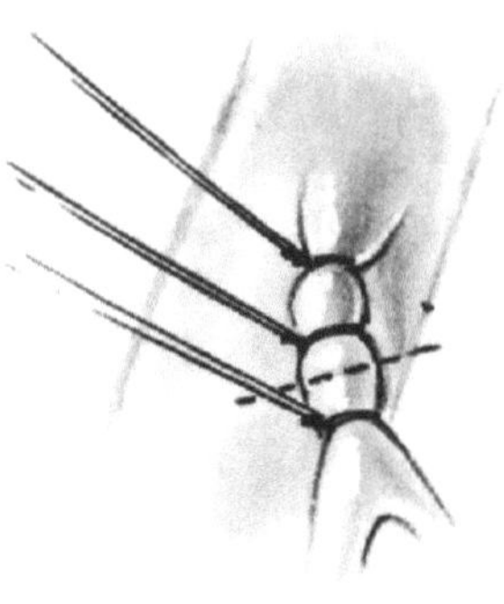

Fig. 4-9

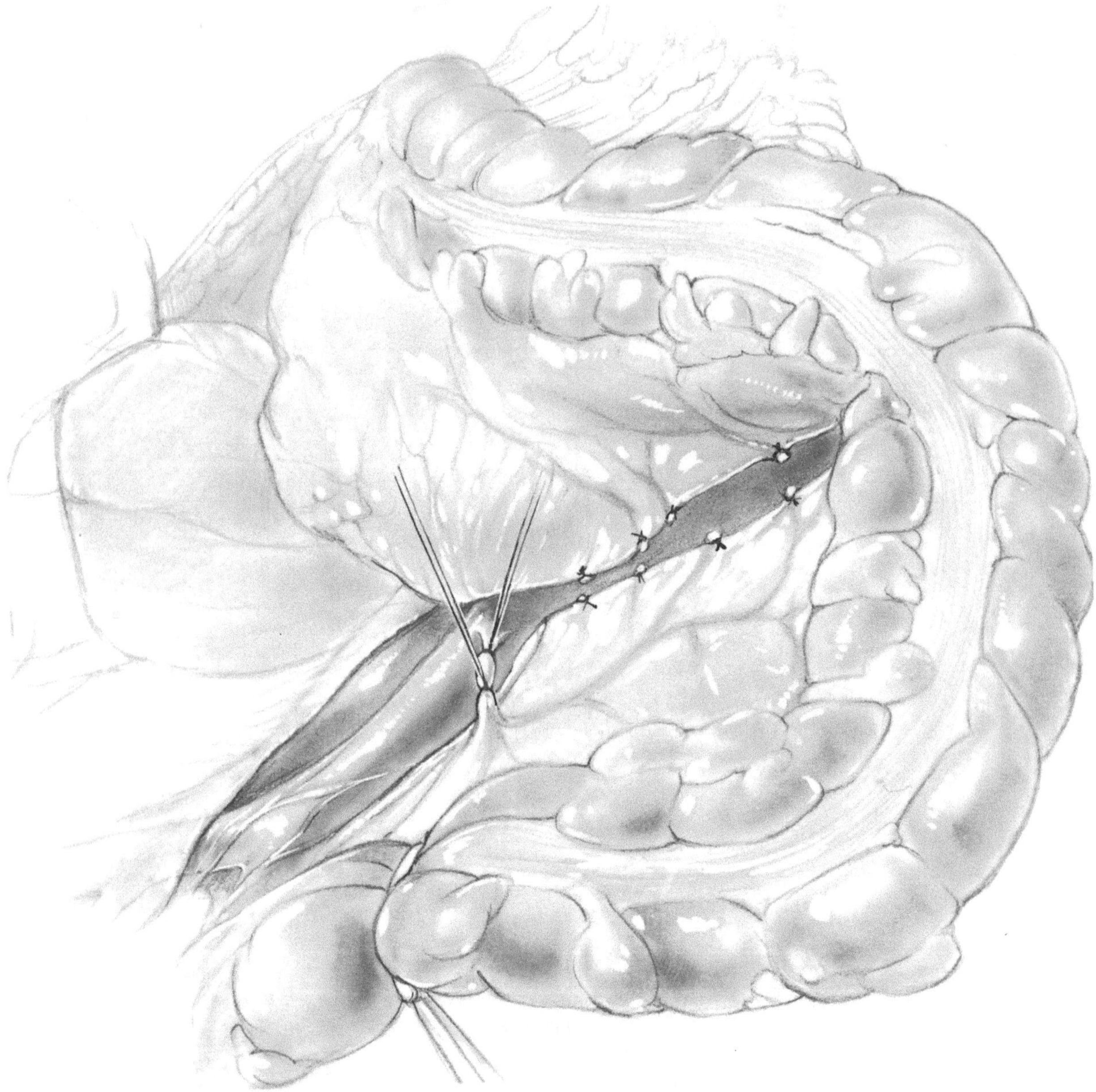

Fig. 4-10

## Insertion of Wound Protector

Insert a Wound Protector ring drape or moist laparotomy pads into the abdominal cavity to protect the subcutaneous panniculus from contamination when the colon is opened.

## Division of Colon and Rectum

Expose the point on the proximal colon selected for division. Apply an Allen clamp to the specimen side. Divide the colon after applying a Doyen or other type of nontraumatic clamp to avoid contamination. Completely clear the areolar tissue and fat from the distal centimeter of the proximal colon so the serosa is exposed throughout its circumference. Handle the distal end of the specimen in the same manner by applying an Allen clamp to the specimen side. Now divide the upper rectum and remove the specimen. Suction the rectum free of any contents. Apply no clamp. Use fine PG or PDS sutures to control any bleeding from the rectal wall. Completely clear surrounding fat and areolar tissue from a cuff of rectum 1 cm in width so seromuscular sutures may be inserted accurately.

## End-to-End Two-Layer Anastomosis, Rotation Method

There are eight steps to the end-to-end two-layer anastomosis, rotation method.

1. Check the *adequacy of the blood supply* of both ends of the bowel. Confirm that a *cuff of at least 1 cm of serosa* has been cleared to the areolar tissue and blood vessels at both ends of the bowel.
2. *Rotate the proximal colonic segment* so the mesentery enters from the right lateral margin of the anastomosis. Leave the rectal segment undisturbed **(Fig. 4–11)**.
3. If the diameter of the lumen of one of the segments of bowel is significantly narrower than the other, *make a Cheatle slit*, 1–2 cm long, on the antimesenteric border of the narrower segment of bowel (see Figs. 2–10, 2–11).

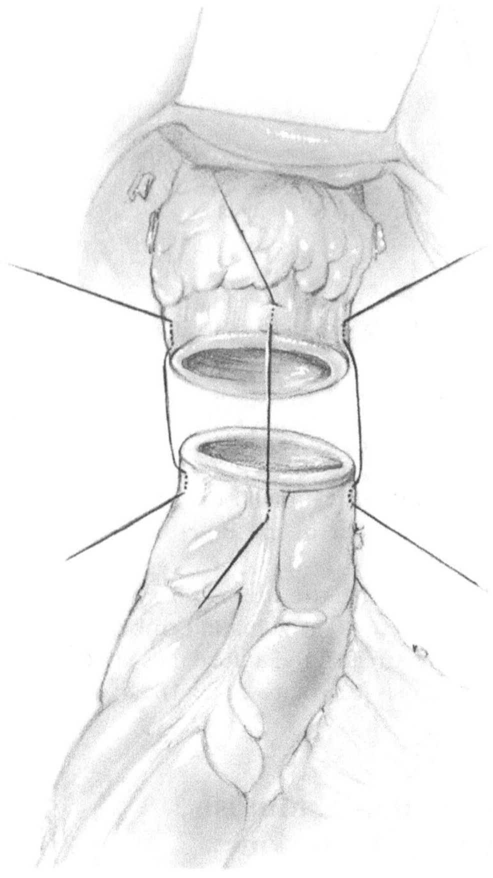

Fig. 4–11

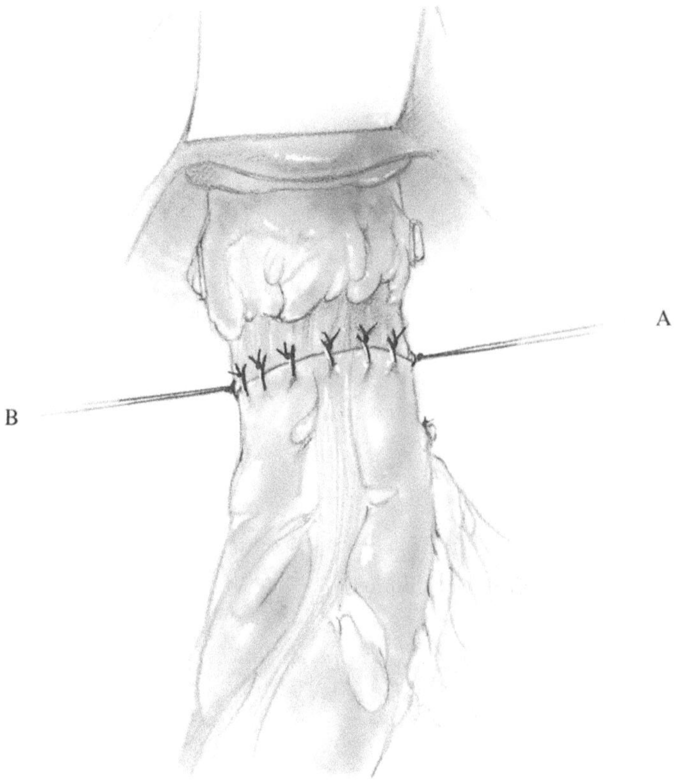


Fig. 4–12

4. *Insert the first layer of seromuscular sutures.* If the rectal stump is not bound to the sacrum and if it can be rotated easily for 180°, it is more efficient to insert the anterior seromuscular layer as the first step of the anastomosis.
5. Insert interrupted 4-0 silk atraumatic Lembert seromuscular guy sutures, first to the lateral border of the anastomosis and then to the medial border. Using the technique of successive bisection, place the third Lembert suture on the anterior wall halfway between the first two (Fig. 4–11). Each stitch takes about 5 mm of tissue (including the submucosa) from the rectum and then from the descending colon.
6. After all the anterior sutures have been inserted, *tie them and cut all the suture tails* except for those of the two end guy sutures, which should be grasped in hemostats **(Fig. 4–12)**. Pass a hemostat underneath the suture line, grasp the right lateral stitch (**Fig. 4–13**, A), and rotate the anastomosis 180° **(Fig. 4–14)**.
7. Place a double-armed 5-0 Vicryl or PG *suture in the middle of the deep mucosal layer* **(Fig. 4–15a)**. Complete this layer with a continuous locked suture through the full thickness of the bowel **(Fig. 4–15b)**. Then, with the same two needles and

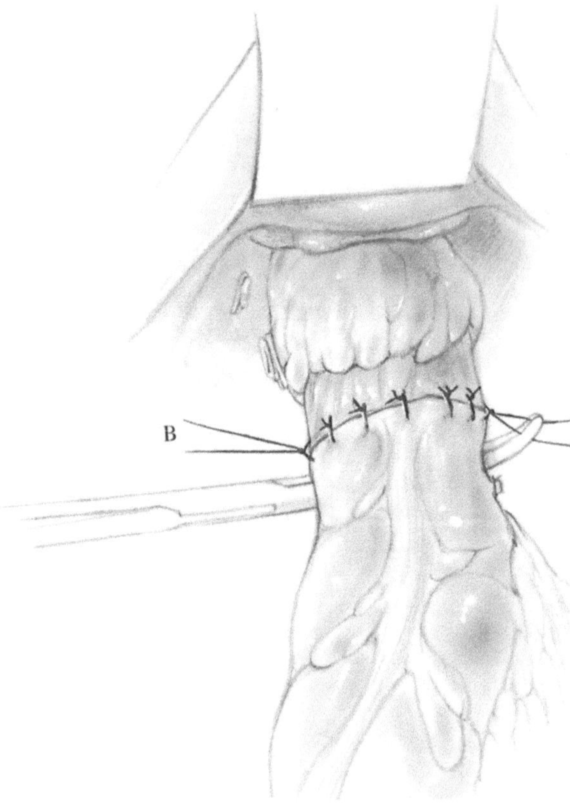


Fig. 4–13

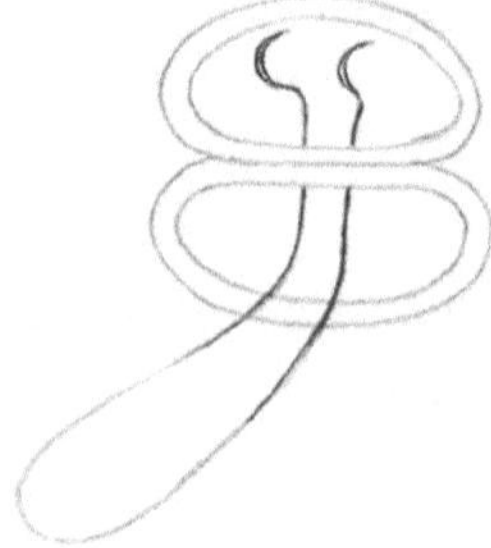

Fig. 4–15a

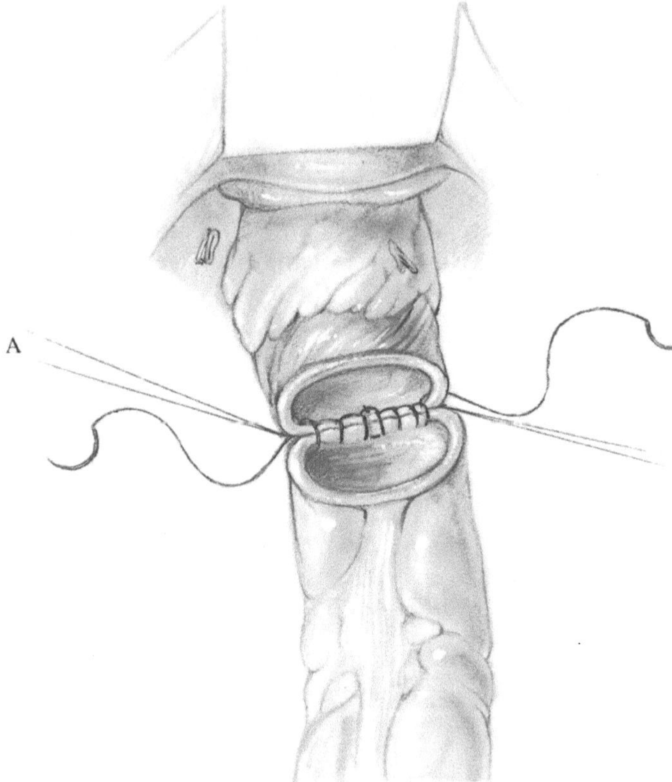


Fig. 4–15b

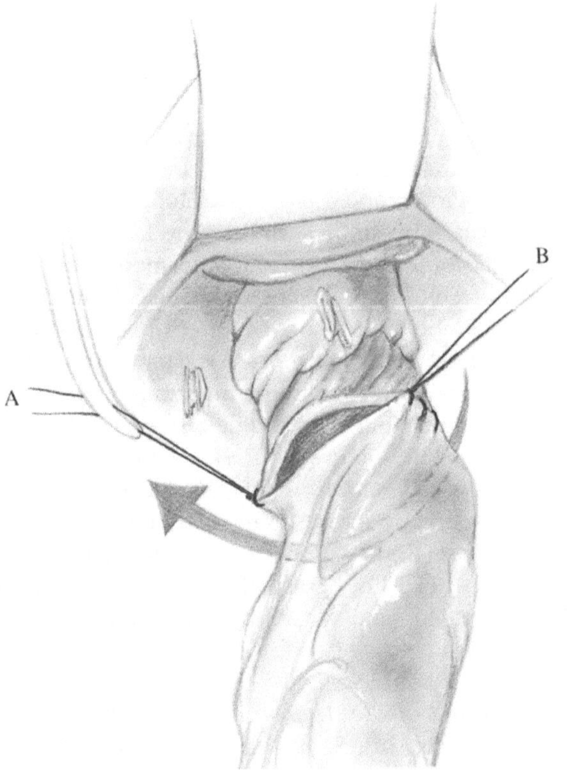


Fig. 4–14

using a continuous Connell or Cushing suture, complete the remainder of the mucosal approximation **(Fig. 4–16)**.

8. Approximate the *final seromuscular layer* with interrupted 4-0 atraumatic Lembert silk sutures **(Fig. 4–17)**. After all the suture tails are cut, permit the anastomosis to rotate back 180° to its normal position.

## End-to-End Anastomosis, Alternative Technique

When the rectum and colon cannot be rotated 180° as required for the method described above, an alter-

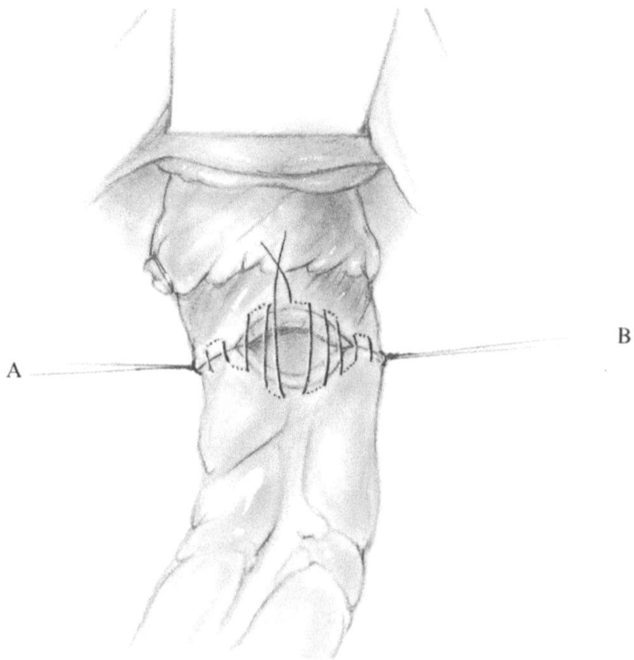


Fig. 4–16

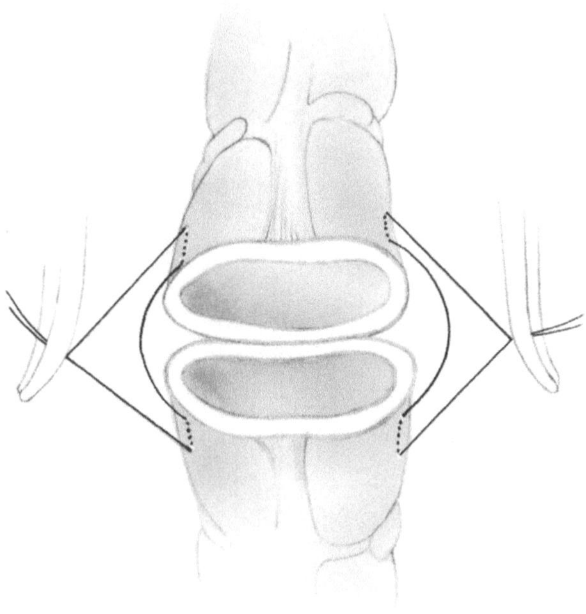

Fig. 4–18

native technique must be used in which the posterior seromuscular layer is inserted first. To do this, insert a seromuscular suture of 4-0 silk into the left side of the rectum and the proximal colon. Do not tie this suture; grasp it in a hemostat and use it as the left guy suture. Place a second, identical suture on the right lateral aspects of the rectum and proximal colon and similarly hold it in a hemostat **(Fig. 4–18)**.

Insert interrupted 4-0 silk seromuscular Lembert sutures **(Fig. 4–19)** to complete the posterior layer by successive bisection. As each suture is inserted, attach it to a hemostat until the layer is completed. At the conclusion of the layer, tie all the sutures and

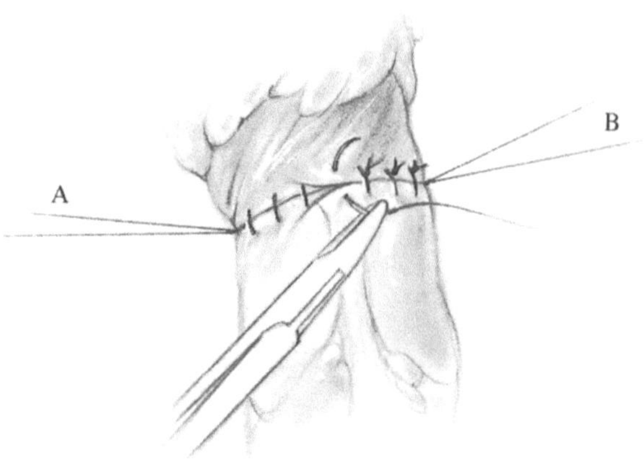


Fig. 4–17

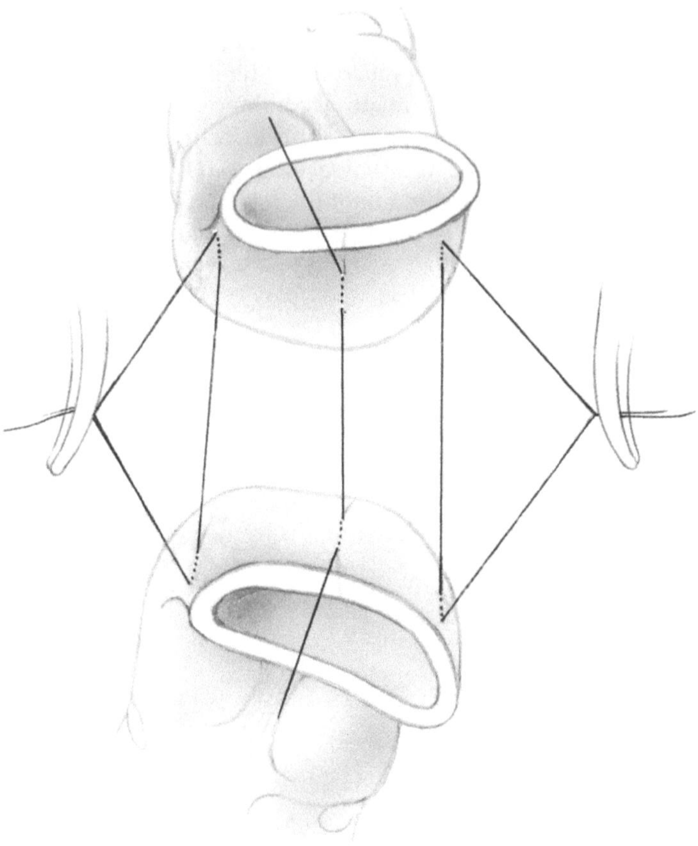

Fig. 4–19

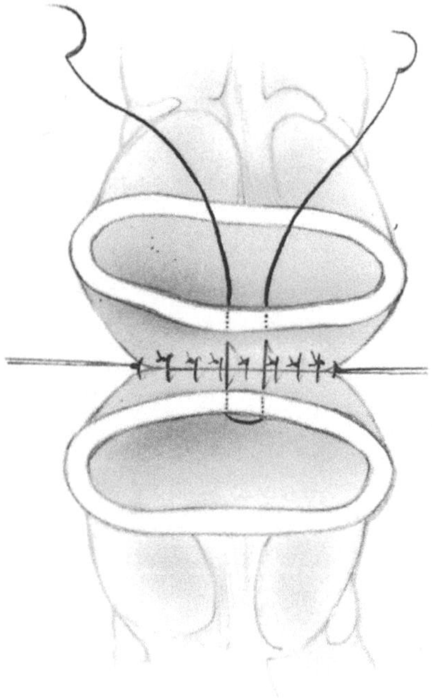

Fig. 4–20

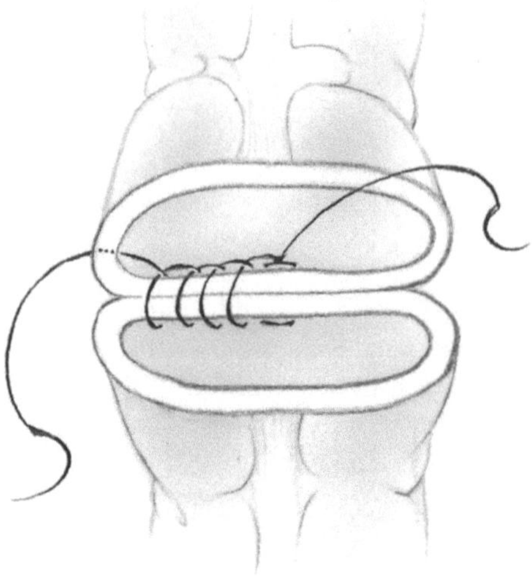

Fig. 4–22

cut all the tails except for those of the two lateral guy sutures. Begin the posterior mucosal layer with a double-armed atraumatic suture of 5-0 Vicryl. Insert the suture in mattress fashion in the midpoint of the posterior layer of mucosa and tie it **(Fig. 4–20)**. Use one needle to initiate a continuous locked suture, taking bites averaging 5 mm in diameter and going through all coats of bowel **(Fig. 4–21)**. Continue this in a locked fashion until the left lateral margin of the anastomosis is reached **(Fig. 4–22)**. At this point pass the needle from the inside to the outside of the rectum and hold it temporarily in a hemostat.

Grasp the remaining needle and insert a continuous locked suture of the same type, beginning at the midpoint and continuing to the right lateral margin of the bowel. Here, pass the needle through the rectum from inside out **(Fig. 4–23)**.

Standing on the left side of the patient, use the needle on the right lateral aspect of the anastomosis to initiate the anterior mucosal layer. Insert continuous sutures of either the Cushing or Connell type to a point just beyond the middle of the anterior layer. Then grasp the needle emerging from the left lateral margin of the incision and insert a similar

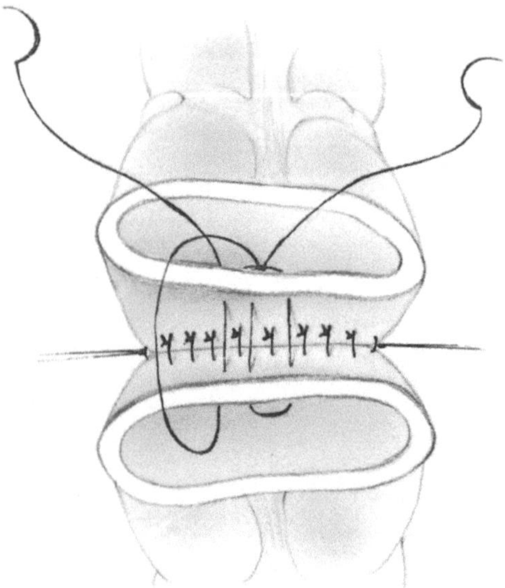

Fig. 4–21

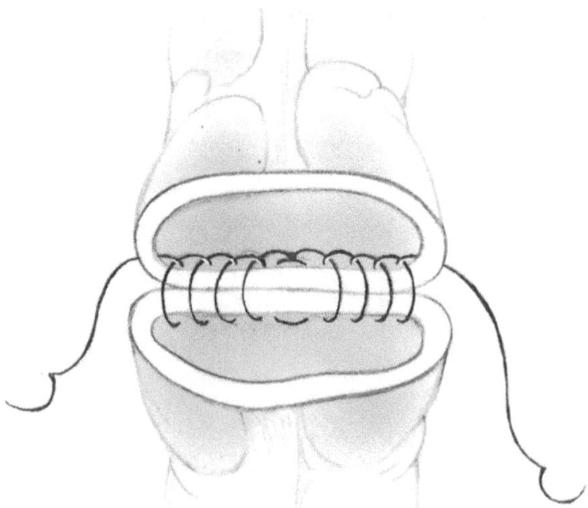

Fig. 4–23

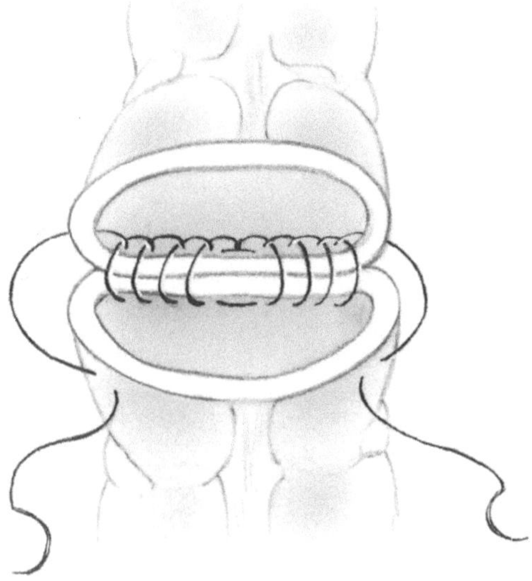

Fig. 4-24

continuous Connell or Cushing stitch. Complete the anterior mucosal layer by tying the suture to its mate and cutting the tails of these sutures **(Fig. 4–24, 4–25)**.

Complete the anterior seromuscular layer by inserting interrupted 4-0 silk atraumatic Lembert sutures **(Fig. 4–26)**. Now carefully rotate the anastomosis to inspect the integrity of the posterior layer. Test the diameter of the lumen before closing the mesentery by invaginating the colon through the lumen gently with the thumb and forefinger. Then close the mesentery with continuous 2-0 PG sutures **(Fig. 4–27)**. Leave the peritoneal defect in the left paracolic gutter unsutured.

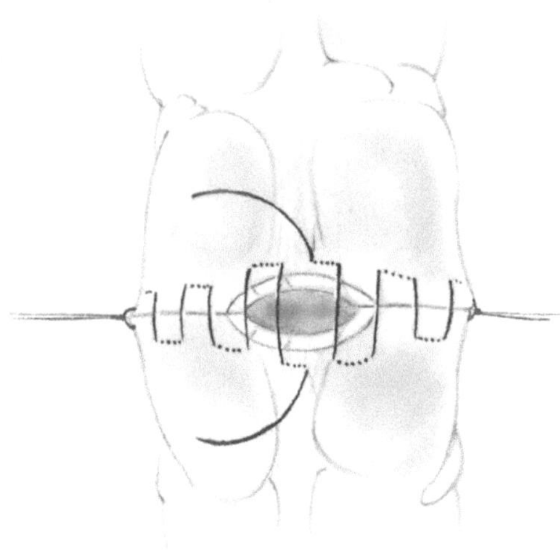

Fig. 4-25

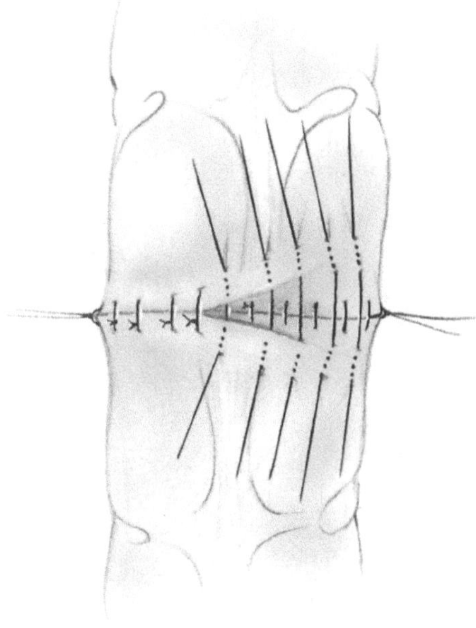

Fig. 4-26

## Stapled Colorectal Anastomosis

To construct a stapled colorectal anastomosis, first close the proximal descending colon with a 55/3.5 mm linear stapling device **(Fig. 4–28)**. Apply an Allen clamp to the specimen side and divide the colon flush with the stapler. Remove the stapler **(Fig. 4–29)** and replace the Allen clamp with an umbilical tape ligature covered with a sterile rubber glove **(Figs. 4–30, 4–31)**. Alternatively, divide the colon with a cutting linear stapler. Then direct attention to the rectum, a segment of which was previously cleared of surrounding fat and vascular tissue. Use the 55/3.5 mm linear stapling device (Fig. 4-28) to apply a layer of staples to this segment of rectum. Do not remove the specimen; retain it so mild upward traction on it can stabilize the rectum during application of the stapling device (Fig. 4-29).

Make a stab wound on the antimesenteric border of the proximal colon at a point 5-6 cm proximal to the staple line. A scalpel blade or electrocautery may be used to make this incision. Make a second stab wound in the anterior wall of the rectal stump at a point 1 cm distal to the staple line already in place **(Fig. 4–32)**. Approximate the two stab wounds opposite each other, placing the proximal colonic segment anterior to the rectal stump. Insert the linear cutting stapling device, with one fork in the rectal stump and the other in the proximal colonic

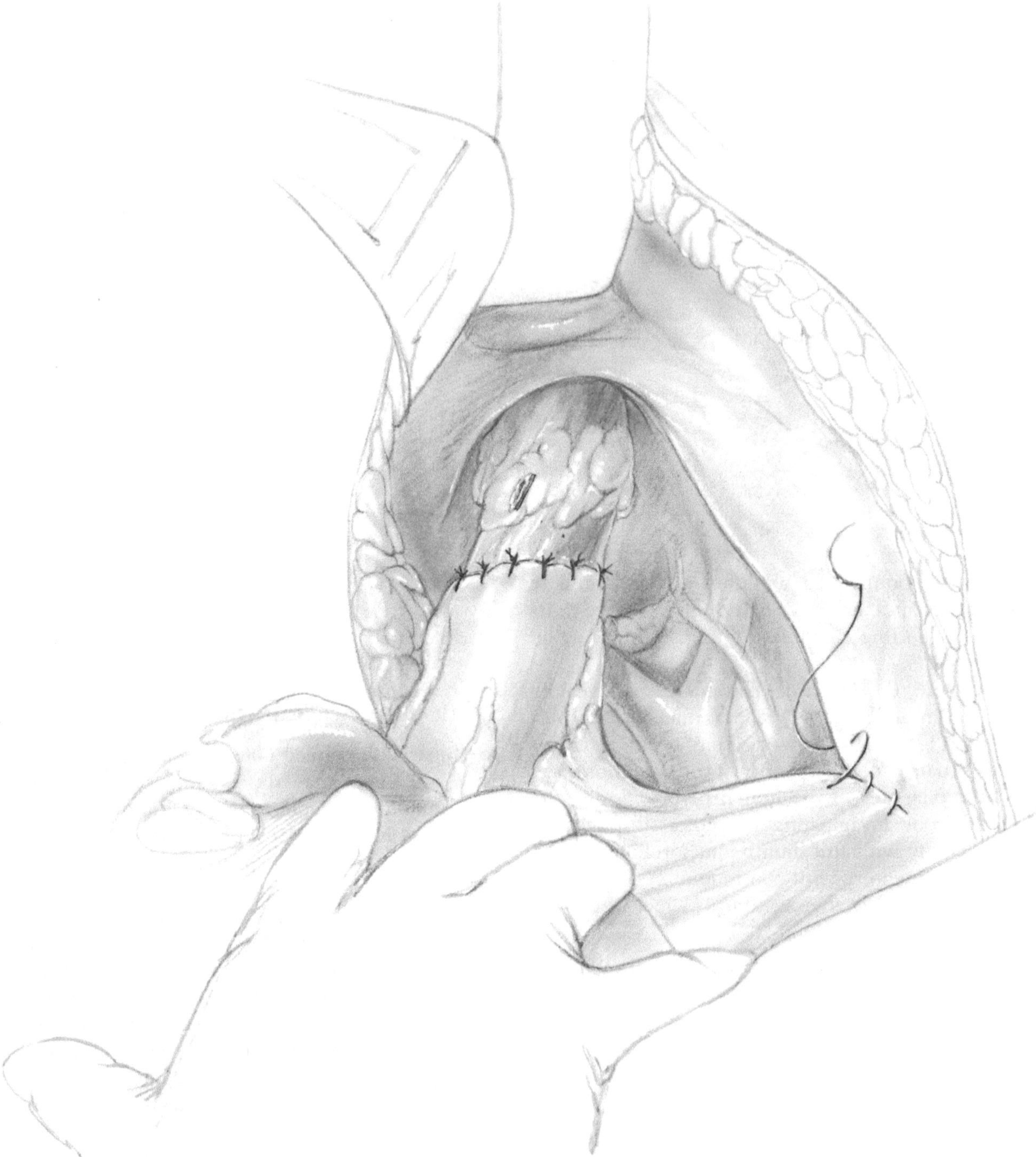

Fig. 4–27

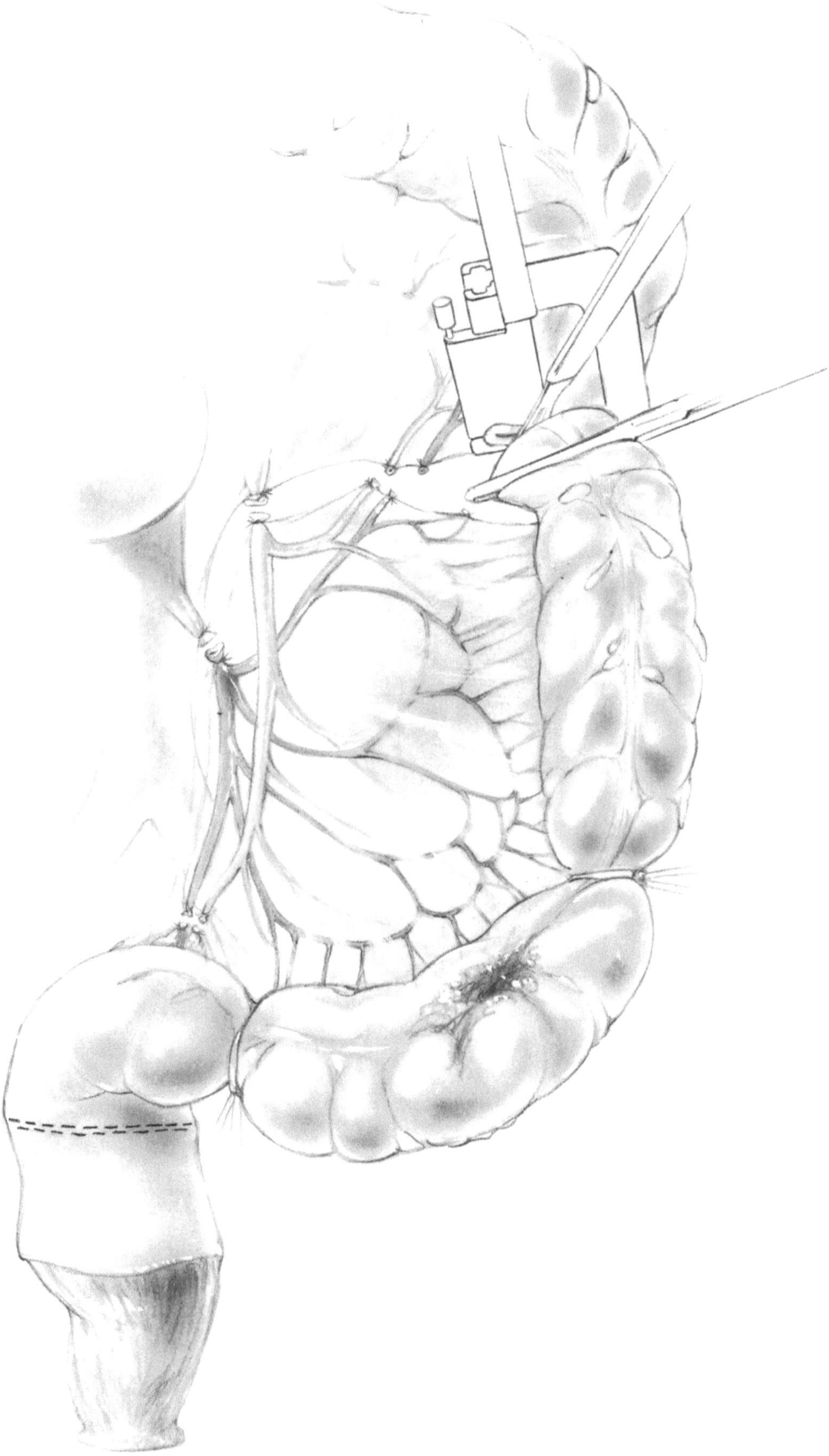

Fig. 4-28

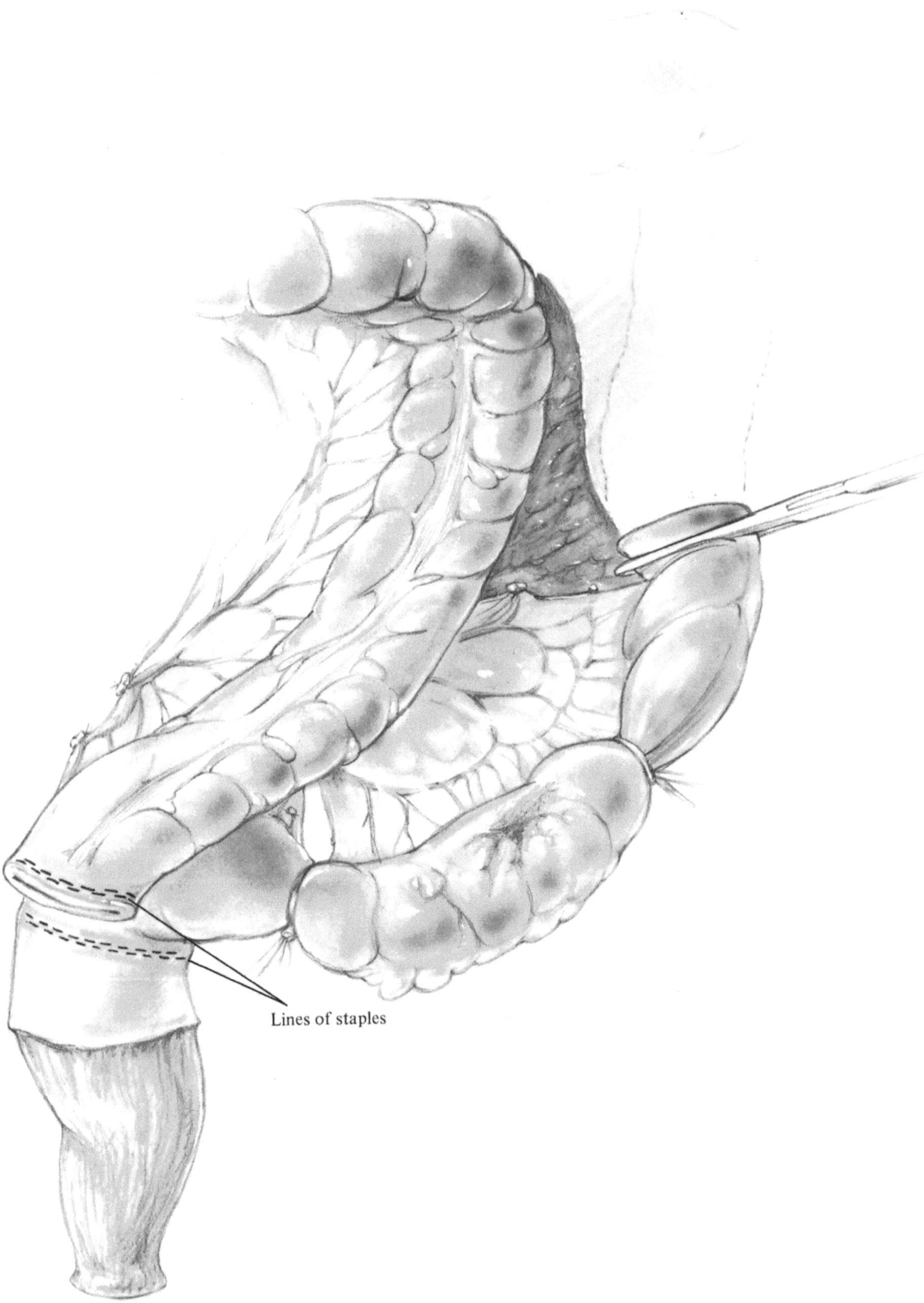


Fig. 4-29

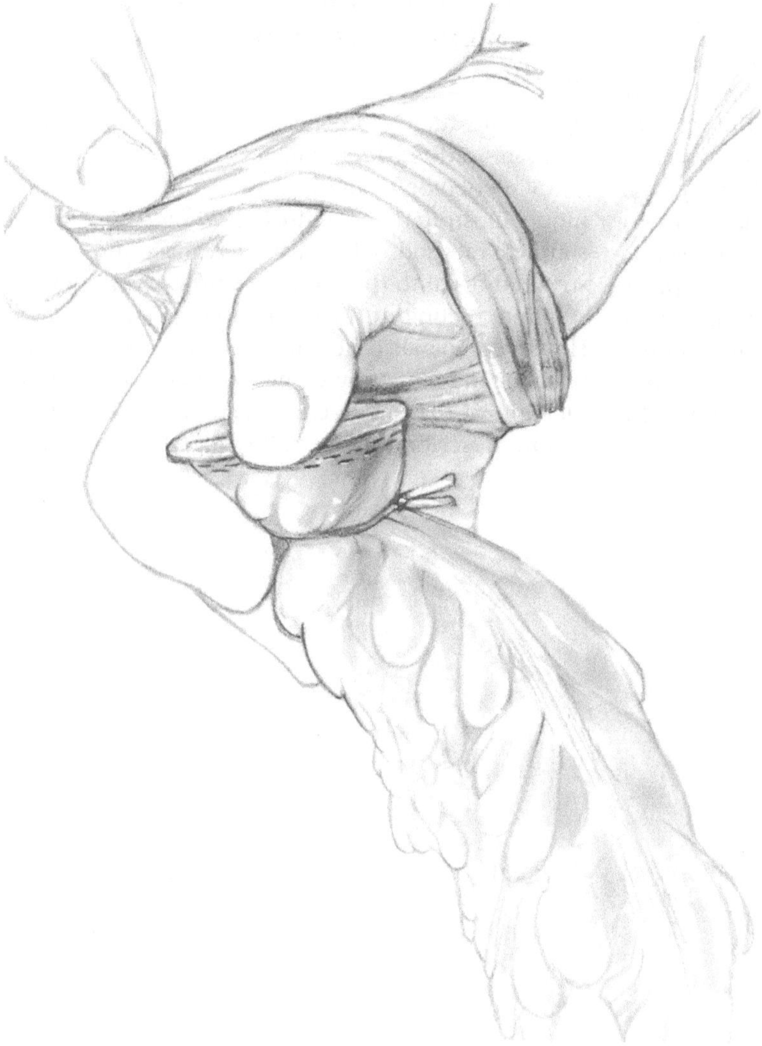

Fig. 4-30

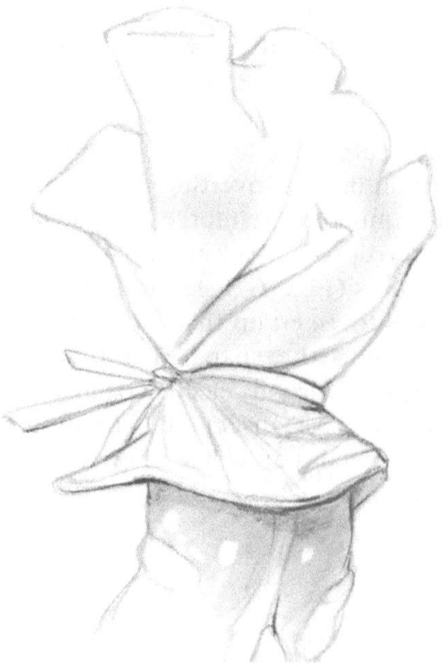

Fig. 4-31

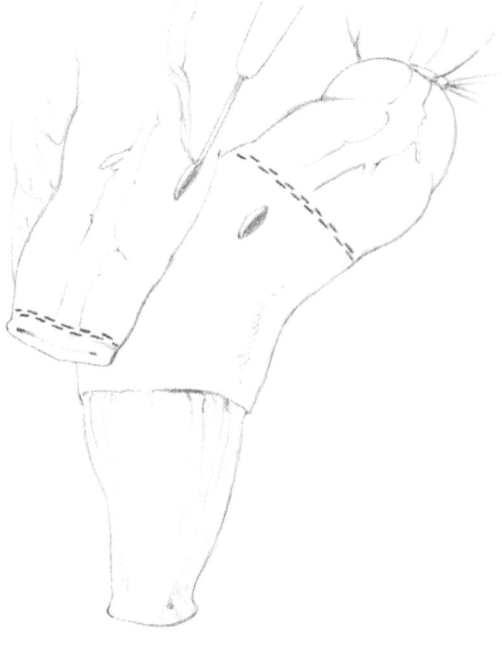

Fig. 4-32

segment **(Fig. 4–33)**. Allis clamps or guy sutures may be used to approximate the rectum and colon in the crotch of the stapler. Fire and remove the stapler; then carefully inspect the staple line for any defects or bleeding. Close the remaining defect with a continuous inverting 4-0 PG atraumatic suture to the mucosa. Reinforce this closure with a layer of interrupted 4-0 silk atraumatic seromuscular Lembert sutures **(Fig. 4–34)**. Carefully inspect all the staple lines to ascertain that the staples have closed properly into the shape of a B. Bleeding points may require careful electrocoagulation or fine suture ligatures. Transect the rectosigmoid just above the rectal staple line (Fig. 4-34) and remove the specimen.

## Stapled Colocolonic Functional End-to-End Anastomosis: Chassin's Method

When the lumen of one segment of bowel to be anastomosed is *much* smaller than the other, as in many ileocolonic anastomoses, the stapling technique illustrated in Figures 2-21 and 2-23 is the simplest method. When a stapled anastomosis is constructed distal to the sacral promontory, the circular stapling technique (see Chapter 45) is preferred. However, for all other intraperitoneal anastomoses of small and large bowel, we have developed a modification of the end-to-end anastomosis. This modification, described in the following steps, avoids the

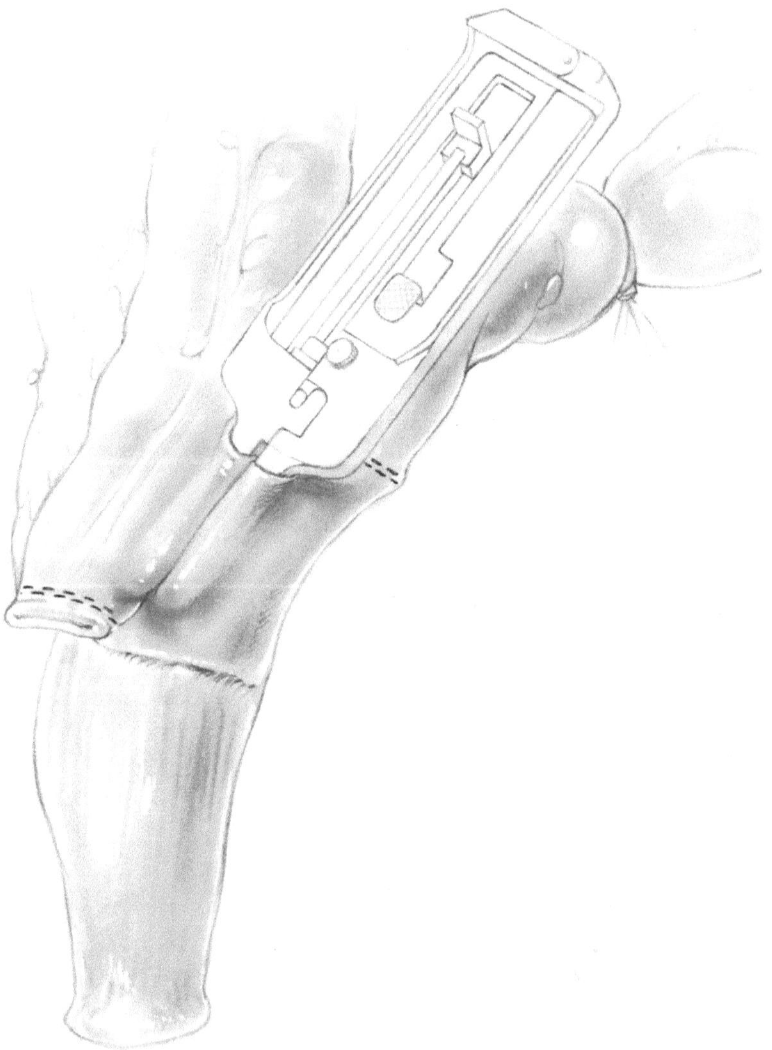

Fig. 4-33

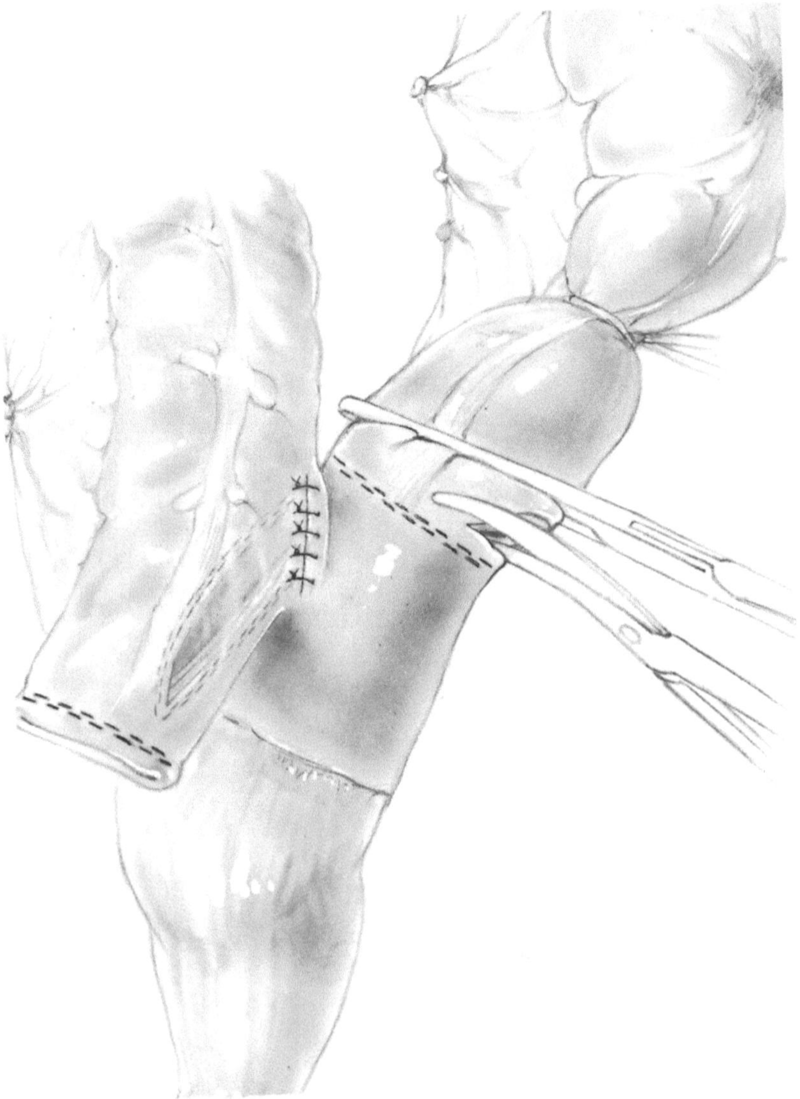

Fig. 4–34

possibility that six rows of staples are superimposed, one on the other, as may happen with the Steichen method.

1. Align the two open ends of bowel to be anastomosed side by side with the antimesenteric borders of each in contact.

2. Insert the linear cutting stapling instrument, placing one fork in each lumen **(Fig. 4–35)**. Draw the mesenteric borders of the bowel in the direction opposite to the location of the stapler. Avoid bunching too much tissue in the crotch of the stapling device. Lock and fire the instrument.

3. After unlocking the stapling instrument, withdraw it from the bowel. Apply Allis clamps to the extremities of the GIA staple line (**Fig. 4–36**, point A, shows the first extremity).

4. Place the 90 mm linear stapler in the proper position and fire it **(Fig. 4–37)**. Excise the redundant bowel with Mayo scissors and lightly electrocoagulate the everted mucosa.

5. Remove the linear stapler **(Fig. 4–38)** and carefully inspect the entire anastomosis for the proper B formation of staples.

6. Finally, insert a single 4-0 atraumatic silk seromuscular Lembert suture at the base of the anastomotic staple line (Fig. 4-38). This prevents any undue distracting force from being exerted on the stapled anastomosis.

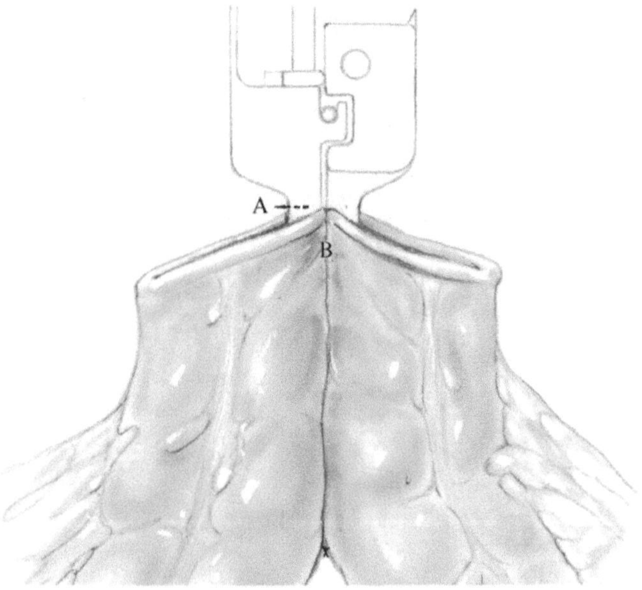

Fig. 4-35

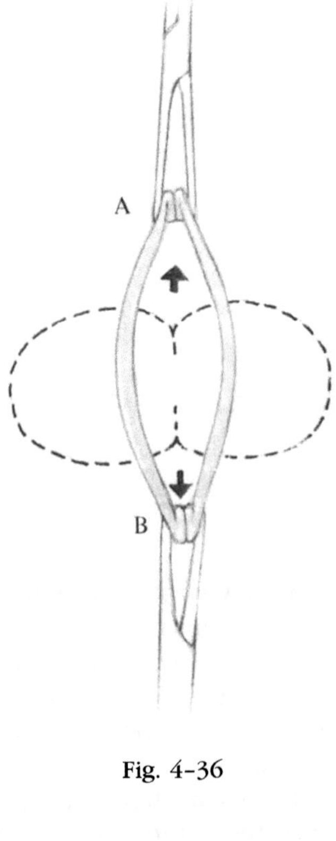

Fig. 4-36

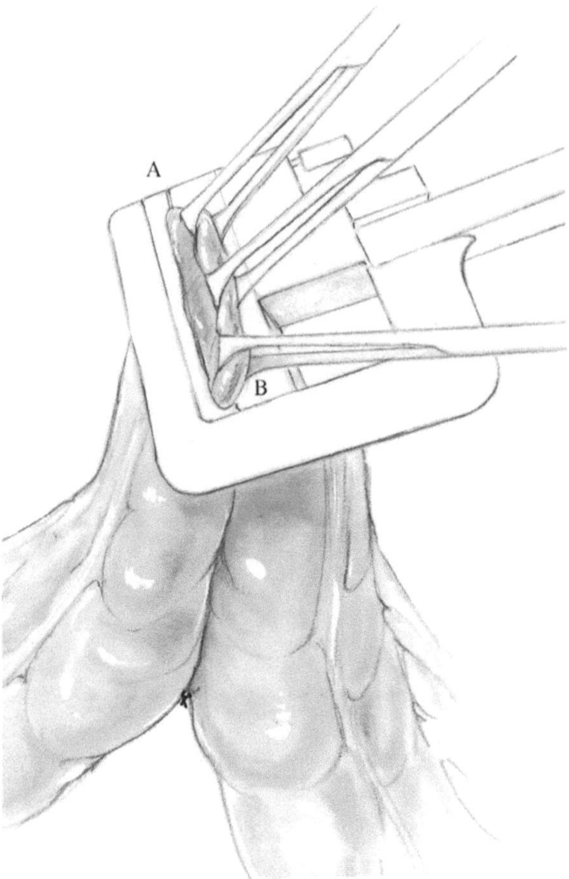

Fig. 4-37

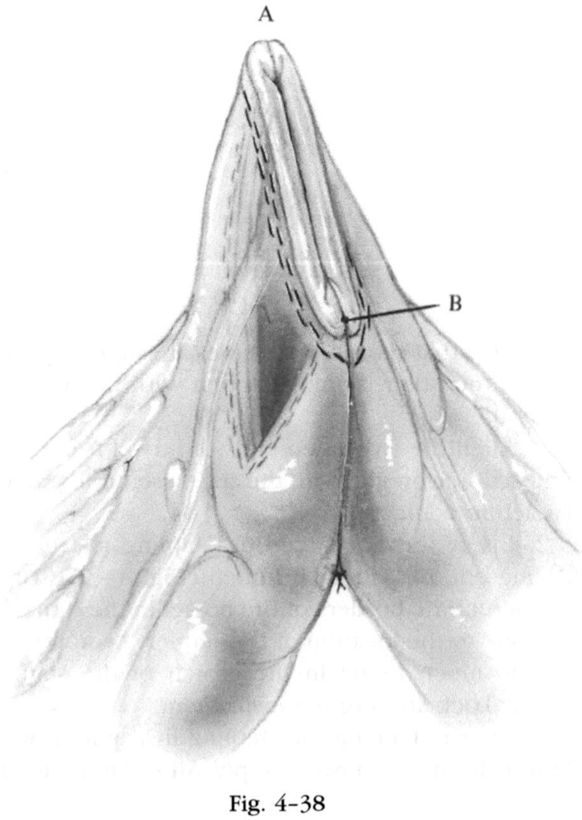

Fig. 4-38

## Closure

Discard all contaminated surgical gloves and instruments. Irrigate the abdomen. Most surgeons prefer to close the defect in the mesocolon (Fig. 4-27). A continuous suture of 2-0 PG is suitable for this purpose, although the defect is usually so large that omitting this step does not seem to lead to internal bowel herniation. Close the abdominal incision in routine fashion without placing any drains in the peritoneal cavity.

# POSTOPERATIVE CARE

See Chapter 2.

# COMPLICATIONS

See Chapter 2.

# REFERENCES

Bergamaschi R, Arnaud JP. Intracorporeal colorectal anastomosis following laparoscopic left colon resection. Surg Endosc 1997;11:800.

Weiss EG, Wexner SD. Laparoscopic segmental colectomies, anterior resection, and abdominoperneal resection. In Scott-Conner CEH (ed) The SAGES Manual. Fundamentals of Laparoscopy and GI Endoscopy. New York, Springer-Verlag, 1999, pp 286–299.

# 5 Laparoscopic Left Hemicolectomy

Steven D. Wexner

## INDICATIONS

Endoscopically unresectable colonic polyp

Crohn's colitis (limited segmental in selected cases)

Diverticulitis

Volvulus

Colonic carcinoma

## PREOPERATIVE PREPARATION

### Mechanical Bowel Preparation

Sodium phosphate 90 ml on the day before the surgery

### Administration of Prophylactic Antibiotics

Oral antibiotics (neomycin and metronidazole) on the day before the surgery, and intravenous antibiotics at induction of anesthesia

### Other Perioperative Steps

Sequential compression stockings and subcutaneous heparin or low molecular weight heparin for venous thrombosis prophylaxis

## PITFALLS AND DANGER POINTS

Injury to inferior epigastric vessels, left ureter, and spleen

Inadequate mobilization of colon and resection margin

Tenuous blood supply to the distal or proximal margins

Tension on the anastomosis

## OPERATIVE STRATEGY

Although laparoscopic left hemicolectomy is technically demanding that necessitates successful completion of a challenging learning curves. The requisite learning is limited not only to the techniques and methods, but as importantly to appropriated patient selection. Moreover some preoperative evaluation(s) may be valuable to facilitate the procedure. Specifically, computed tomography (CT) scan can be useful in assessing the extent of the disease; water soluble contrast enema and/or small bowel series may be helpful to anatomically localize any stenosis or fistula tract in patients with inflammatory processes. Colonoscopy with biopsy is widely performed to determine the pathology, however it may not always accurately detect the anatomical site. Intraoperative localization can be both difficult and time consuming, particularly when the surgical indication is an endoscopically unresectable adenoma or a small carcinoma. Therefore, it is advisable to perform the endoscopic tattoo marking (India ink injection) that allows extraluminal recognition of the tumor site in these patients. Thus preoperative endoscopic marking can facilitate lesion location and thus direct port placement and operative strategy. However on some occasions, such as with diverticulitis or segmental Crohn's colitis, a water soluble contrast enema may provide more useful data.

Preoperative placement of ureteric stents may be indicated when severe pelvic and/or retroperitoneal inflammatory processes are anticipated.

## OPERATIVE TECHNIQUE

### Room Setup and Patient Positioning

The video monitors should be placed near the patient's left shoulder and the patient's right knee, because a right hand dominant surgeon typically stands on the patient's right side, with the assistant on the opposite side and the camera operator on the same side cephalad to the surgeon at the commence of the surgery. The light sources, electrosurgical units, camera system, insufflator and pressure monitor are on the patient's right side. The patient should be secured to the operating table allowing various positioning including steep Trendelenburg and lateral rotation during the procedure.

The patient is placed in the modified lithotomy position allowing the access to the perineum but not interfering with the mobility of the surgical instruments. Both arms are tucked to the sides (adducted) enabling flexibility in the surgeon's position around the operating table. Well positioned and carefully padded Allen stirrups (Allen Medical, Bedford Heights, OH) are used perineal nerve injuries and the adducted arms are also carefully padded to prevent any brachial or other upper extremity plexopathy, neuropathy, or pressure injury.

If cystoscopy and bilateral ureteric catheters are not being utilized then a sterile bladder catheter is placed after which rectal irrigation is undertaken. Irrigation is accomplished through a mushroom tipped catheter initially with normal saline and then with povidone iodine.

## Trocar Placement

The Hasson (open) technique is used to place a 12-mm port through a supraumbilical incision. After achieving a 15 mm Hg pneumoperitomeum, a 30-degree, angled 10-mm diameter laparoscope is introduced through this port. The port is secured to the fascia by suture materials on both sides of the port. Following camera insertion into the abdominal cavity, an exploration commences with a view at the entire abdomen. Anatomy, resectability, adhesions, and concomitant conditions are assessed.

Place two trocars in the right lateral to the rectus muscle. Each trocar should be placed under direct vision and in the lateral to the rectus muscle in order to give a mechanical advantage during dissection and evade inadvertent injury to the epigastric vessels. It is essential that these accessory trocars should be placed at least a hand-spread width from each other to avoid instrument crowding. Additional one or two trocars may be placed in the left paraumbilical or suprapubic, and suprapubic midline, if necessary for adequate mobilization of the splenic flexure. Proposed sites of port placement are shown in **Figure 5–1**.

Intraoperative colonoscopy can be performed to localize the diseased segment after the establishment of the pneumoperitoneum and the trocar placement.

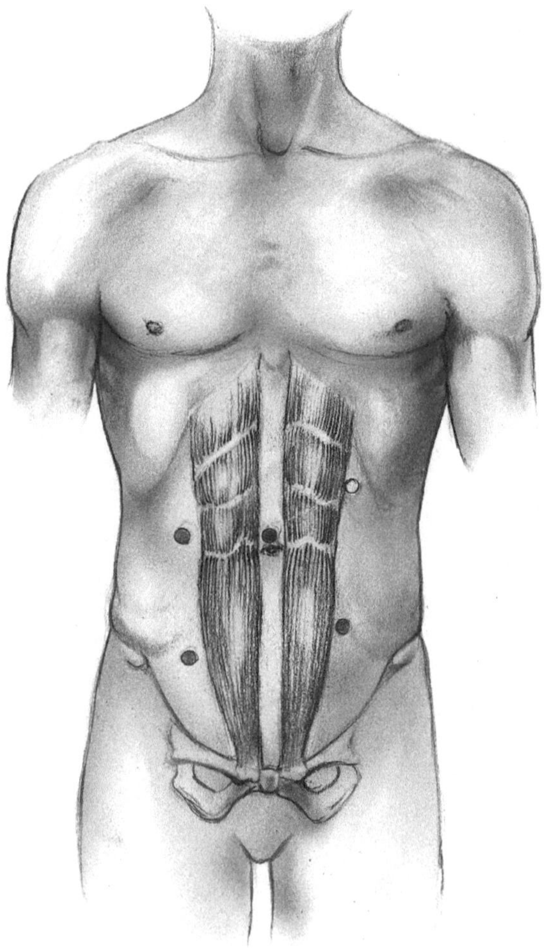

Fig. 5–1

## Mobilizing the Left Colon and Identification of the Left Ureter

We typically perform the "lateral-to-medial" technique. Following positioning of the patient to right side tilted down, start with the mobilization of the left colon from the left lateral sidewall, along with the white line of Toldt **(Fig. 5–2)**. The surgeon uses the two-right side ports for instrumentation. The surgeon grasps the bowel gently with an atraumatic forceps (Babcock clamp is preferred), and medially retracts it. This maneuver typically starts at the level of the sigmoid colon using either an electrocautery or the ultrasonic scalpel. The ultrasonic scalpel has amongst its several advantages in improved visualization as vessels and tissue are dissected without production of smoke. Then the dissection should be carried out on the plane between posterior aspect of the colonic mesentery and Gerota's fascia.

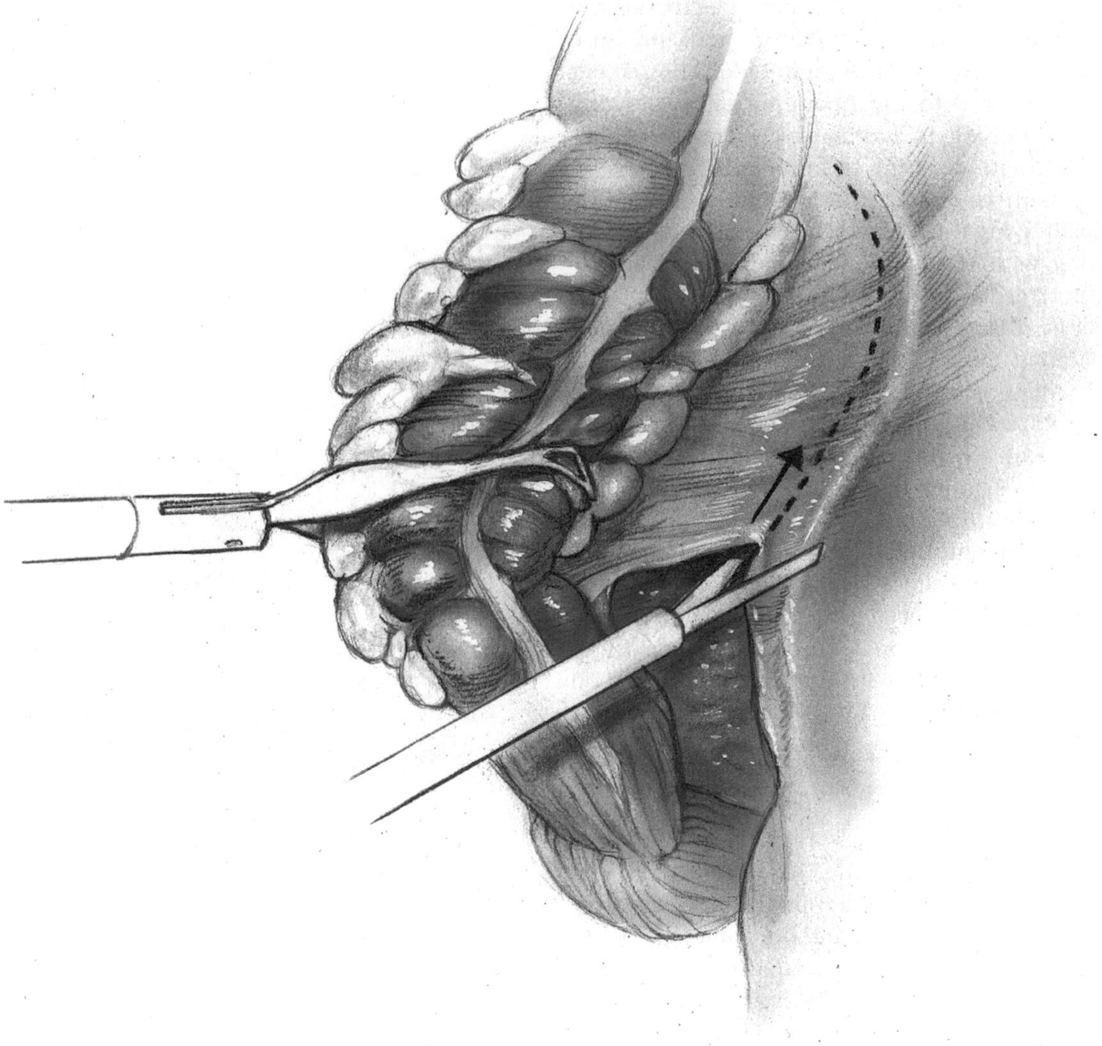

Fig. 5-2

As the sigmoid colon and the distal descending colon are medially mobilized, it is crucial to identify the left ureter prior to any vascular division. The left ureter is usually identified in the left iliac fossa overlying the iliac vessels. Again, preoperative indwelling of ureteric stents can be useful to assist this step especially in patients with inflammatory processes, giving tactile and visual sensation to the surgeon. If the surgeon fails to identify the left ureter at this point in the laparoscopic procedure, conversion to a laparotomy is considered.

## Dissecting the Splenic Flexure and Isolation of the Transverse Mesentery

The operating table is placed in the reverse Trendelenburg position and kept tilted down on the right side. Dissection then proceeds to the proximal colon to the proximal colon to the splenic flexure and distal to middle portion of the transverse colon. The surgeon must insure a sufficient resection margin and adequate mobilization to enable a tension-free anastomosis. This maneuver requires great attention

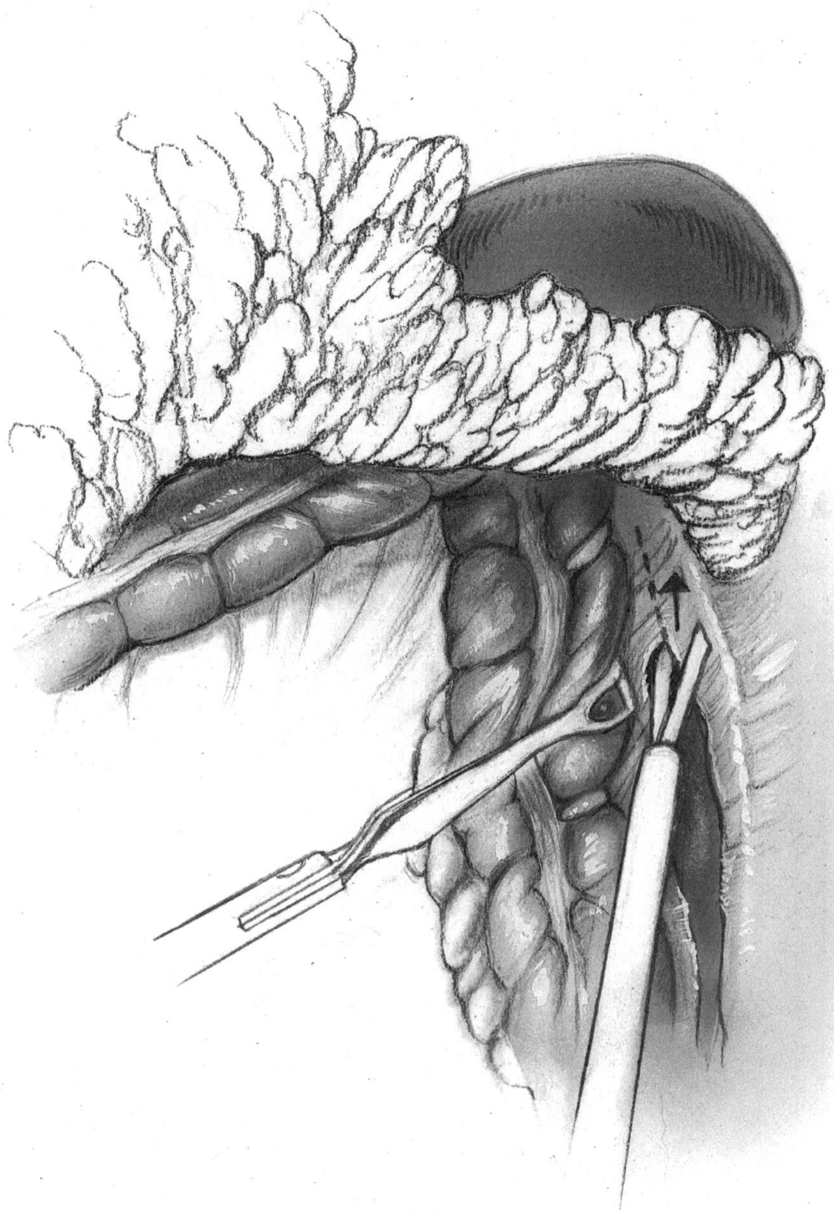

Fig. 5-3

not to traumatize the spleen **(Fig. 5–3)**. The surgeon can move to the position between the patient's legs, a position from which we believe it is technically superior to dissect the splenic flexure. The surgeon may place the additional trocars as previously described, in the suprapubic midline or left paraumbilical so that he or she can face both the splenic flexure and the monitor on the patient's shoulder in a straight line. The dissection should be continued as close to the bowel as possible, staying laterally and on the plane between Gerota's fascia and the mesentery.

Once the most cephalad portion of attachments at the splenic flexure are mobilized then the greater omentum is separated from the transverse colon **(Fig. 5–4)**. The division of the gastrocolic ligament may be necessary if the dissection is carried up to midtransverse colon. This maneuver is performed with cautery, clips, or the ultrasonic scalpel **(Fig. 5–5)**. Caudal and medial retraction of the transverse

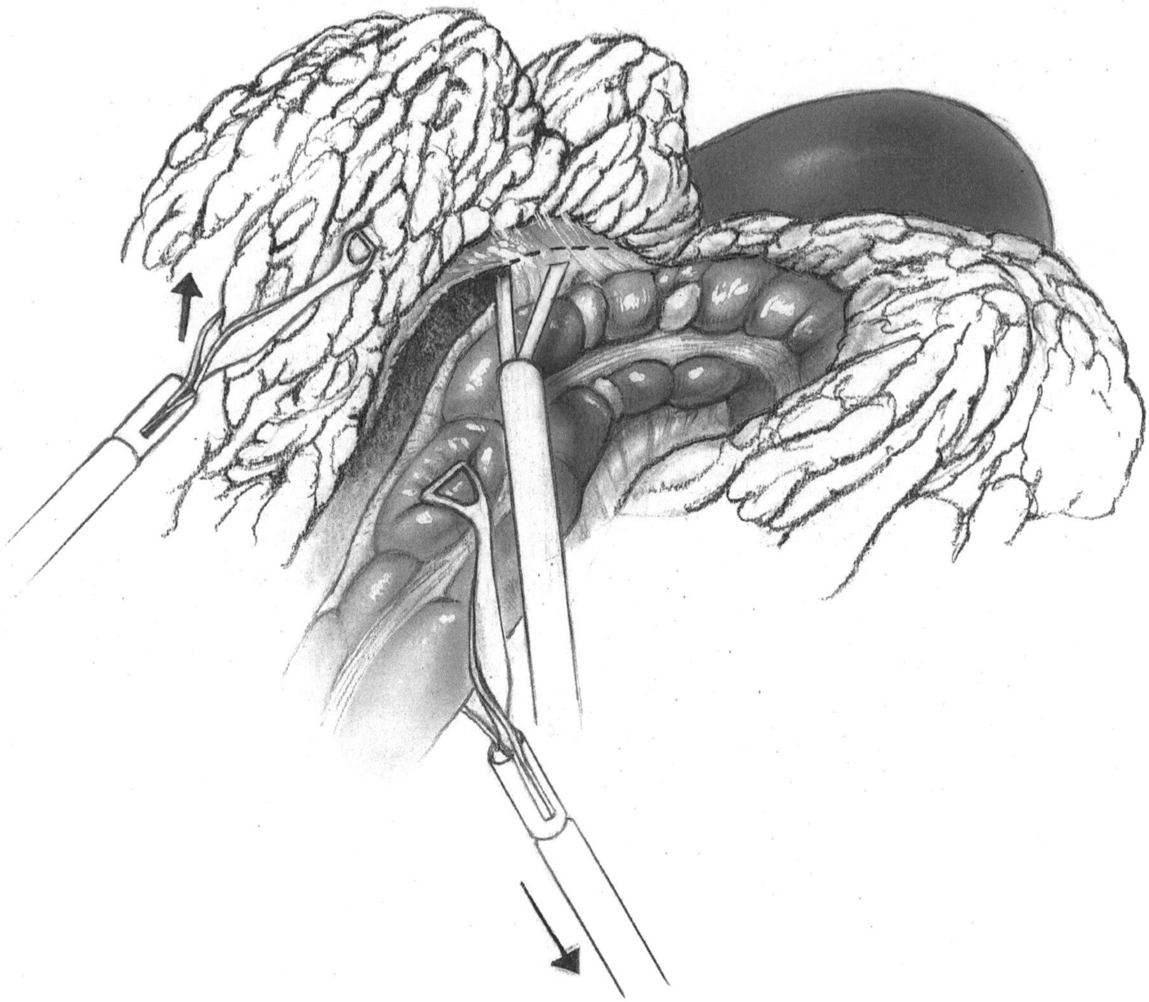

Fig. 5-4

colon facilitates the isolation of the transverse mesentery. Any injuries to the pancreas body or tail must be carefully avoided.

## Identification and Transection of the Mesentric Vessels

Once the left colon is completely mobilized, next phase is to identify and transect the inferior mesenteric vessels. The surgeon moves back to the patient's right side and uses the right-side ports. Providing gentle contertraction with the Babcock clamp, inferior mesenteric vascular arcade is exposed and identified within the sigmoid mesentery as "bow-stringing" **(Fig. 5–6)**. Windows are created within the mesentery skeltonizing the vessels, after which a vascular stapler or clips is applied. The respective instrument must be accurately applied to avoid any injury to the ureters, which lies just behind the sigmoid mesentery. The left ureter and the gonadal vessels may have to be gently reflected laterally to avoid being transected with the inferior mesenteric pedicle. Once assured that the left ureter is not incorporated, the stapler is fired and the vessels are divided close to their origins. It is crucial to visualize the distal tips of stapler application to insure that any extraneous tissue is not incorporated. The inferior mesenteric vein can also be transected allowing the proximal colon further reach towards to the pelvis. Vacular division may be extended to the left branch of the middle colic vessels depending upon the pathology and the location of diseased

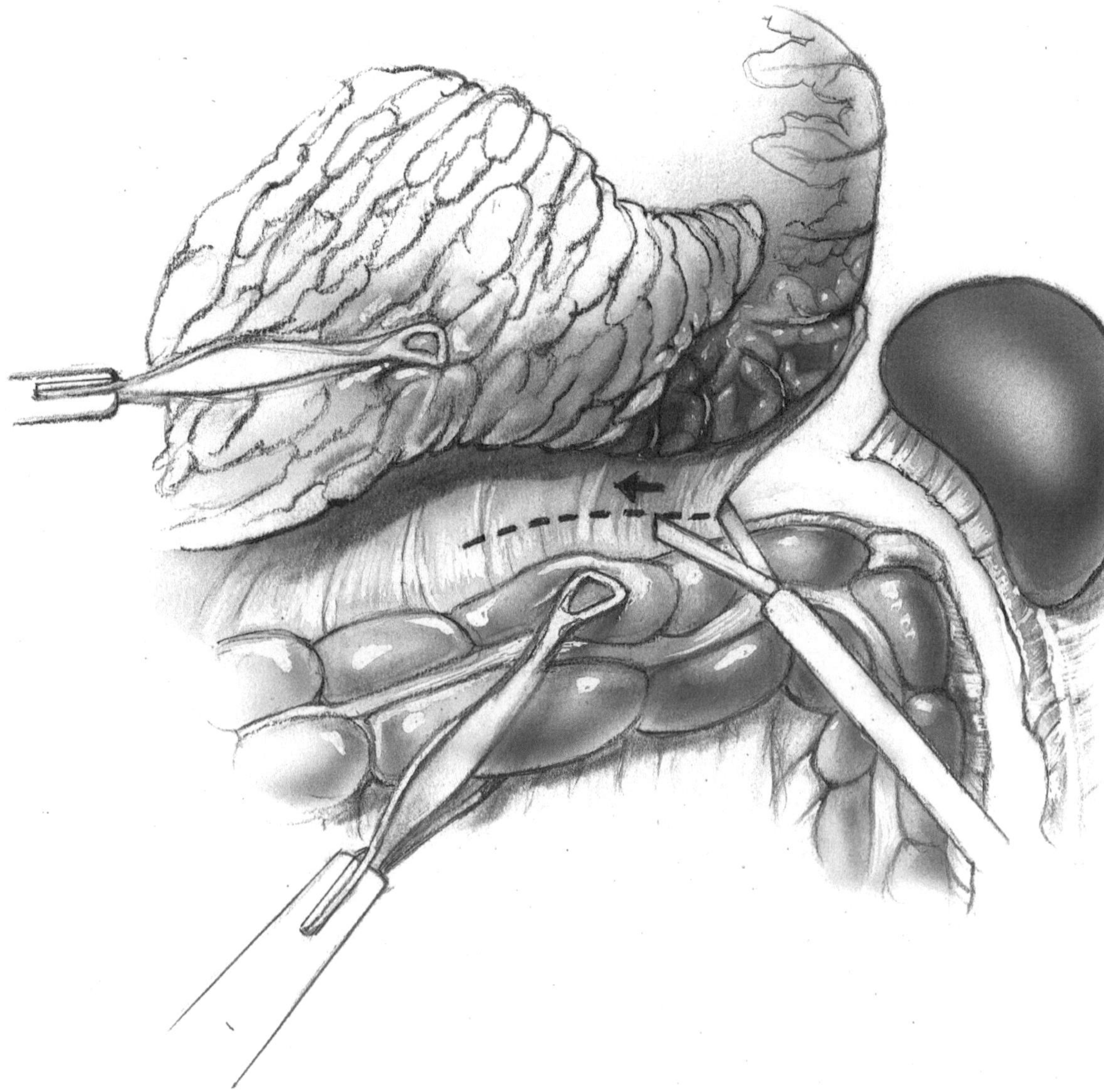

Fig. 5-5

segment. Similar contertraction is performed, giving an adequate tension to the transverse mesentery.

The dissection of the remaining mesentery is then initiated from the transected vascular pedicle, using clips, a cautery, the ultrasonic scalpel, or an alternate energy source. This dissection can be close to the bowel or along the root of the mesentery based on the indication for surgery.

After the transection has been accomplished, grasp the assumed proximal margin of the colon and gently deliver it down to the pelvis in order to assure that adequate length of the colon has been mobilized for performing a tension-free anastomosis. The anatomical blood supply to the proximal margin of the colon needs to be evaluated as well.

## Transection of the Distal Colon or Rectosigmoid Junction

To obtain the adequate distal margin, the dissection of the bowel may be extended over the sacral promontory and into the presacral space as necessary. Termination of the colonic teniae or the sacral promontory is the landmark of the rectosigmoid junction. The vessels in the posterior mesorectum occasionally require control by clips or a vascular stapler to

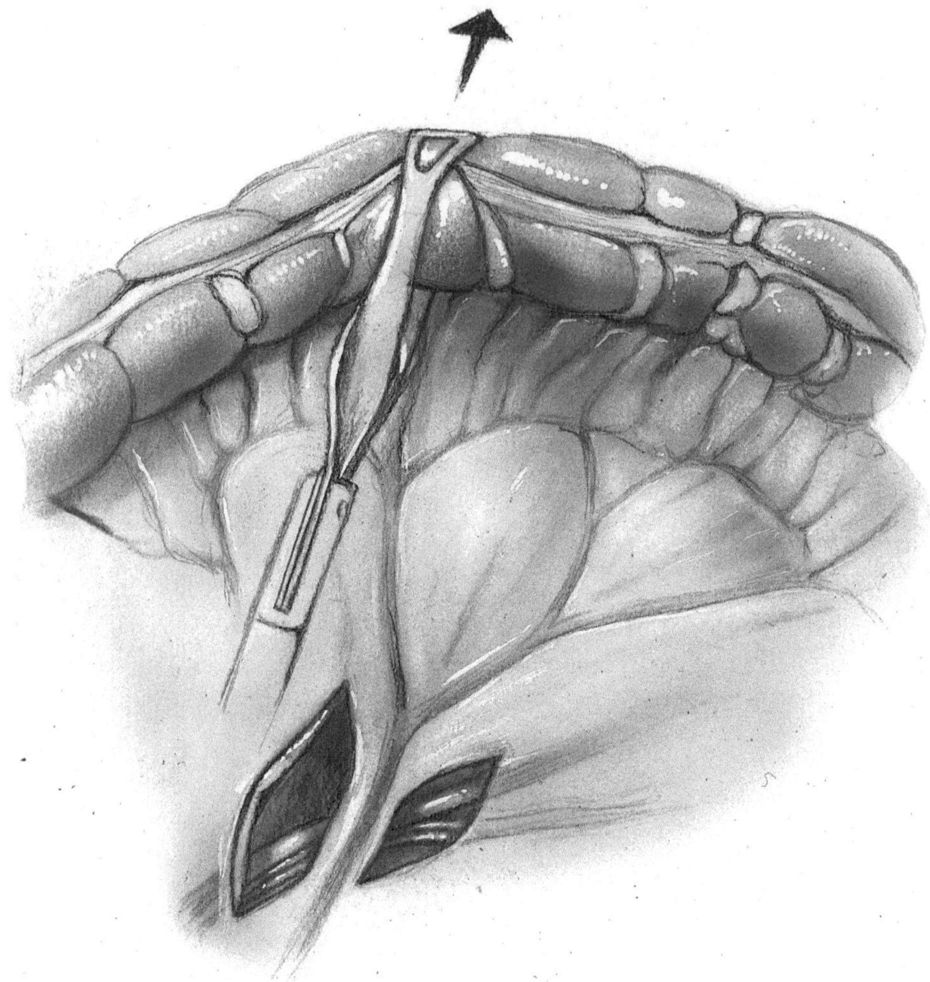

Fig. 5-6

achieve ideal hemostasis. Verification of the distal level of the bowel transection must be done prior to the application of the linear bowel stapler. This may be performed by the flexible endoscope into the rectum while occluding the proximal colon with a Babcock clamp.

The 10-12 mm port in the right lower quadrant is exchanged with the 18 mm port using Seldinger technique. The 45-60 mm bowel stapler is then introduced through this port and the bowel is transected at prechosen resection margin, insuring that no extraneous tissue is incorporated **(Fig. 5-7)**. More than one application of the stapler may be necessary to accomplish the bowel transection. Assess the length of mesentery to insure a tension-free anastomosis in the following phase. If more length is necessary, further scoring of the peritoneum overlying the mesentery or transection of the inferior mesenteric vein may be necessary. If it is divided, proximal ligation at the duodenum with either clips or a stapler are preferred.

## Exteriorization of the Left Colon

Once the left colon has been completely mobilized, a trial reach to the intended level of anastomosis is undertaken. The preoperative proximal margin can be marked with clips to facilitate the extracorporeal component of the operation. The bowel is then exteriorized through either the left lateral or the suprapubic midline incision and a 10-12 mm port is placed in the left lower quadrant position (if this port has not been placed prior to this point). A Babcock clamp is then used to gently hold the proximal colon in order to deliver it from the abdominal cavity. The incision is enlarged along the trocar length; typically

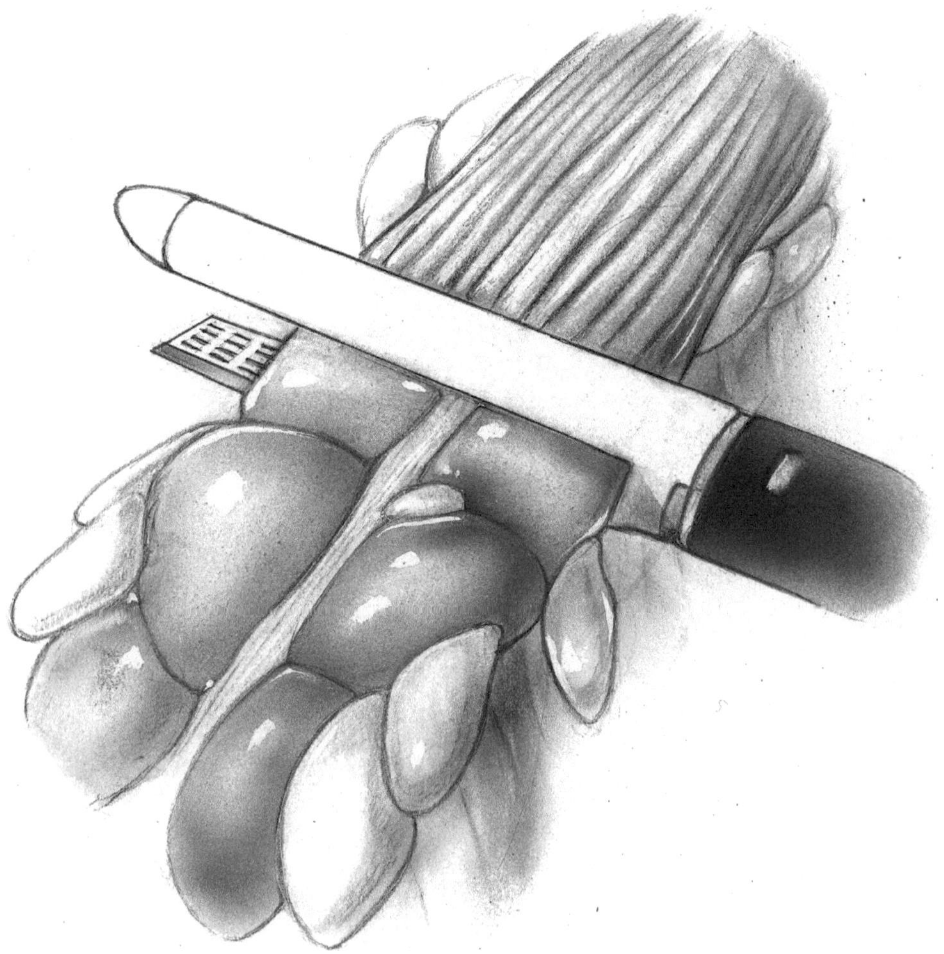

Fig. 5–7

5-cm incision is adequate for this maneuver. A wound protector may assist in minimizing potential contamination.

Once the diseased segment has been completely exteriorized **(Fig. 5–8)**, the proximal colonic resection proceeds with conventional surgical techniques. After an adequate resection margin has been obtained, a purse string clamp is applied on the normal proximal bowel and the diseased segment is then transected **(Fig. 5–9)**. After the purse string clamp is removed, assess the vascularity of the resection margin is verified.

## Performing the Anastomosis

If the distal margin is in the descending colon, the anastomosis can be extracorporeally performed using stapling devices for a functional end to end anastomosis or alternatively using the handsewn technique. The bowel is then replaced into the abdominal cavity.

In the much more common scenario, the distal margin involves the rectosigmoid junction. In this setting the anastomosis is performed intracorporeally. The anvil of the 29 or 33 mm circular stapler is placed into the proximal margin of the bowel, and the purse string suture is then secured **(Fig. 5–10)**. The edge of the proximal bowel with anvil is appropriately trimmed by removing the attached appendices. The proximal bowel with the anvil is then returned into the abdominal cavity and the incision is closed after which a pneumoperitoneum is reestablished.

The laparoscopic phase is resumed as the surgeon moves between the legs to introduce the 29 or 33 mm circular stapling device into the rectum. A

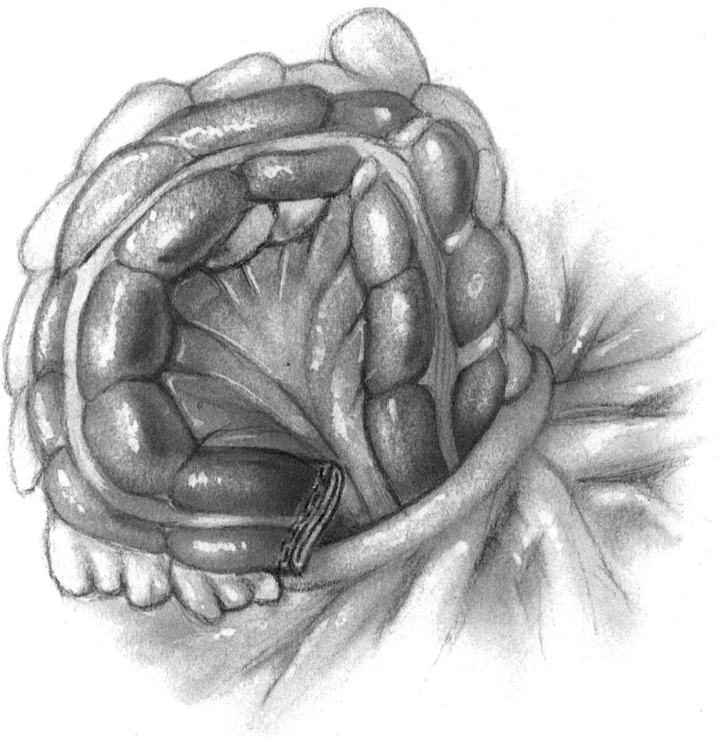

Fig. 5-8

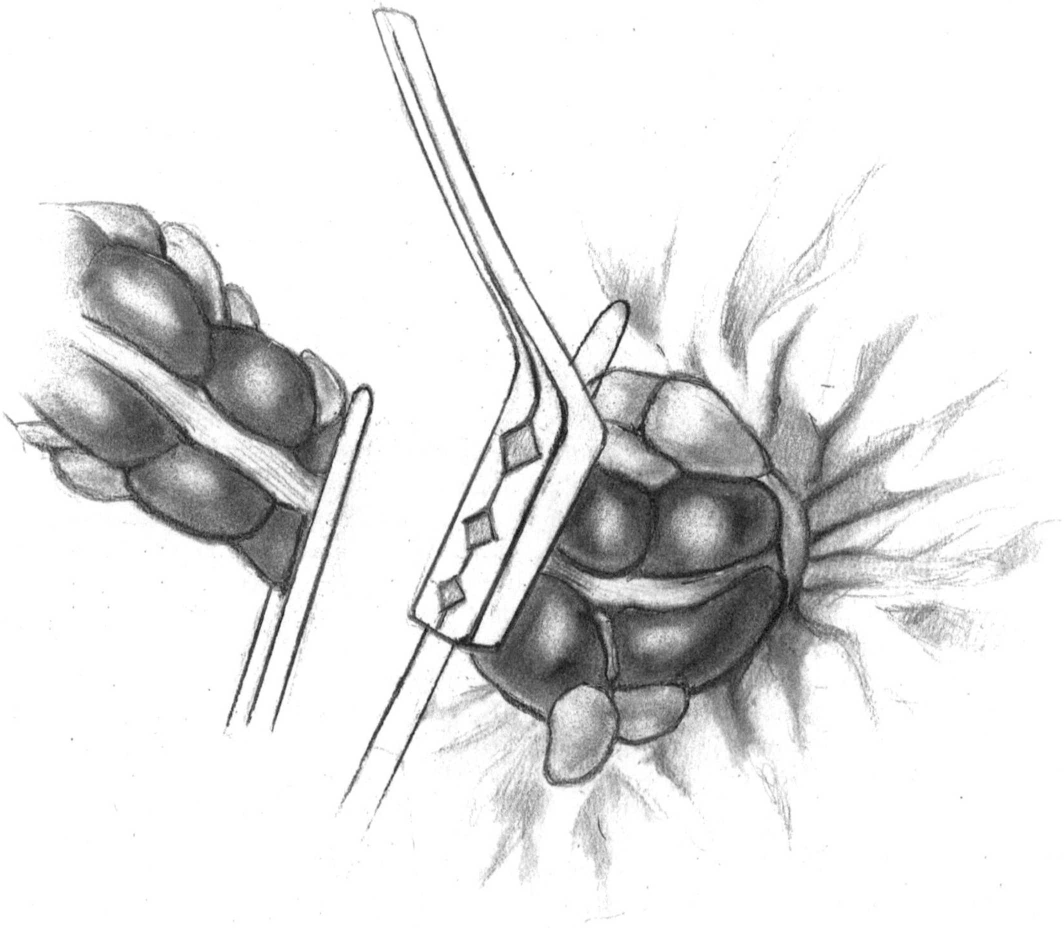

Fig. 5-9

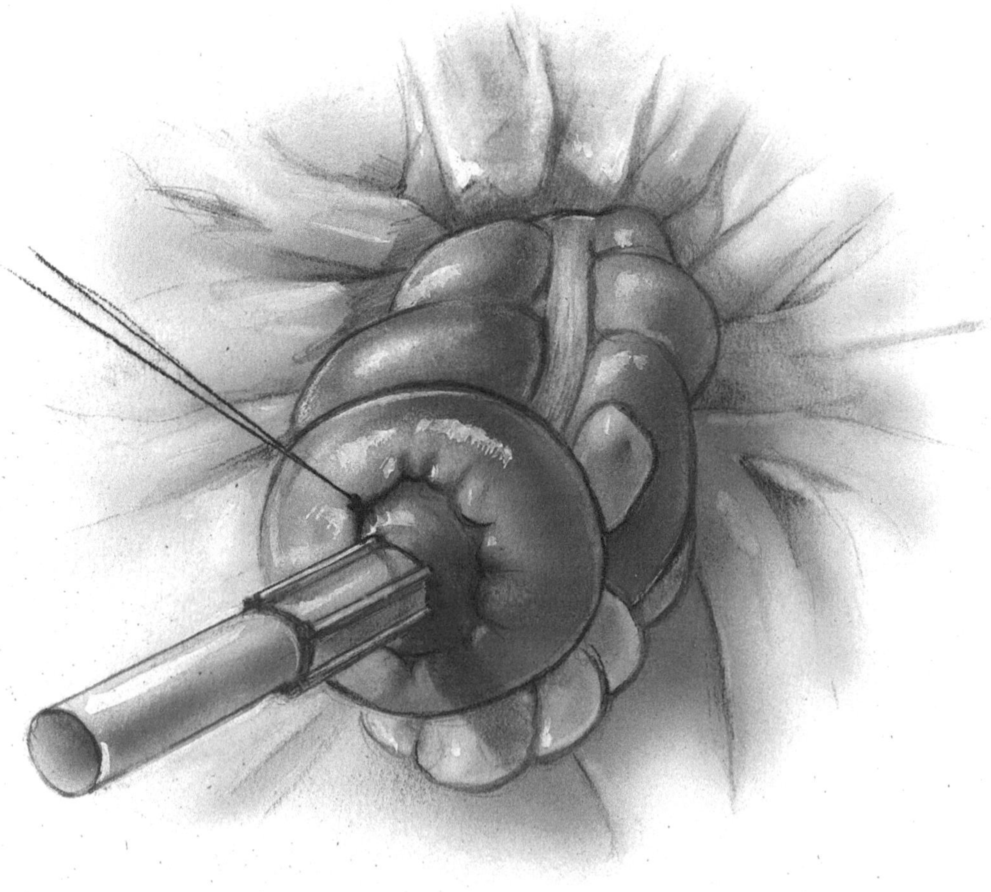

Fig. 5–10

Babcock clamp through the right lower quadrant port can help stabilize the distal stump of the bowel adjacent to the staple line. With slight pressure against the top of the stump, the spike is made to protrude **(Fig 5–11)**. The anvil holder is used in order to deliver the anvil into pelvis and then to approximate it to the trocar and the shaft of the circular stapler **(Fig. 5–12)**. Switch the position of the camera to the right lower quadrant port so that the team can circumferentially visualize both the distal and proximal portion of the anastomosis. While closing the stapler, any extraneous tissue must be reflected away and the surgeon must verify that there is no tension and proper alignment prior to the firing. The stapler is then fired verifying that both mesentery and bowel are oriented in their appropriate anatomical position. To check the integrity of the anastomosis, a noncrushing clamp is once again gently placed on the proximal bowel, in conjunction with transanal endoscopy with air insufflation into the water-filled pelvis. The abdominal team then verifies that no air leaks are present.

## Closure of the Wound

After irrigation of the wounds, each wound is closed by reapproximating the fascia. The skin may be then closed by either staples or subcuticular sutures.

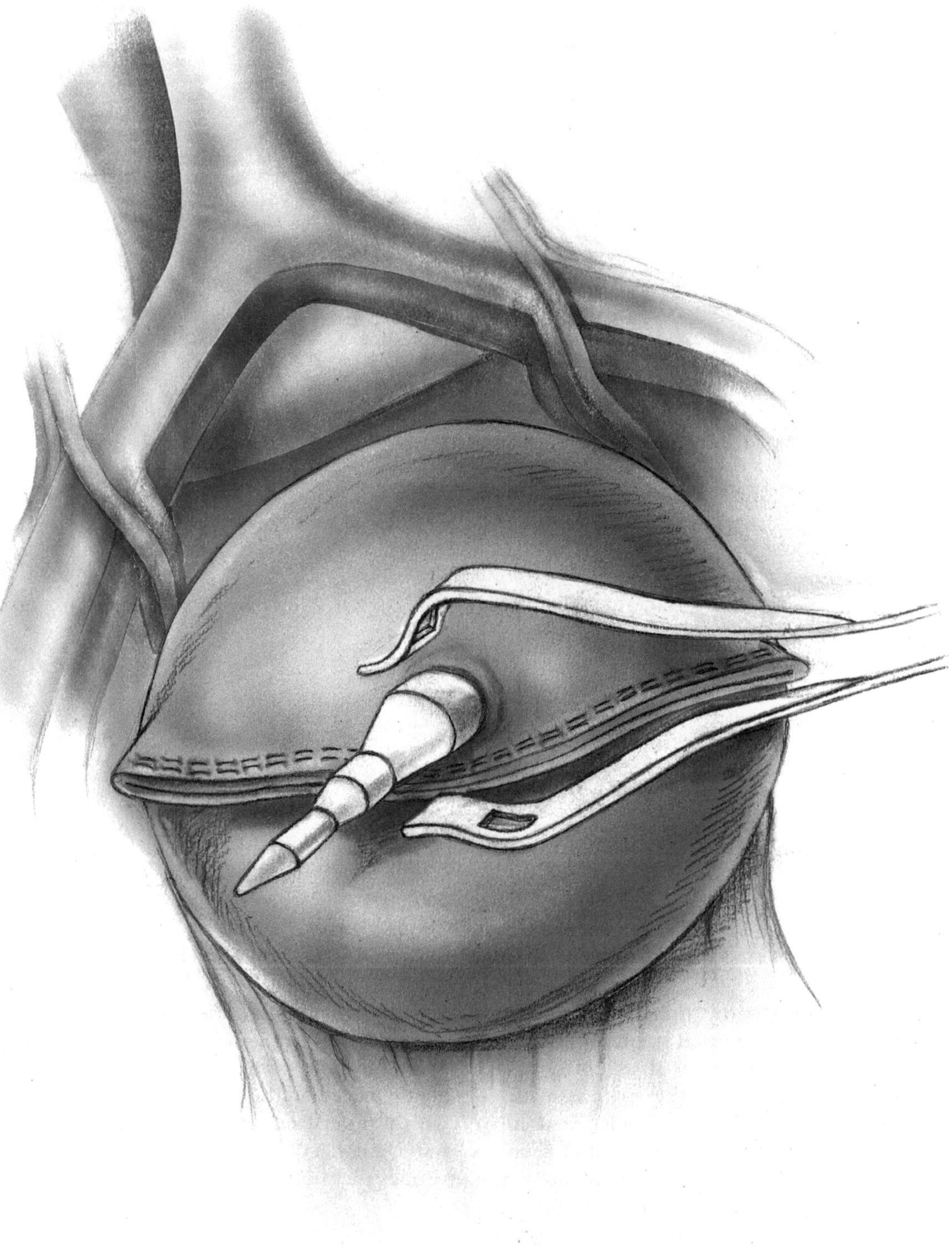

Fig. 5-11

Fig. 5-12

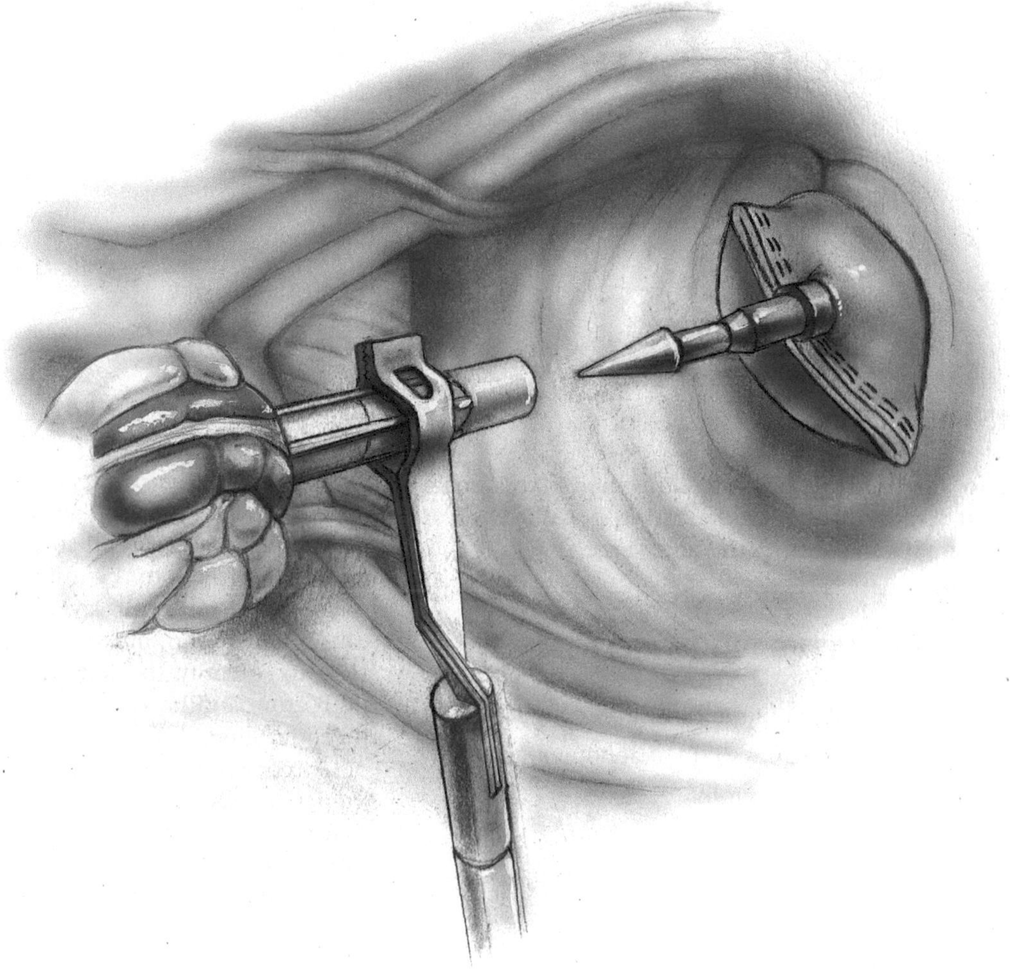

## POSTOPERATIVE CARE

Intravenous antibiotics are postoperatively continued for three doses unless significant fecal contamination or an abscess is encountered during the surgery.

Oral intake can be initiated on the day of surgery, and then advanced to a regular diet as the patient tolerates feeding. In general the regimen begins in the clear liquid and then advanced to solid food.

## COMPLICATIONS

Postoperative ileus or small bowel obstruction

Wound infection

Anastomotic leak

Anastomotic stenosis

Port site herniation

## REFERENCES

Zucker KA. Laparoscopic left hemicolectomy and sigmoidectomy. In: Bruce MacFadyen BV, Jr. (ed) Laparoscopic Surgery of the Abdomen. New York. Springer-Verlag. 2003: 369–379.

Milsom JW, Bohm B. Proctosigmoidectomy. In: Laparoscopic Colorectal Surgery New York: Springer-Verlag 1995: 148–166.

Resimann P, Salky BA, Pfeifer J, Edye M, Jagleman DG, Wexner SD: Laparoscopic surgery in the management of inflammatory bowel disease. Am J Surg 1996; 171: 41–51.

Coller JA, Bruce CJ. Laparoscopic sigmoid resection for diverticular disease. In: Wexner SD (ed) Laparoscopic Colorectal Surgery. New York. Wiley-Liss 1999: 141–157.

Wexner SD, Moscovitz ID. Laparoscopic colectomy in diverticular and Crohn's disease. Surg Clin North Am. 2000; 80(4): 1299–1319.

Jacobs M. Laparoscopic left colectomy. In: Philips EH, Rosenthal RJ (ed) Operative Strategy in Laparoscopic Colorectal Surgery. New York: Springer-Verlag. 1995: 230–235.

# 6 Low Anterior Resection for Rectal Cancer

## INDICATIONS

Low anterior resections are performed to treat malignant tumors of the middle and upper thirds of the rectum, 6–14 cm from the anal verge.

## PREOPERATIVE PREPARATION

Mechanical and antibiotic bowel preparation

Computed tomography (CT) of abdomen and pelvis

Endorectal ultrasonography

Other staging studies as indicated

See Chapter 1

## PITFALLS AND DANGER POINTS

Anastomotic failure

Presacral hemorrhage

Trauma to rectal stump during presacral dissection

Ureteral damage

## OPERATIVE STRATEGY

### Prevention of Anastomotic Complications

Anastomotic complications are rare when the resection is high and the anastomosis is intraperitoneal (see Chapter 4). Conversely, a low anterior resection with a colorectal anastomosis below the peritoneal reflection is clinically and radiographically much more prone to leak. The low colorectal anastomosis offers additional difficulty for several reasons.

1. *Anatomic exposure is often difficult*. This is especially true in men, whose pelvis is narrow, and obese patients. Difficulty with exposure often requires the surgeon's hand to be held at an awkward angle, so it is easy to make small tears in the rectum when inserting sutures.

2. *It is easy to mistake mucosa for the muscular layer* owing to the lack of serosal cover over the retroperitoneal rectum. If sutures or staples are erroneously inserted into the mucosal instead of the submucosal and muscular layers, the anastomosis will leak because the mucosa itself has little tensile strength. Identify the longitudinal muscle covering the rectum and be sure to incorporate this layer in the suture line.

3. *The diameter of the rectal ampulla frequently measures in excess of 5–6 cm*, and the lumen of the proximal colon, after proper bowel preparation, is often half this size. The anastomotic technique used must be capable of correcting this disparity.

4. When the surgeon has not achieved perfect hemostasis in the pelvis, *a hematoma forms in the presacral space*. It frequently becomes infected and develops into an abscess, which may erode through the colorectal suture line.

5. If the pelvic peritoneal floor is closed above the colorectal anastomosis, deadspace may surround the anastomosis, which is especially conducive to leakage in the anastomosis. The peritoneal pelvic floor is not resutured after the colorectal anastomosis is completed.

6. Do not leave any empty space in the hollow of the sacrum behind a low anastomosis. For most low anterior resections, we free the attachments of the splenic flexure (see Figs. 4-4 to 4-8) so the descending colon has sufficient redundancy that relaxed colon fills the sacral space behind the anastomosis. If this step cannot be accomplished, fill the empty space in the pelvis by lengthening the omentum sufficiently that it can be delivered to the presacral space.

7. We have virtually eliminated leakage by adopting the side-to-end (Baker) colorectal anastomosis. This permits the diameter of the anastomosis to be exactly equal to that of the lumen of the

commodious rectal ampulla. Healthy-sized bites of tissue may be enclosed in the sutures with no danger of postoperative stenosis. In effect, at the conclusion of the anastomosis, *the rectal ampulla has been invaginated into the side of the proximal colon* (see Fig. 6-23). Placing the anastomosis within 1 cm of the closed end of the proximal colon eliminates the danger of developing a blind-loop syndrome.

8. Following a low anastomosis we routinely insert a closed suction drain into the presacral space, bringing it out through a puncture wound in the left lower quadrant.

9. Although the use of staples for low colorectal anastomoses has been demonstrated to be safe by numerous studies, it is important to observe all the precautions described below to ensure uneventful healing.

## Which Colorectal Anastomosis: Sutured, Circular Stapled, or Double Stapled?

Sutured colorectal anastomoses, described below, have been demonstrated to be safe when performed with delicacy of technique by a skilled surgeon on well dissected healthy tissues. Lesions 9–10 cm from the anal verge can generally be removed and a sutured colorectal anastomosis performed. However, when the surgeon resects lesions lower than 10 cm from the anal verge, suturing the colorectal anastomosis can be difficult. Insertion of the circular stapler into the rectum allows construction of a safe colorectal stapled anastomosis with greater ease for the surgeon than is true for the sutured anastomosis.

If the cancer resection has left a rectal stump situated so low in the pelvis that even insertion of the purse-string suture becomes difficult (lesions at 6–8 cm), use the Roticulator 55 mm linear stapler (U.S. Surgical Corp.) to close the proximal edge of the rectal stump rather than a purse-string suture. Passing the circular stapler into the rectum then permits construction of a circular colorectal anastomosis through the linear staple line closing the proximal edge of the rectal stump. This method is especially suitable for the lowest colorectal anastomoses.

## Extent of Lymphovascular Dissection

Goligher (1975) advocated routine ligation of the inferior mesenteric artery at the aorta not only for lesions of the descending colon but also for rectal cancer. When this is done, the entire blood supply of the proximal colon must come through the marginal artery all the way from the middle colic artery **(Fig. 6–1)**. Although this proves adequate in most patients, there is a danger that the surgeon may not recognize those patients whose blood supply is not sufficient. We believe the risk of this occurring is greater than the benefits that may accrue to the patient by routinely amputating the extra 3 cm of inferior mesenteric artery. It is important that the blood supply to the proximal colon undergoing anastomosis not only be adequate but be optimal before this segment is used in a low colorectal anastomosis. Consequently, in the usual case of rectal cancer we transect the inferior mesenteric artery just distal to the origin of the left colic vessel **(Fig. 6–2)**. Even if only the ascending branch of the left colic artery is preserved, there usually is vigorous arterial pulsation in the mesentery of the descending colon. For obese patients, transillumination of the mesentery is helpful for identifying the junction between the inferior mesenteric and left colic arteries.

If the inferior mesenteric artery is ligated proximal to the takeoff of the left colic artery, be sure always to liberate the splenic flexure and resect most of the descending colon unless it can be proven that the circulation through the marginal artery at a lower level is vigorous. This can be accomplished only by demonstrating pulsatile flow from a cut arterial branch at the proposed site of the transection of the colon. *Poor blood flow leads to poor healing.*

In the usual rectal cancer case the sigmoid colon is removed and the descending colon is used for anastomosis. This generally requires liberation of the splenic flexure, which can be accomplished in a few minutes once the surgeon has mastered the technique.

## Indications for Complementary Colostomy or Loop Ileostomy

When there is difficulty constructing a low colorectal anastomosis and it is likely the surgeon has created a less-than-perfect anastomosis, a complementary diverting right transverse loop colostomy or loop ileostomy should be constructed. It may be closed as early as 2 weeks after the low anterior resection if a barium enema shows a normal anastomosis.

## Presacral Dissection: Prevention of Hemorrhage

Contrary to what apparently is a widely held perception, radical cancer surgery does not require stripping the tissues from the sacrum down to the periosteum. Dissection of the perirectal tissues prox-

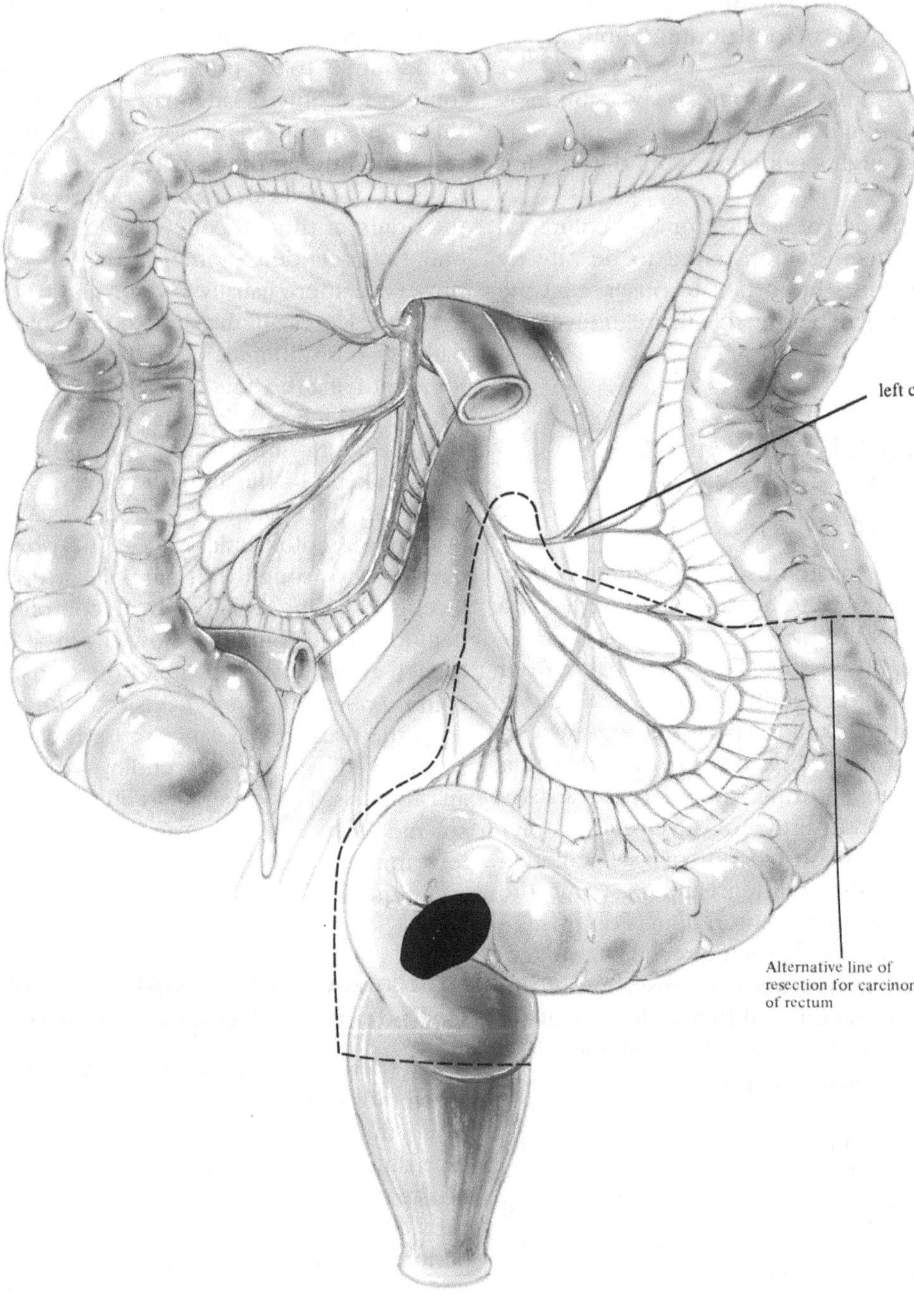
left colic a.
Alternative line of resection for carcinoma of rectum

Fig. 6-1

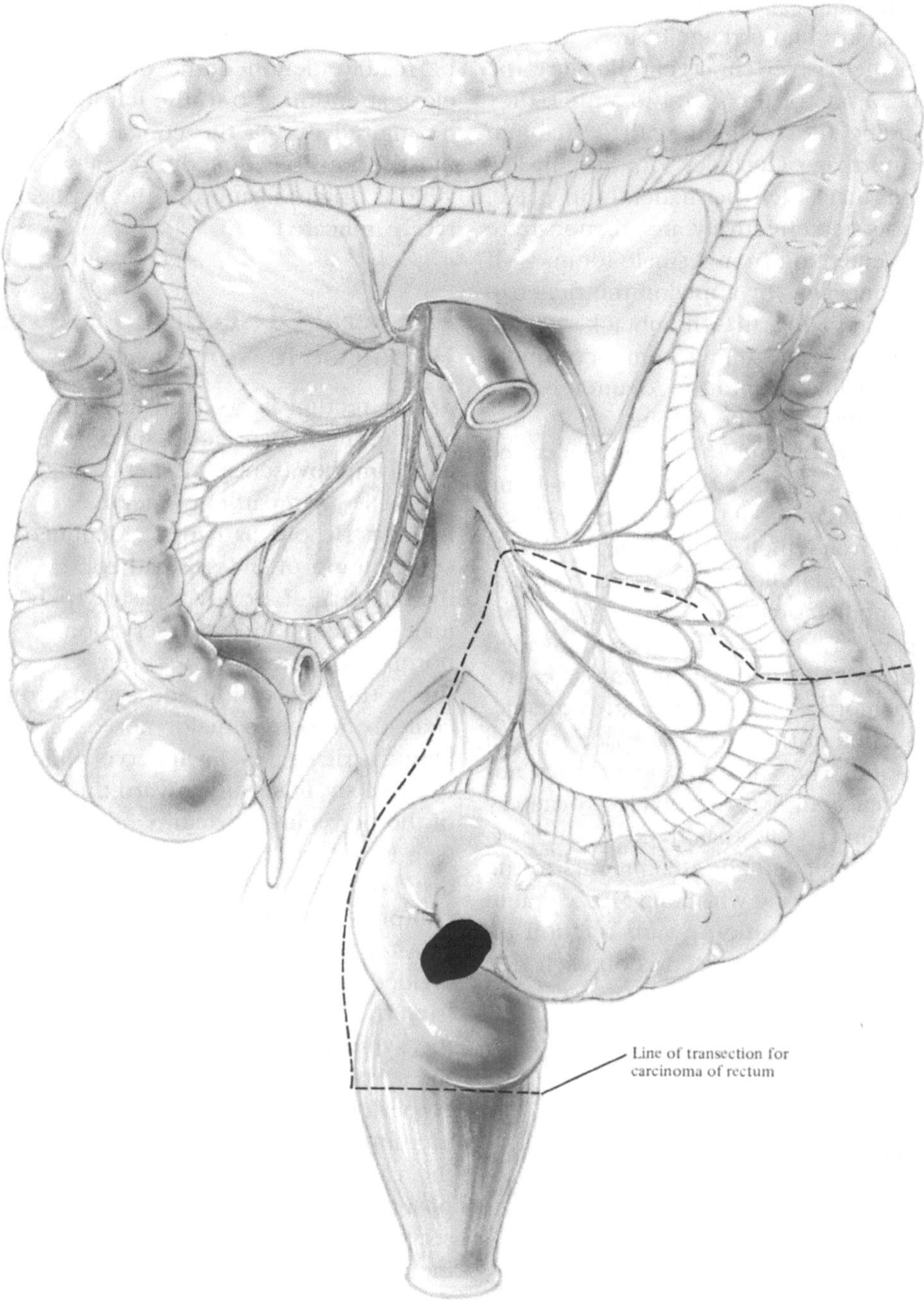


Fig. 6–2

imal to the carcinoma is necessary for removal of *tumor emboli* in the lymph nodes and lymphatic channels. If tumor has widely invaded the mesorectum and presacral tissues, it is generally beyond cure by radical surgery.

There is a network of veins lying on the presacral periosteum that drain into the sacral foramina (see Fig. 6–8b). When these veins are torn by blunt dissection, clamping or ligation to control the hemorrhage that results often is impossible, as the torn vessel retracts into the foramen. The massive venous hemorrhage that follows may not be stemmed by ligating the hypogastric arteries. Most intraoperative fatalities during total proctectomy are caused by this type of presacral venous hemorrhage.

Nivatvongs and Fang (1986) described a method for controlling massive hemorrhage from a torn presacral branch of the basivertebral vein. Because the blood pours out of one of the sacral foramina, they proposed occluding the foramen with a titanium thumbtack (Hemorrhage Occluder Pin; Surgin, Placentia, CA, USA), that is left permanently in place. To accomplish this step effectively, first demonstrate that the blood is emerging from a single foramen. If the bleeding is controlled by applying the fingertip to one foramen, applying the thumbtack will be effective. In some cases stuffing some cottonoid Oxycel (oxidized cellulose) into the foramen before inserting the thumbtack may be helpful.

If the surgeon cannot *quickly* control lacerated presacral veins with a stitch, a thumbtack, or bone wax, the bleeding area should be covered with a sheet of Surgicel over which a large gauze pack is placed, filling the sacral hollow. This practice almost always controls the hemorrhage.

Unless the presacral vessels are directly invaded by a bulky tumor of the mid-rectum, massive presacral venous hemorrhage is entirely preventable. Blunt hand dissection of the presacral space is not a desirable technique. The surgeon's hand does not belong in this area until scissors or electrocautery dissection under direct vision has freed all the perirectal tissues from any posterior attachments to the sacrum. This should be done with long Metzenbaum scissors combined with gentle upward traction on the rectum. As the scissors are inserted on each side of the midline, the perirectal tissues can easily be lifted in an anterior direction *without removing the thin layer of endopelvic fascia that covers the presacral veins*. When the presacral dissection stays in the proper plane, the presacral veins are hidden from view by this layer of fascia (see Fig. 6-8a). Occasionally, branches of the middle sacral vessels enter the perirectal tissues from behind and can be divided by electrocautery.

This dissection is easily continued down to the area of the coccyx, where the fascia of Waldeyer becomes somewhat dense as it goes from the anterior surfaces of the coccyx and sacrum to attach to the lower rectum (see Fig. 6-10). Attempts to penetrate this fascia by blunt finger dissection may rupture the rectum rather than the fascia, which is strong. This layer must be incised sharply with scissors or a scalpel, after which one can see the levator diaphragm. When the posterior dissection has for the most part been completed, only *then* should the surgeon's hand enter the presacral space to sweep the dissection toward the lateral pelvic walls. This maneuver helps define the lateral ligaments. The dissection should be bloodless.

Other points of hemorrhage in the pelvic dissection may occur on the lateral walls. They can usually be readily identified and occluded by ligature. Pay close attention also to the left iliac vein, which may be injured during the course of the dissection. As most serious bleeding during pelvic dissections is of venous origin, ligation of the hypogastric arteries is rarely indicated.

## Presacral Dissection: Preservation of Hypogastric Nerves

As the rectum is elevated from the presacral space and the anterior surface of the aorta cleared of areolar and lymphovascular tissue, a varying number of preaortic sympathetic nerves of the superior hypogastric plexus can be identified. They are the contribution of the sympathetic nervous system to the bilateral inferior hypogastric (pelvic) plexuses. In male patients their preservation is necessary for normal ejaculation. After they cross the region of the aortic bifurcation and sacral promontory, they coalesce into two major nerve bundles, called the hypogastric nerves. Each nerve, which may have one to three strands, runs toward the posterolateral wall of the pelvis in the vicinity of the hypogastric artery (see Figs. 6-4, 6-6). With most malignancies of the distal rectum these nerves can be preserved without compromising the patient's chances of cure.

After the inferior mesenteric artery and vein are divided and the lymphovascular tissues are elevated from the bifurcation of the aorta by blunt dissection, the sympathetic nerves remain closely attached to the aorta and need not be damaged if the dissection is performed gently. At the promontory of the sacrum, if the rectum is dissected as described above, the right and left hypogastric nerves can be seen posterior to the plane of dissection and can be preserved provided there is sufficient distance separating them from the tumor. There also seems to be diminution in the incidence of bladder dysfunction after nerve preservation.

## Ureteral Dissection

To prevent damage to the ureters, these delicate structures must be identified and traced well down into the pelvis. The normal ureter crosses the common iliac artery, at which point this structure bifurcates into its external and internal branches. Because the ureter and a leaf of incised peritoneum are often displaced during the course of dissection, if the ureter is not located in its usual position the undersurfaces of both the lateral and medial leaves of peritoneum should be inspected. The identity of the ureter can be confirmed if pinching or touching the structure with forceps results in typical peristaltic waves. If doubt exists, the anesthesiologist may be instructed to inject indigo carmine dye intravenously, which strains the ureter blue unless the patient is oliguric at the time of injection. The ureter should be traced into the pelvis beyond the point at which the lateral ligaments of the rectum are divided.

## OPERATIVE TECHNIQUE

### Incision and Position

Patients who have lesions within 14 cm of the anal verge should be placed in the same modified lithotomy position utilizing Lloyd-Davies or Allen leg rests, as described in Chapter 7 for abdominoperineal proctectomy **(Figs. 6–3a, 6–3b)**. The second assistant stands between the patient's abducted thighs for the pelvic portion of the operation, and the surgeon works from the patient's left. In this position the surgeon may judge, after the tumor is mobilized, whether an anterior anastomosis, abdominoperineal proctectomy, or end-to-end anastomosis with the EEA stapling device is suitable. These techniques are best done with the patient in this position. A midline incision, extending from a point about 6 cm below the xiphoid process down to the pubis, is used.

### Exploration and Evisceration of Small Bowel

Palpate and inspect the liver. A moderate amount of metastasis is not a contraindication to a conservative version of the anterior resection. Explore the remainder of the abdomen and then eviscerate the small bowel into a plastic intestinal bag or moist gauze pads.

### Mobilization of Sigmoid

Expose the left lateral peritoneal gutter. Occlude the lumen of the colon by ligating the distal sigmoid with umbilical tape. Draw the sigmoid colon medially to expose and divide several congenital attachments between the mesocolon and the posterolateral parietal peritoneum with scissors **(Fig. 6–4)**. Extend the incision in the peritoneum cephalad as far as the splenic flexure.

Identify the left ureter and tag it with a Silastic loop for later identification. Use scissors to continue the peritoneal incision along the left side of the rectum down to the rectovesical pouch. Identify the course of the ureter well down into the pelvis. Now retract the sigmoid to the patient's left and make an incision on the right side of the sigmoid mesocolon. The incision should begin at a point overlying the bifurcation of the aorta and should continue in a caudal direction along the line where the mesosigmoid meets the right lateral leaf of peritoneum in the presacral space. After the right ureter has been identified, carry the incision down toward the rectovesical pouch **(Figs. 6–5, 6–6)**.

If the exposure is convenient, incise the peritoneum of the rectovesical pouch, or the rectouterine pouch in female patients (Fig. 6-5). If the exposure is not convenient, delay this step until the presacral dissection has elevated the rectum sufficiently to bring the rectovesical pouch easily to the field of vision.

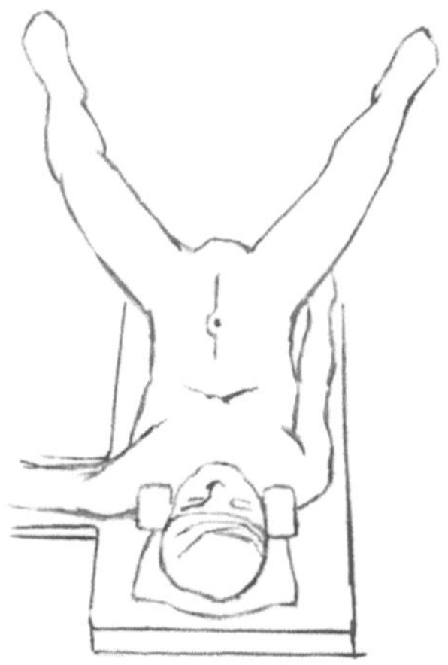

Fig. 6-3a

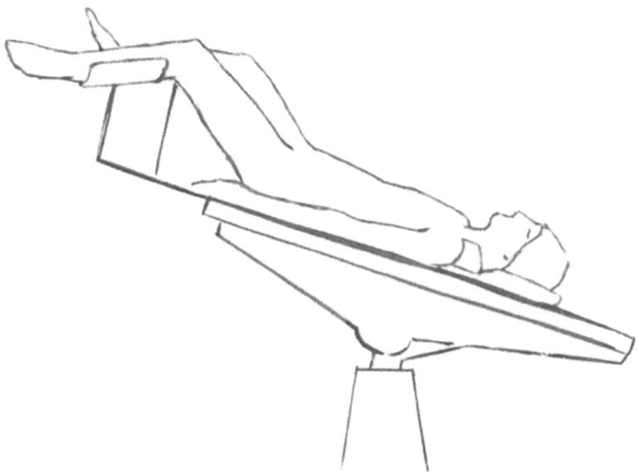

Fig. 6-3b

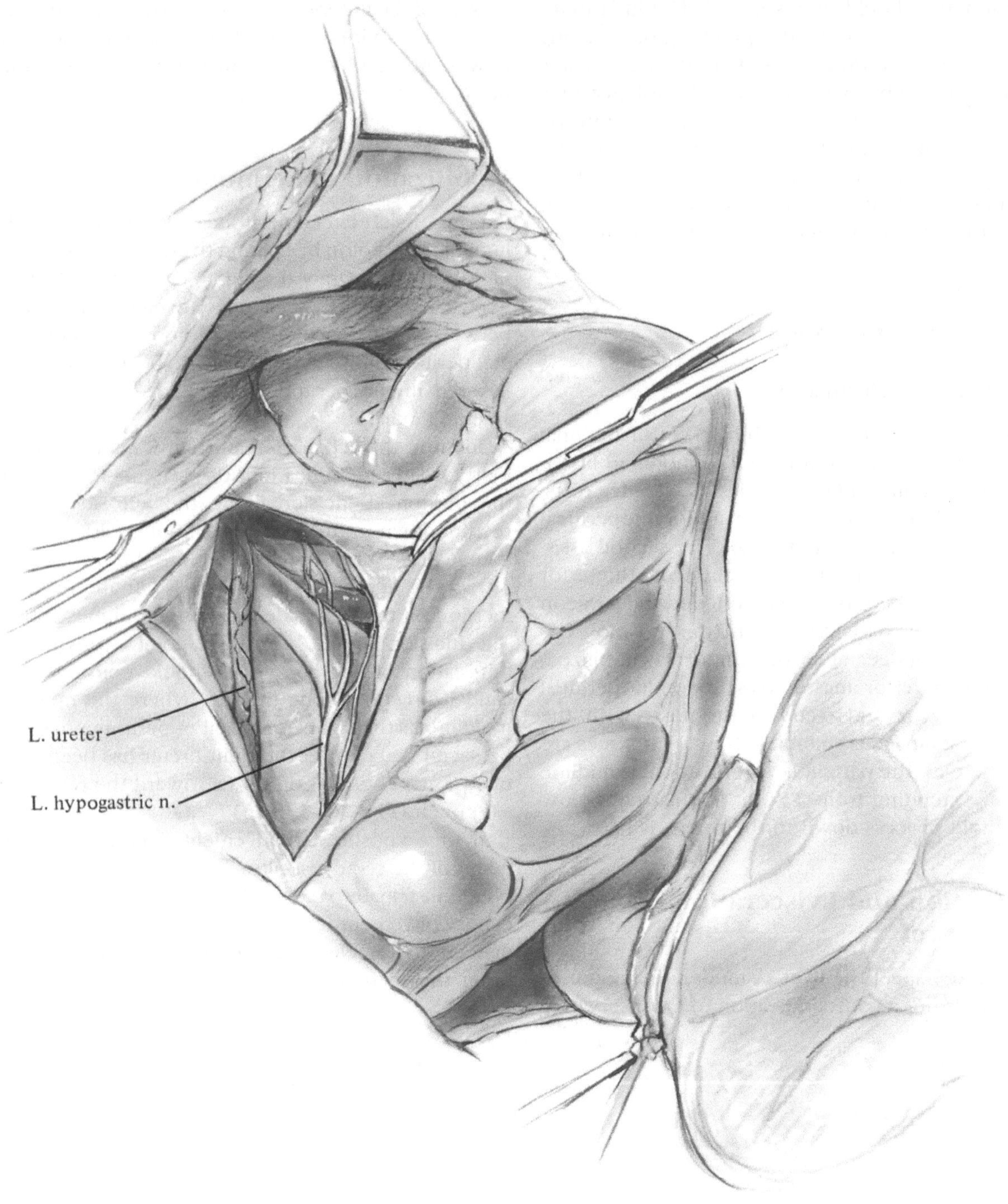


Fig. 6-4

## Lymphovascular Dissection

Apply skyward traction to the colon and gently separate the gonadal vein from the lateral leaf of the mesocolon, allowing it to fall posteriorly. Insert an index finger between the deep margin of the mesosigmoid and the bifurcation of the aorta to feel the pulsation of the inferior mesenteric artery lying superficial to the finger. In markedly obese patients this vessel may be divided and ligated at the level of the aortic bifurcation without further dissection. In most patients, however, it is simple to incise the peritoneum overlying the origin of the inferior mesenteric artery and to sweep the areolar and lym-

Fig. 6-5

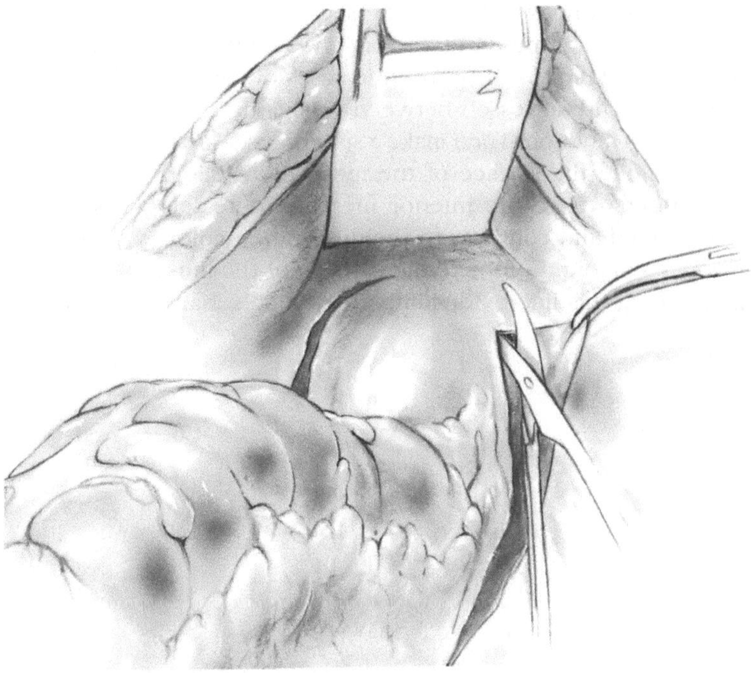

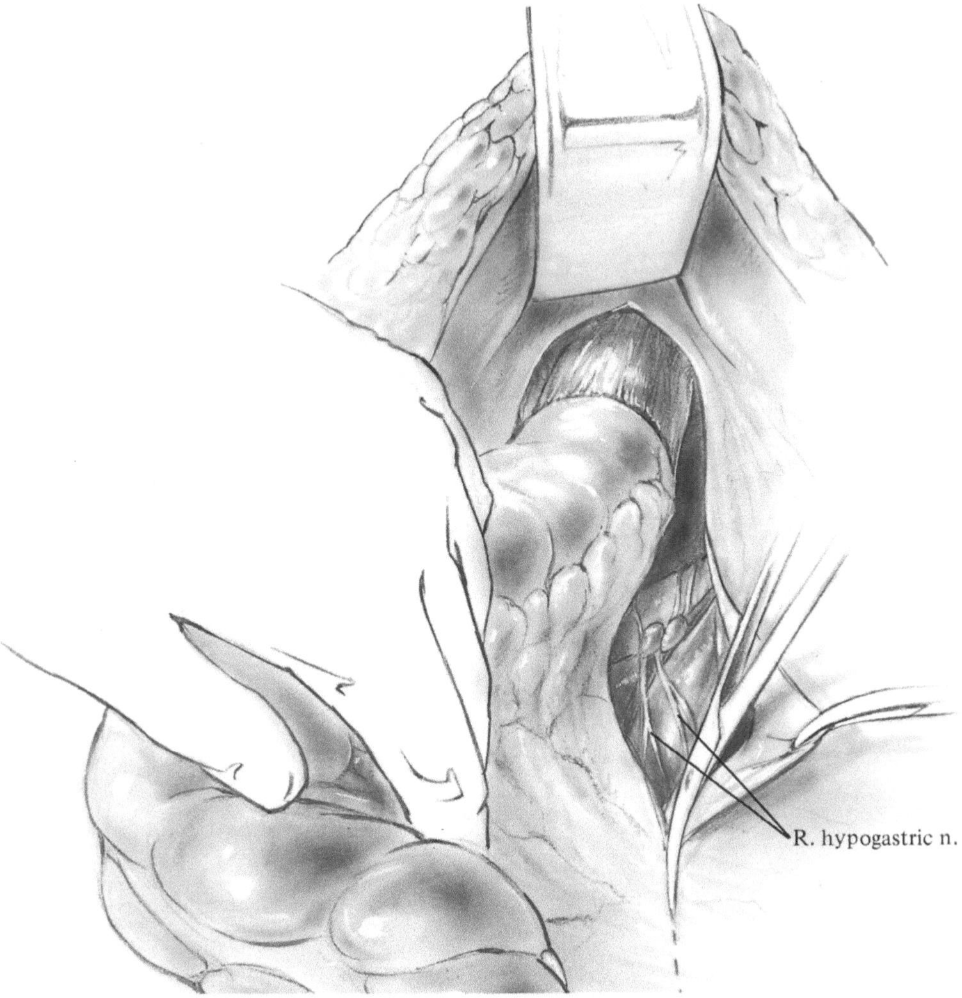


Fig. 6-6

phatic tissue downward until one sees the point at which the inferior mesenteric artery gives off the left colic branch **(Fig. 6–7)**. In routine cases divide the inferior mesenteric vessels between 2-0 ligatures just distal to this junction. Then make a superficial scalpel incision along the surface of the mesocolon: Begin at the point where the inferior mesenteric vessels were divided and continue to the descending colon or upper sigmoid. Complete the division of the mesentery along this line by dividing it between serially applied Kelly hemostats and then ligating with 2-0 silk or PG (Fig. 6–7). In nonobese patients it is feasible to incise the peritoneum up to the point where a vessel is visualized and then apply hemostats directly to each vessel as it is encountered. With this technique, the surgeon encounters only one or two vessels on the way to the marginal artery of the colon.

Sweep the mesosigmoid and the lymphovascular bundle distal to the ligated inferior mesenteric vessels

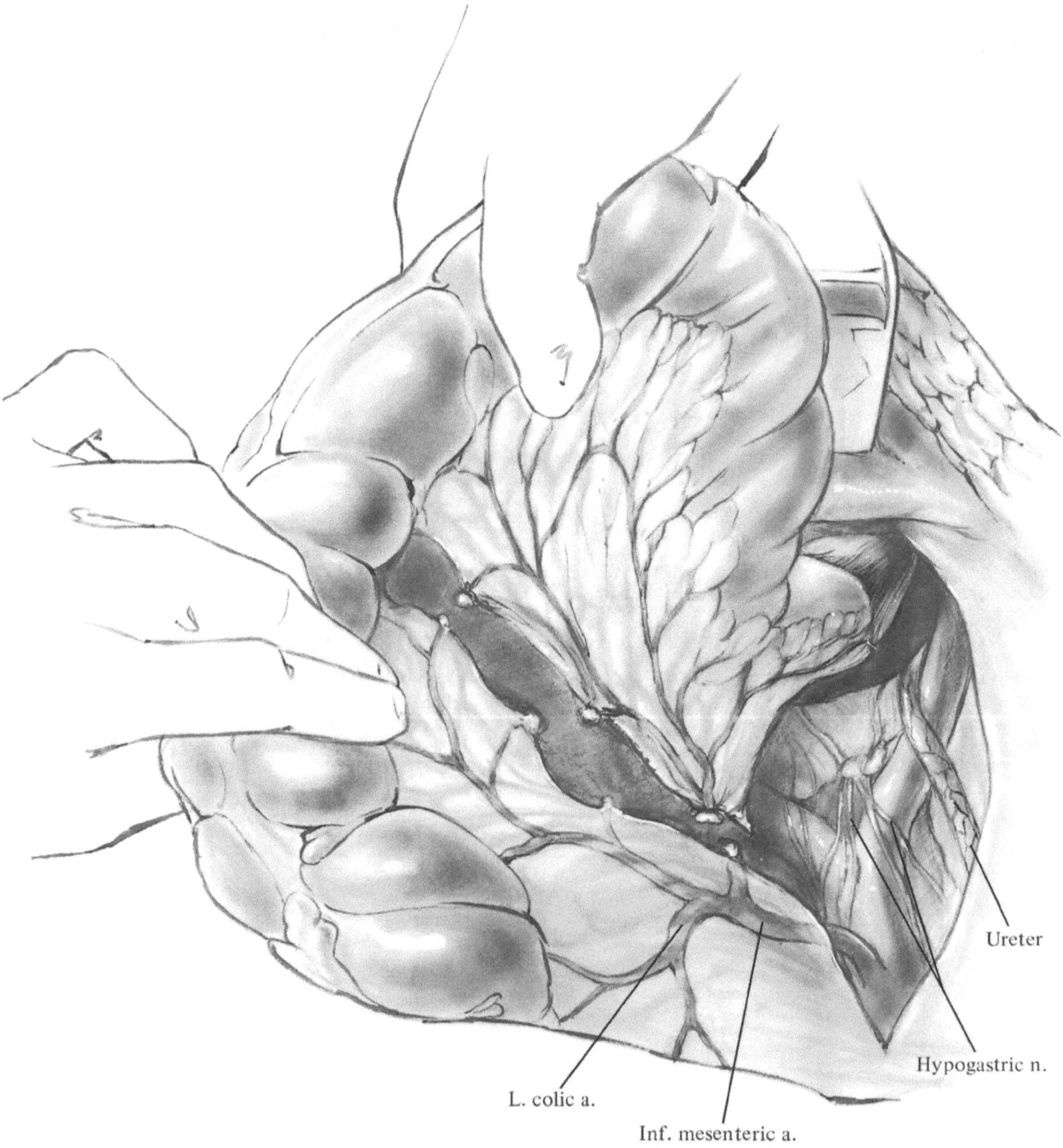


Fig. 6–7

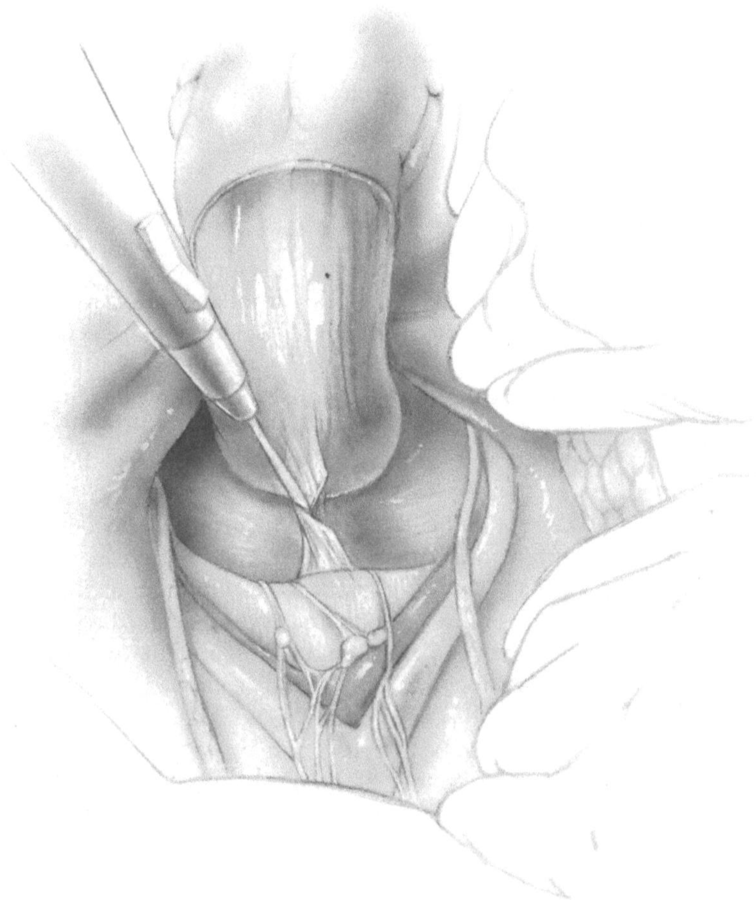

Fig. 6–8a

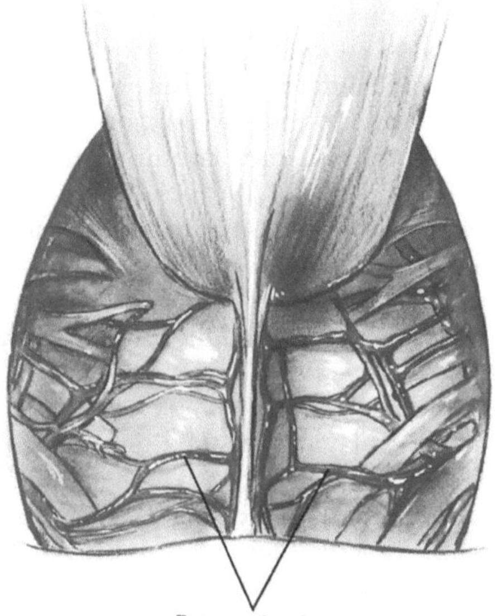


Fig. 6–8b

off the anterior surfaces of the aorta and common iliac vessels by blunt dissection. Leave the preaortic sympathetic nerves intact. To minimize the time during which the patient's abdomen is exposed to possible fecal contamination, do not divide the descending colon at this stage.

## Presacral Dissection

With the lower sigmoid on steady upward retraction, it becomes evident that there is a band of tissue extending from the midsacral region to the posterior rectum and mesorectum. On either side of this dense band there is only areolar tissue. Stoutly resist any tendency to insert a hand into the presacral space. Instead, use long, closed Metzenbaum scissors as a blunt dissector **(Fig. 6–8a)**. Insert it first to the right of the midline behind the rectum; by gently elevating the mesorectum the proper presacral plane is then entered. Repeat this maneuver identically on the left side of the midsacral line. Then direct attention to the remaining band of tissue, which contains branches of the middle sacral artery, and divide it with the electrocautery (Fig. 6–8a).

At this time the surgeon sees a thin layer of fibroareolar tissue covering the sacrum. If a shiny layer of sacral periosteum, ligaments, or the naked presacral veins can be seen **(Fig. 6–8b)**, the plane of dissection is *too deep*, presenting a danger of major venous hemorrhage. Elevate the distal rectum from the lower sacrum with gauze in a spongeholder. If the dissection has been completed properly, as described, note that the preaortic sympathetic nerves divide into two major trunks in the upper sacral area and then continue laterally to the right and left walls of the pelvis (see Figs. 6-4, 6-6). Gently dissect these nerves from the posterior wall of the specimen unless the nerves have been invaded by tumor.

Now insert a hand into the presacral space, with the objective not of penetrating more deeply toward the coccyx but, rather, of extending the presacral dissection laterally to the right and to the left, so the posterior aspect of the specimen is elevated from the sacrum as far as the lateral ligaments on each side. Place the lateral ligament on the left side on stretch by applying traction to the rectum toward the right. Place a right-angle Mixter clamp underneath the lateral ligament and divide the tissue with electrocautery **(Fig. 6–9)**.

Carry out a similar maneuver to divide the right lateral ligament. Before dividing each lateral ligament, recheck the position of the respective ureter and hypogastric nerve to be certain they lie away from the point of division. Then divide the fascia of Waldeyer, which extends from the coccyx to the posterior rectal wall **(Fig. 6–10)**.

Now direct attention to the anterior dissection. Use a Lloyd-Davies bladder retractor to pull the bladder (in women, the uterus) in an anterior and caudal direction. If the peritoneum of the rectovesical pouch has not already been incised, perform this maneuver now, thereby connecting the incisions in the pelvic peritoneum previously made on the right and left sides of the rectum **(Fig. 6–11a)**. Apply one or more long hemostats or forceps to the posterior lip of the incised peritoneum of the rectovesical pouch. Place traction on these hemostats to draw the peritoneum and Denonvilliers' fascia in a cephalad and posterior direction, and use Metzenbaum scissors dissection to separate the rectum from the seminal vesicles and prostate **(Fig. 6–11b)**. Use blunt finger dissection to further separate the rectum from the posterior wall of the prostate. Finally, secure hemostasis in this region by cauterizing multiple bleeding points.

In female patients the anterior dissection is somewhat simpler. With a Harrington retractor elevating the uterus, use scalpel dissection to initiate the plane of dissection separating the peritoneum and fascia of Denonvilliers from the posterior lip of the cervix until the proximal vagina has been exposed. Some surgeons routinely perform bilateral salpingooophorectomy in women who have rectal and sigmoid cancer because the ovaries are sometimes a site of metastatic deposit. Whether this step is of value has not been ascertained. We do not perform this maneuver in the absence of visible metastasis to the ovaries.

## Pelvic Hemostasis

The entire pelvic dissection, if properly performed, entails minimal blood loss. Although hemostatic clips may control clearly identified vessels along the lateral wall of the pelvis, they are not useful in the presacral area. Here the vessels consist of thin-walled veins, which are easily torn by metallic clips at the time of application or during the act of sponging the area later.

Except in the case of a small, clearly defined bleeding point that can be held in a forceps, electrocautery may also be hazardous, as the coagulating tip may act as a scalpel and convert the bleeding point to a major venous laceration. Here a ball-tipped electrode is safer than one with a blade or pointed tip.

See the discussion above, under Operative Strategy, concerning the use of a thumbtack to control massive presacral bleeding localized to a single foramen. Almost invariably, presacral bleeding results from a tear in one or more of the veins that drain into a sacral foramen. When hemorrhage occurs, the area of bleeding should be covered by a sheet of topical hemostatic agent over which pressure is applied with a large gauze pack. Place omentum between the pack and the anastomosis. If the area of bleeding is only 1–2 cm in diameter, removing the gauze pack may be attempted at a later stage in the operation, leaving a small patch of hemostatic agent. Unless this maneuver produces complete hemostasis, replace the gauze pack in the presacral space and leave it there for 24–48 hours. Then remove it by relaparotomy under general anesthesia.

## Mobilization of Proximal Colon

If the previously selected point on the descending colon does not easily reach down into the pelvis, mobilize the remainder of the descending colon by incising first the peritoneum in the paracolic gutter and then the "renocolic" ligament. Liberate the entire splenic flexure according to the steps described in Chapter 4. Considerable additional length may be obtained by dividing the transverse branch of the left colic artery (Fig. 6–1). Completely clear the fat and mesentery from a 1 cm width of serosa at the point selected for dividing the descending colon.

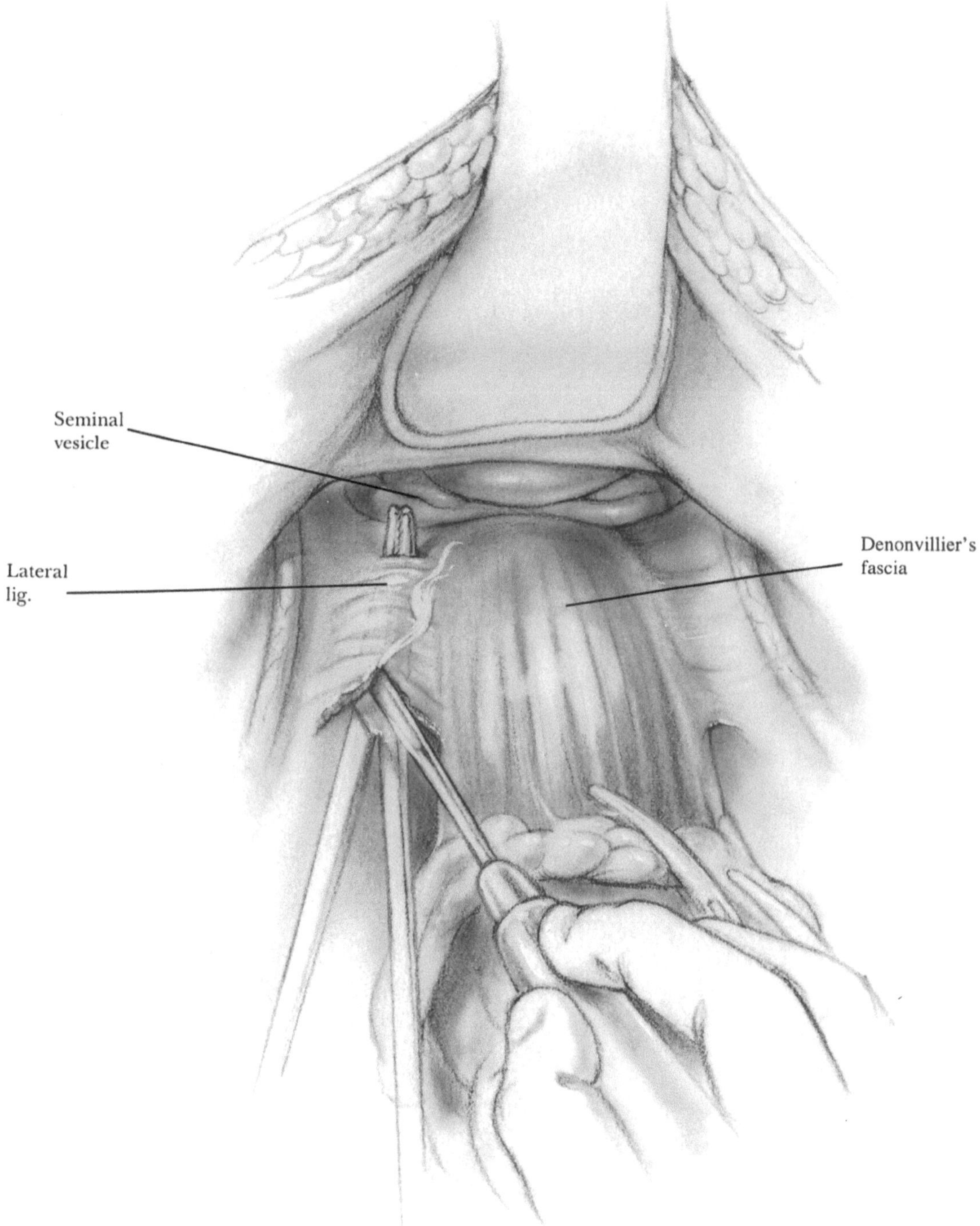


Fig. 6–9

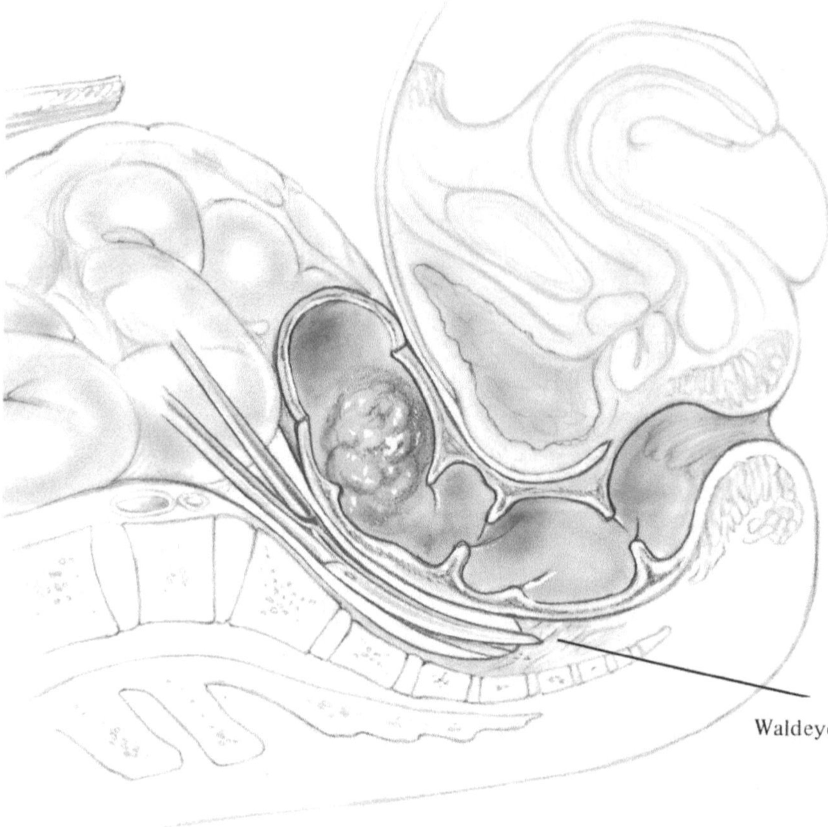


Fig. 6–10

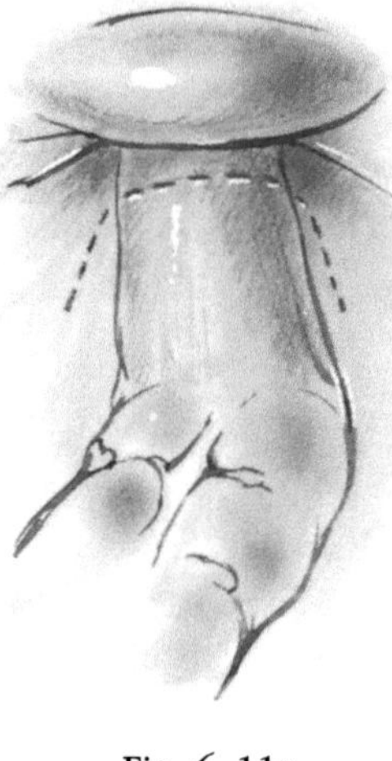

Fig. 6–11a

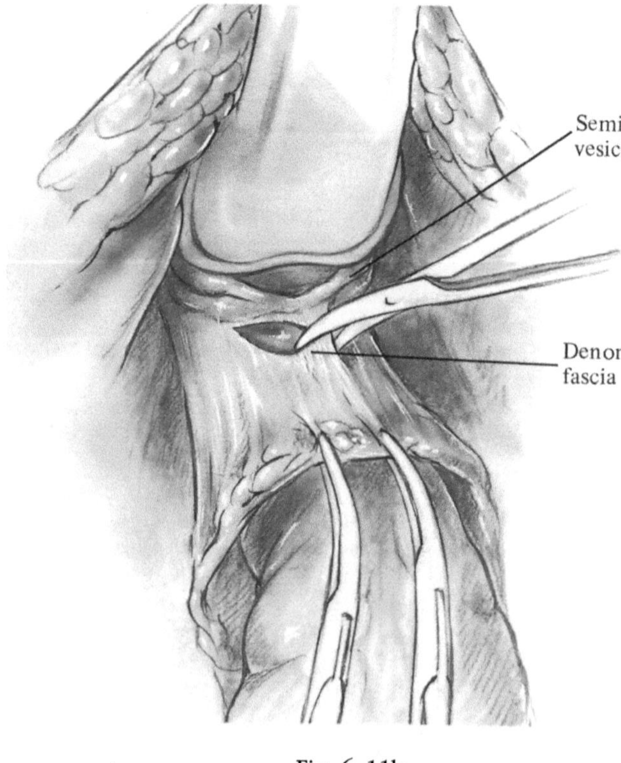


Fig. 6–11b

## Preparation of Rectal Stump

When the rectum is divided at a low level, the mesorectum is no longer a single pedicle traveling along the posterior surface of the rectum. Rather, it fans out into multiple branches. Select a point 4–5 cm distal to the lower border of the tumor and seek the plane between the muscularis of the rectum and the surrounding blood vessels. This plane can sometimes be palpated with the finger; and at other times a large blunt-nosed hemostat can be insinuated into it. In most patients this vascular layer can be divided by electrocoagulation after passing a right-angle clamp between the vasculature and the rectal wall.

Well delineated longitudinal muscle fibers should now be visible all around the lower rectum at the site selected for the anastomosis. At this time place a large right-angle clamp across the entire lumen of the rectum below the tumor.

## Irrigation of Rectal Stump

If there is any question as to the adequacy of the bowel preparation, insert a Foley catheter with a 5 ml bag into the rectum. Attach the catheter to plastic tubing to permit the intermittent inflow and drainage of 500 ml of sterile water. This not only removes retained fecal matter but lyses any shed tumor cells. After the irrigation is completed and the rectum is emptied, remove the catheter and apply a large right-angle clamp distal to the tumor to occlude the rectal lumen.

## Selection of Anastomotic Technique

Use the side-to-end suture technique for a low colorectal anastomosis at or just below the peritoneal reflection. Alternatively, a circular stapling device may be used. At higher levels, the techniques described in Chapter 4 are also suitable. See also the discussion under Operative Strategy, above.

### *Side-to-End Low Colorectal Anastomosis (Baker)*

Turn to the previously cleared area on the descending colon that is to be used for the anastomosis. Apply a 55/3.5 mm linear stapler across this cleared area and fire the staples **(Fig. 6–12)**. Place an Allen

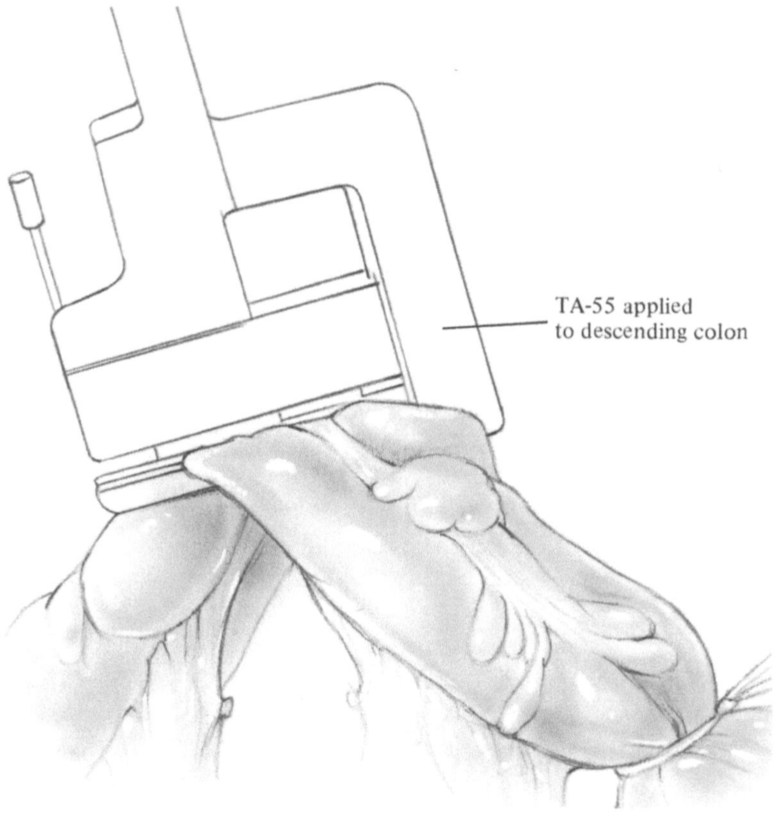


Fig. 6–12

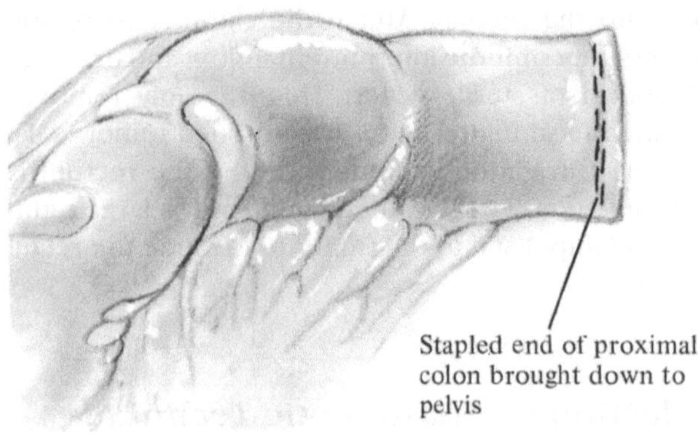


Fig. 6-13

clamp 1 cm distal to the stapler to occlude the specimen side. Divide the colon flush with the stapling device using a scalpel and lightly cauterize the everted mucosa **(Fig. 6–13)**. Ligate the specimen side with umbilical tape. After the Allen clamp is removed, apply a sterile rubber glove over the ligated end and tie the glove in place with another umbilical tape ligature **(Figs. 6–14a, 6–14b)**. Alternatively, divide the colon with a linear cutting stapler. Retain this segment of colon containing the specimen temporarily to provide traction on the rectal stump.

Bring the stapled end of the proximal colon down into the pelvis and line it up tentatively with the rectal stump 4-5 cm beyond the tumor. Place a scratch mark along the antimesenteric border of the descending colon beginning at a point 1 cm proximal to the stapled end and continuing cephalad for a distance equal to the diameter of the rectal stump.

Now insert a lateral guy suture into the left lateral margin of the rectal stump and the proximal colon and hold this suture in a hemostat. Place a second guy suture in a similar fashion between the right lateral margin of the rectum and the colon and hold

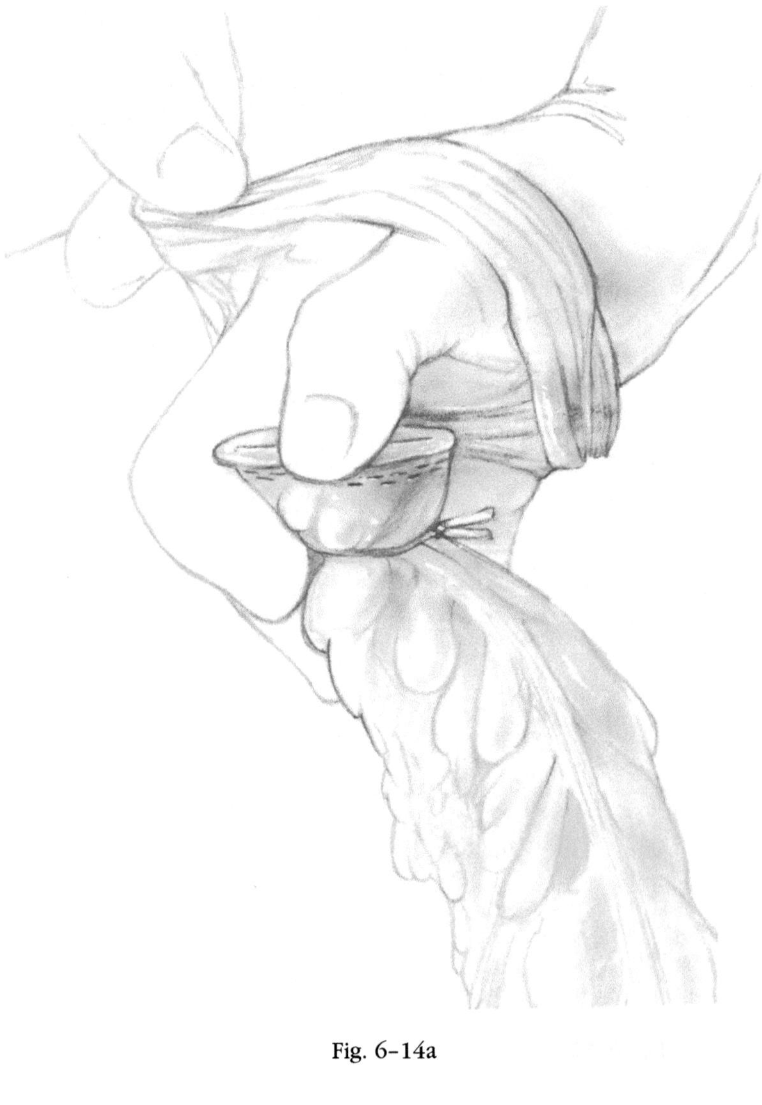

Fig. 6-14a

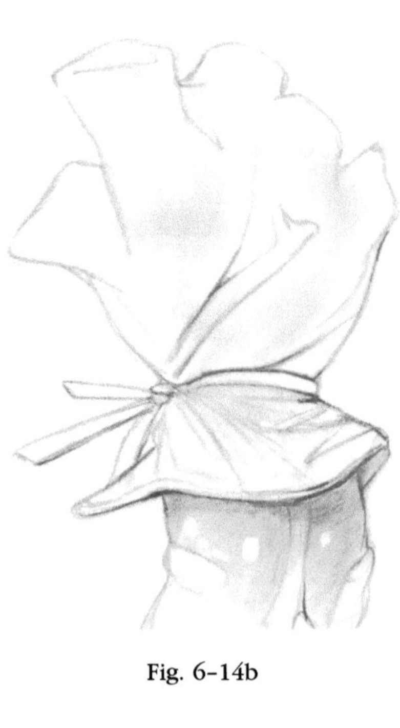

Fig. 6-14b

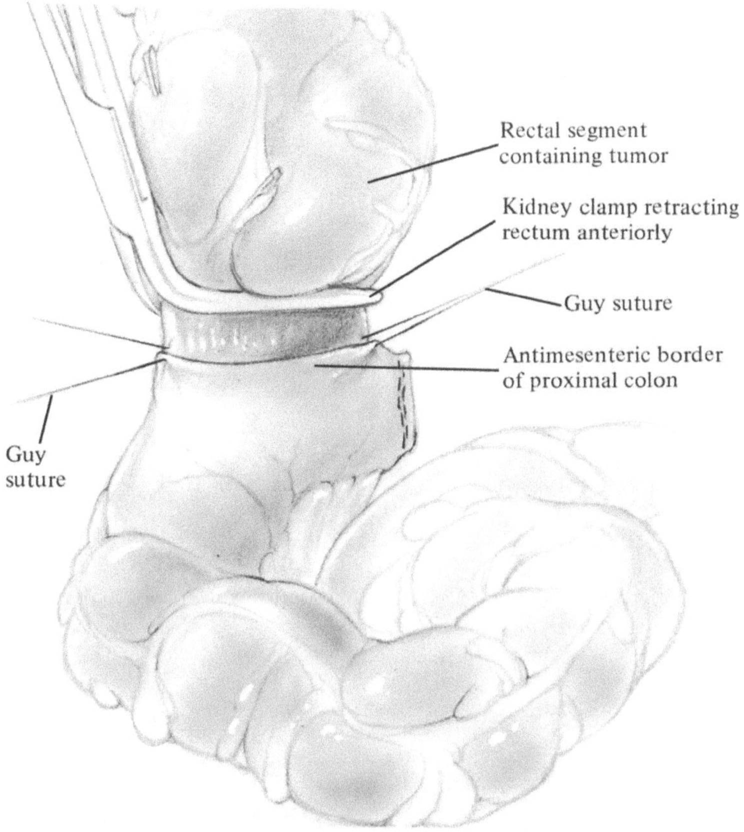


Fig. 6–15

it in a hemostat **(Fig. 6–15)**. Approximate the posterior muscular layer with interrupted 4-0 silk Cushing sutures, taking bites of colon and rectum 5 mm wide. Use a Stratte or a Finochietto angled needleholder (see Glossary) when sewing deep in the pelvis; this facilitates smooth insertion of the curved needle. Insert these sutures 6–7 mm behind the anticipated lines of transection of the colon and rectum. The preferred technique is successive bisection **(Figs. 6–16, 6–17)**. Tie none of these sutures until all have been placed. When the anastomosis is at a very low level, it is convenient to keep the proximal colonic segment well above the promontory of the sacrum until all the posterior seromuscular sutures have been inserted. Be sure these stitches catch the longitudinal muscle of the rectum. If only mucosa is used for anastomosis, failure is likely.

Incise the previous scratch mark in the proximal colonic segment with a scalpel and Metzenbaum scissors **(Fig. 6–18)**. Make a similar incision along a line 6-7 mm proximal to the sutures already placed in the rectum.

If exposure is difficult, it is sometimes helpful to maintain gentle traction on the tails of the Cushing sutures to improve exposure while suturing the mucosa. Then cut the tails of the Cushing sutures successively as the mucosal sutures are inserted. Otherwise, cut all the Cushing sutures at one time, except for the two lateral guy sutures, which should be retained for the moment.

Begin the posterior mucosal closure at the midpoint of the posterior layer using an atraumatic suture of 3-0 PG. Start a continuous locked suture at the midpoint and continue it to the right lateral margin. The second suture of the same material should progress from the midpoint toward the left lateral margin of the suture line **(Fig. 6–19)**.

Divide the anterior wall of the rectum below the large right-angle clamp and remove the specimen. Request an immediate frozen section histologic examination of the distal margin of the specimen to rule out the presence of cancer. If tumor cells are found at the margin, resection of additional rectum is indicated.

Now approximate the anterior mucosal layer by a continuous suture of the Connell or Cushing type **(Fig. 6–20)**. Accomplish this by grasping the needle, which has completed the posterior mucosal layer

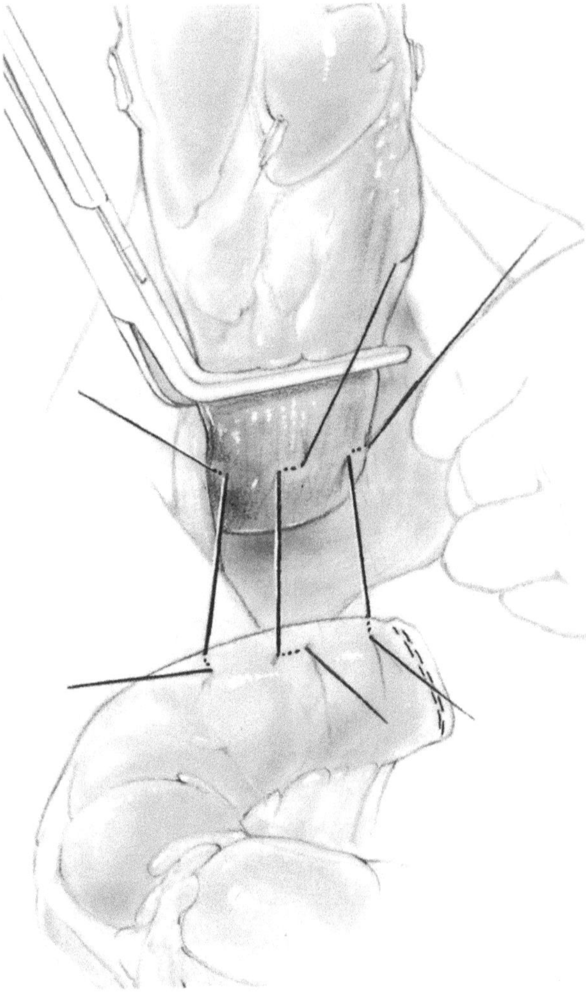

Fig. 6-16

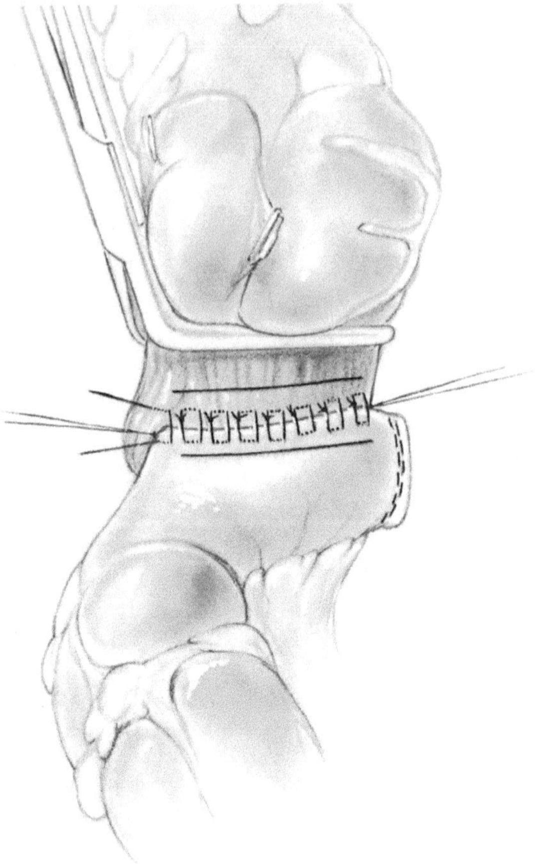

Fig. 6-17

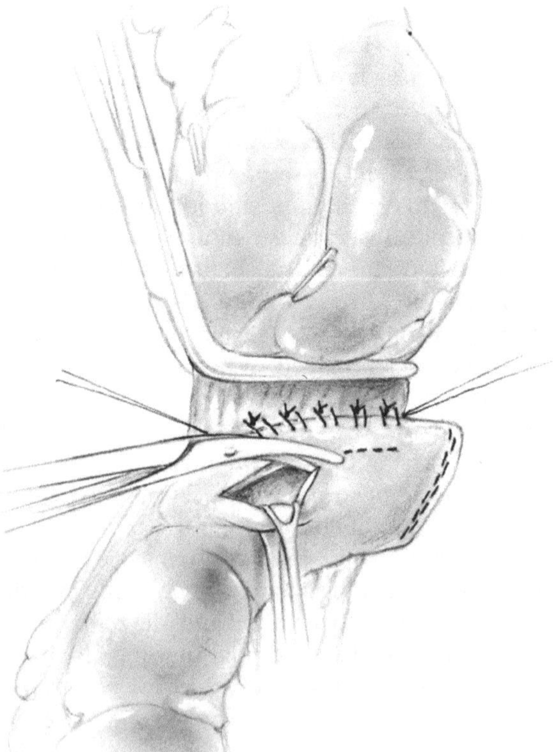

Fig. 6-18

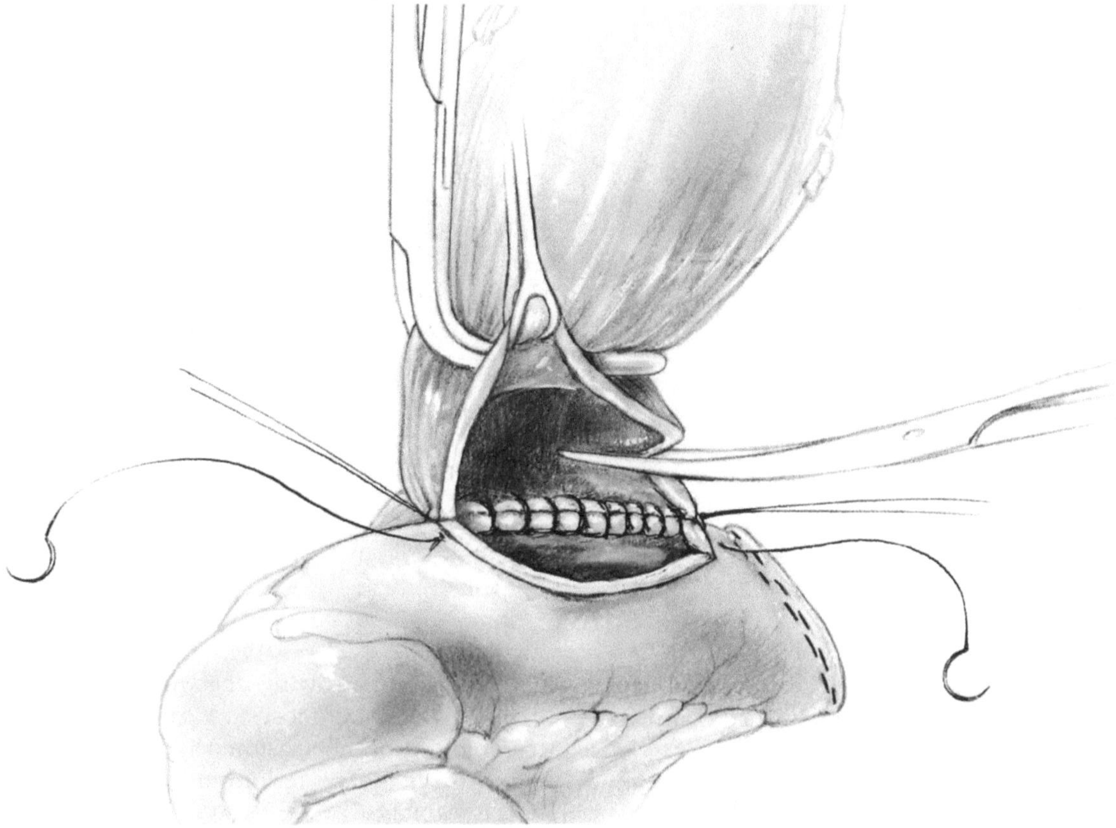

Fig. 6–19

and is now in the lumen at the right margin of the anastomosis, and passing it from inside out through the rectum. The suture line should progress from the right lateral margin toward the midpoint of the anterior layer. When this has been reached, grasp the second needle, located at the left lateral margin of the posterior mucosal layer. Use this needle to complete the anterior mucosal layer from the left lateral

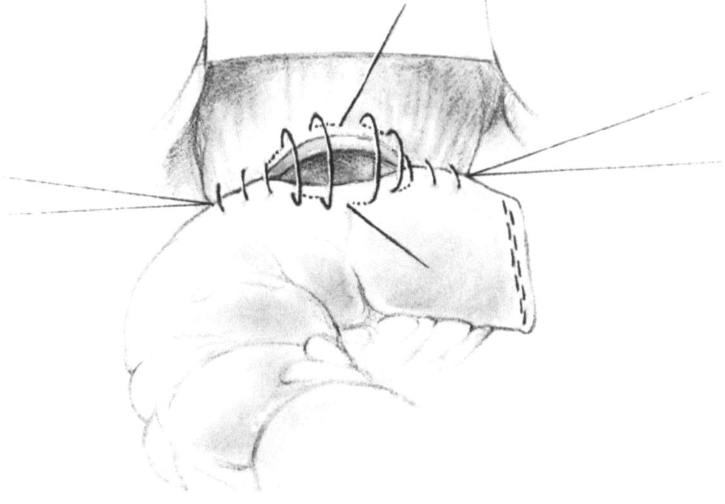

Fig. 6–20

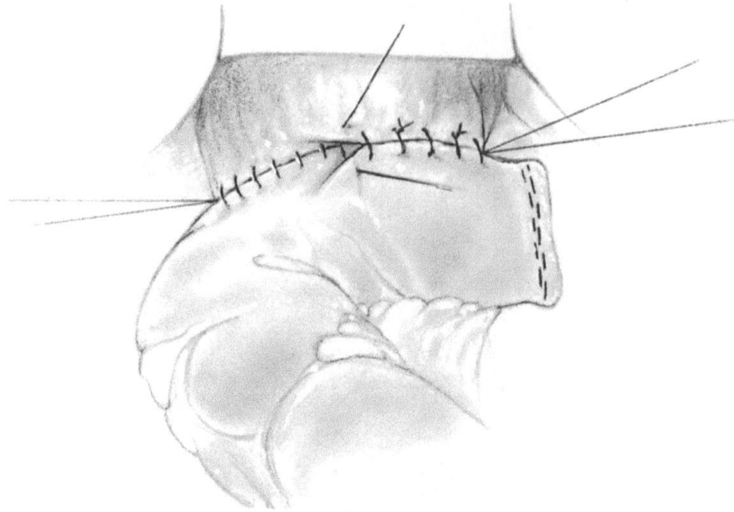

Fig. 6–21

margin to the midpoint where the anterior mucosal layer is terminated with the mucosa completely inverted (Fig. 6–20).

Close the anterior muscular layer with interrupted 4-0 atraumatic silk Lembert or Cushing sutures **(Figs. 6–21, 6–22)**. Insert this row of sutures about 6mm away from the mucosal suture line to accomplish a certain amount of invagination of the rectum into the colon. Because the dimension of the side-to-end lumen is large narrowing does not result. A sagittal section of the anastomosis in **Figure 6–23** illustrates this point. After the anastomosis is completed, carefully inspect the posterior suture line for possible defects, which if present can be corrected by additional sutures.

At this point cut the sutures and thoroughly irrigate the pelvis with a dilute solution of antibiotics. The large defect in the peritoneum need not be

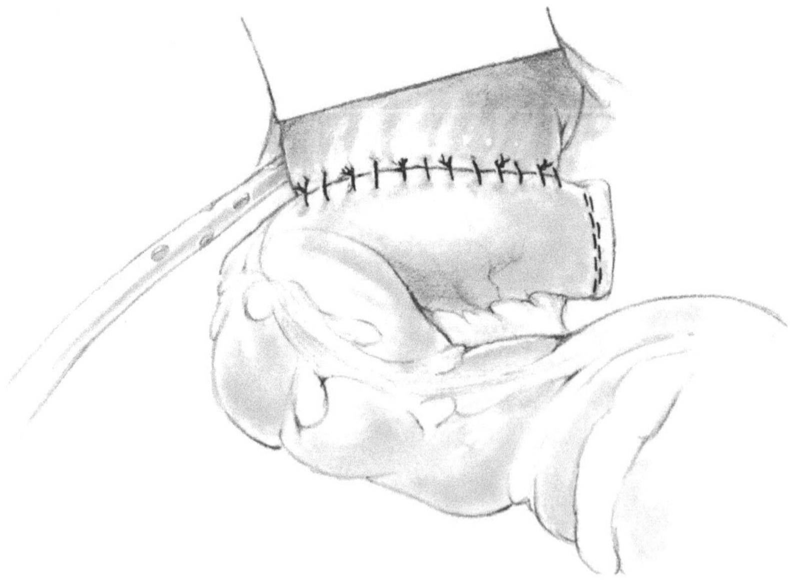

Fig. 6–22

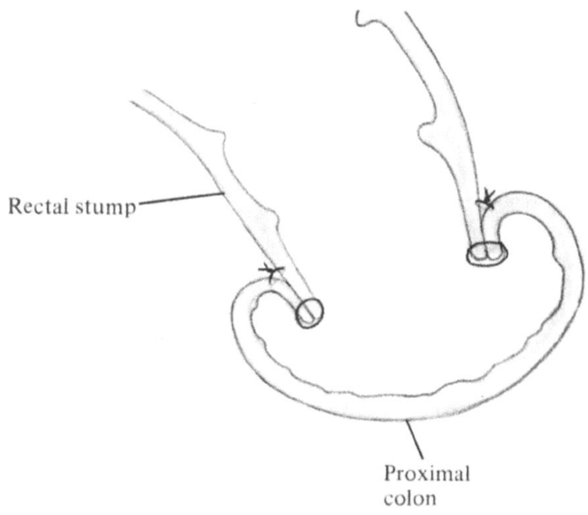


Fig. 6–23

closed. This omission has brought no noticeable ill effect, probably because the defect is so large as not to entrap any small intestine permanently.

Make a final check to ensure there is no tension on the colorectal suture line. If there is, additional proximal colon must be liberated. There must be sufficient slack that the colon *fills up the hollow of the sacrum* on its way to the anastomosis, thereby eliminating any deadspace.

### *Alternative to Colorectal Side-to-End Anastomosis*

When the surgeon does not find it practicable to leave the specimen attached to the rectal stump for purposes of traction (the preferred technique described above), an alternative method may be used for the anastomosis. After the first step in the Baker method (Fig. 6–12) has been completed, remove the specimen by a scalpel incision across the rectum distal to the right-angle clamp. This leaves the rectal stump wide open. To prevent the short rectal stump from retracting beyond the prostate, apply long (30 cm) Allis clamps to the right and left corners of the rectal stump. Then insert a Lloyd-Davies bladder retractor deep to the prostate for exposure.

Bring the previously prepared segment of descending colon down to the sacral promontory. The end of this segment of colon should have already been occluded by application of the linear stapling device. Make an incision on the antimesenteric border of the colon beginning 1 cm from the stapled end and continuing proximally for 4–5 cm, which is the approximate diameter of the rectal ampulla.

Insert a guy suture of atraumatic 4-0 silk from the left lateral wall of the rectal stump to the termination of the incision in the colon. Grasp this suture in a hemostat without tying it. Place a similar suture in the right lateral walls of the rectal stump and colon.

Close the remainder of the posterior wall with interrupted horizontal mattress sutures of atraumatic 4-0 silk. Place the first suture at the midpoint of the posterior layer. Using a curved needle, begin the stitch on the mucosal side of the proximal colon and go from inside out through all layers of colon. Then pass the needle from outside in into the rectal stump. It is vitally important that the muscularis of the rectum be included in this bite. Often the muscularis retracts 1 cm or more beyond the protruding rectal mucosa.

Bring the same needle back from inside out on the rectal stump and then from outside in on the proximal colon. Leave this suture untied but grasp it in a hemostat. When it is tied at a later stage in the procedure, the knot lies on the mucosa of the colon.

Place the second horizontal mattress suture halfway between the first suture and the *left* lateral guy suture by the same technique. Place the third suture so it bisects the distance between the midpoint of the posterior layer and the *right* lateral guy suture. Place the remaining stitches by the technique of successive bisection until this layer is complete **(Fig. 6–24)**.

The colon should slide down against the rectal stump while the assistant holds the ends of all the sutures taut. Tie the sutures and leave the tails long, grasping each again in a hemostat. Retaining the long tails of these stitches and applying mild upward traction improves the exposure for insertion of the mucosal sutures. The remainder of the anastomosis is similar to that described above for the Baker technique.

### *Circular Stapled Low Colorectal Anastomosis*

To use the circular stapling technique for low colorectal anastomosis, place the patient in the Lloyd-Davies position, with thighs abducted, anus exposed, and sacrum elevated on a small sandbag. For tumors situated 6–9 cm above the anal verge, it is necessary to dissect the rectum down to the levator diaphragm, which requires complete division of Waldeyer's fascia posteriorly, dissection of the anterior rectum away from the prostate to the level of the urethra, and division of the lateral ligaments down to the levators.

Unless the patient has a narrow pelvis, the entire levator diaphragm then comes into view **(Fig. 6–25)**.

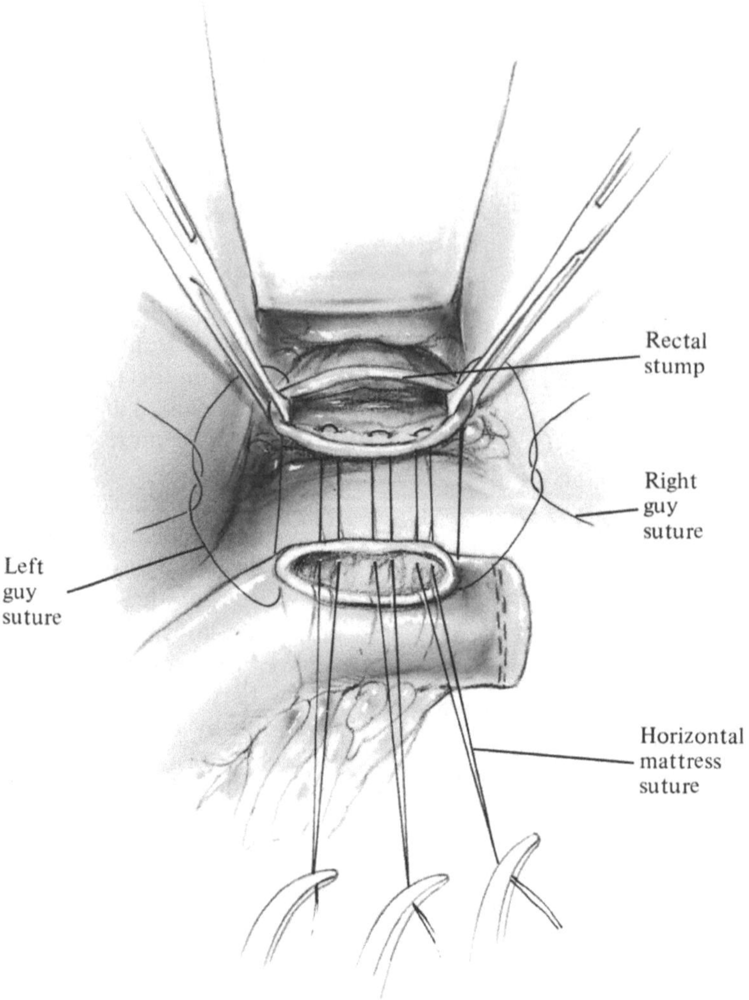


Fig. 6–24

All of the perirectal lymphatics readily peel off the levator musculature. Then follow the posterior wall of the rectum down to the puborectalis muscle, which marks the cephalad margin of the anal canal. Take care not to continue dissecting beyond the puborectalis, as it is easy to enter the intersphincteric plane and liberate the rectum down to the anal verge. An anastomosis to the skin of the anal canal is technically feasible but would result in excision of the internal sphincter together with the specimen because the intersphincteric space is the natural plane of dissection one enters from above.

Place a large right-angle renal pedicle clamp across the rectum about 1 cm beyond the lower edge of the tumor. Then divide the upper colon between Allen clamps at the site previously selected for this purpose. Ligate the cut distal end of the descending colon with umbilical tape and cover it with a sterile rubber glove (Figs. 6–14a, 6–14b). Bring the proximal colon down into the pelvis. There should be sufficient slack in the colon to fill the hollow of the sacrum on its way to the site of the anastomosis. If not, liberate the transverse colon to achieve sufficient slack.

Next, remove the Allen clamp and gently dilate the colon with appropriate sizers or a Foley catheter balloon. Dilating the colon may prove the most frustrating step of the entire operation. Be careful *not to produce any serosal tears* during this maneuver. It is advisable to use the largest cartridge possible to ensure an ample lumen.

Then insert a 2-0 Prolene continuous over-and-over whip-stitch starting at the left margin of the proximal cut end of the colon **(Fig. 6–26a)**. Ascertain that all fat and mesentery have been dissected

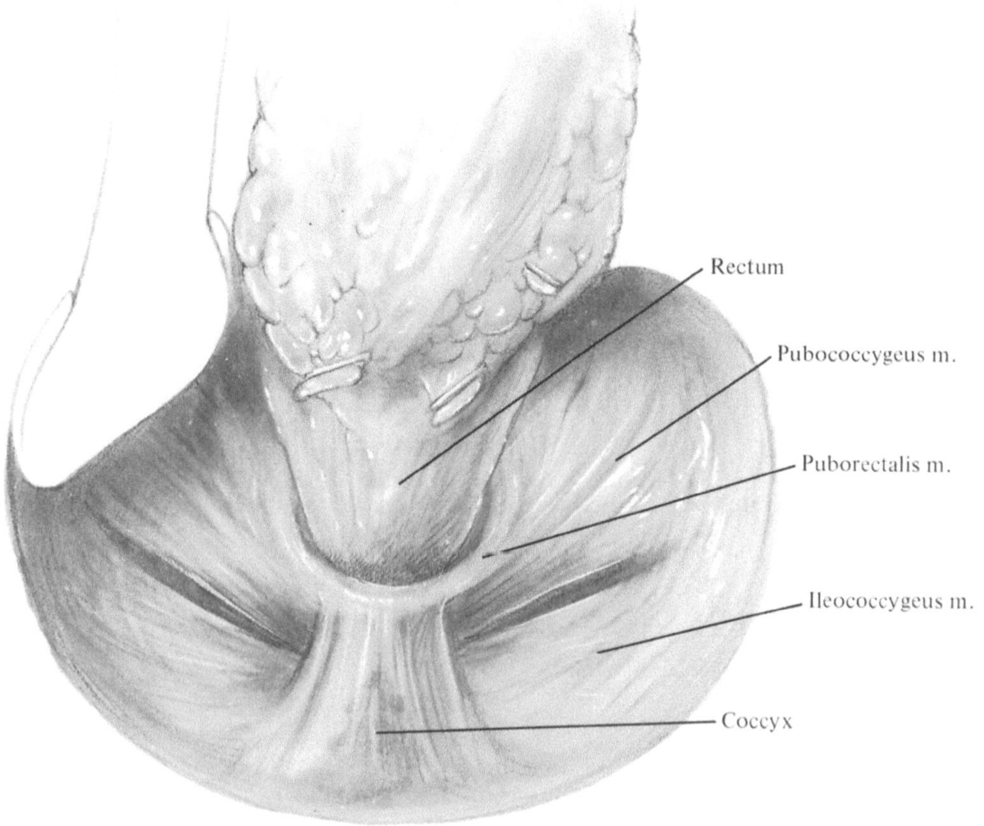


Fig. 6–25

off the distal 1.5 cm of colon so no fat or blood vessels are interposed between the layers of bowel included in the staple line. If blood vessels are trapped in the staple line, firing the stapler may produce significant bleeding in the rectal lumen, which is difficult to control. Alternatively, a purse-string instrument may be used instead of a whip-stitch.

Insert a sterile short proctoscope into the anal canal and aspirate the rectum of its contents. Thoroughly irrigate the rectum with sterile water to wash out any desquamated tumor cells and remove the proctoscope.

Next, insert an over-and-over whip-stitch into the rectal stump. To accomplish this, make an incision through the full thickness of the rectal wall on its left anterolateral aspect, leaving a 4 cm margin beyond the tumor. Place traction on the right-angle clamp to maintain exposure of the lower rectum. Initiate a 2-0 atraumatic Prolene over-and-over whip-stitch at the left lateral corner of the rectal stump **(Fig. 6–26b)**. As this stitch progresses along the anterior wall of the rectum toward the patient's right, divide more

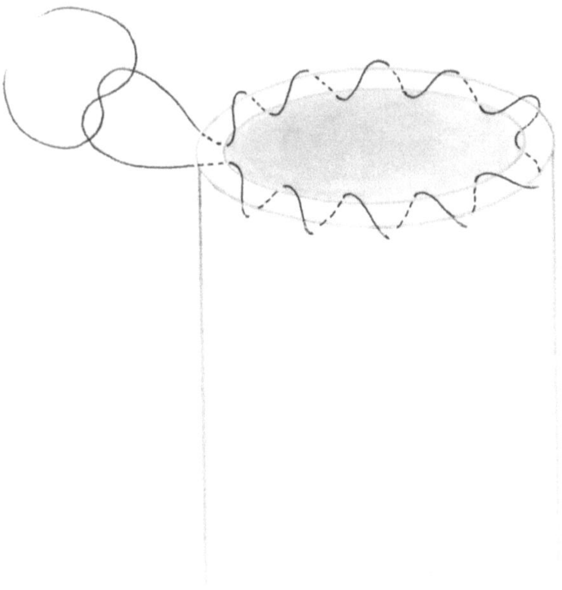

Fig. 6–26a

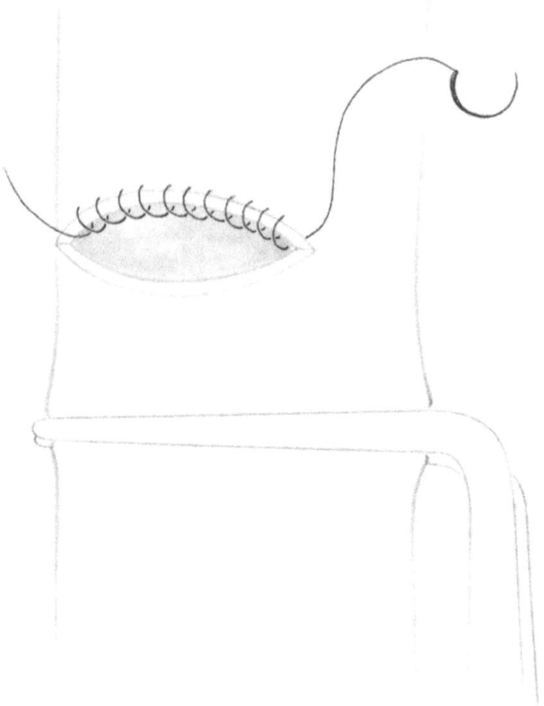

Fig. 6–26b

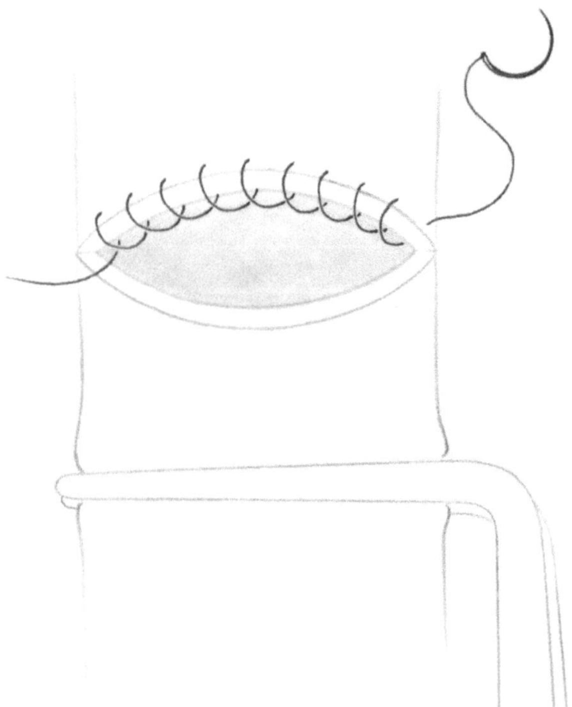

Fig. 6–26c

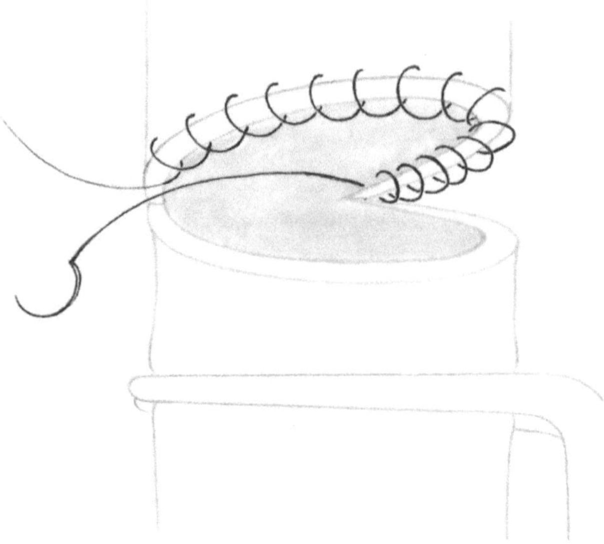

Fig. 6–26d

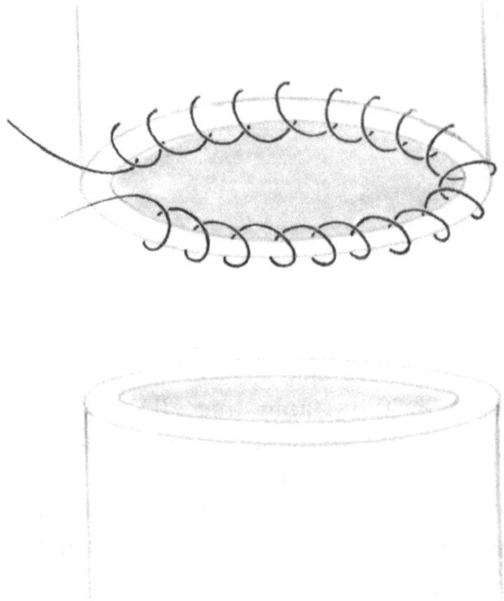

Fig. 6–26e

and more rectal wall **(Fig. 6–26c)**. Continue the same suture circumferentially along the posterior wall of the rectum until the point of origin at the left lateral wall is reached and the specimen is completely detached **(Figs. 6–26d, 6–26e)**. Do not attempt to insert the whip-stitch *after* the specimen has been detached because the rectal stump would retract beyond the prostate and suturing from above would be impossible in the case of tumors of the mid-rectum (6–10 cm above the anal verge). Each bite should contain 4 mm of full-thickness rectal wall, and the stitches should be no more than 6 mm apart to prevent gaps when the suture is tied. A 1.5–2.0 cm width of muscular wall of rectum behind the whip-stitch should be cleared of fat, blood vessels, and

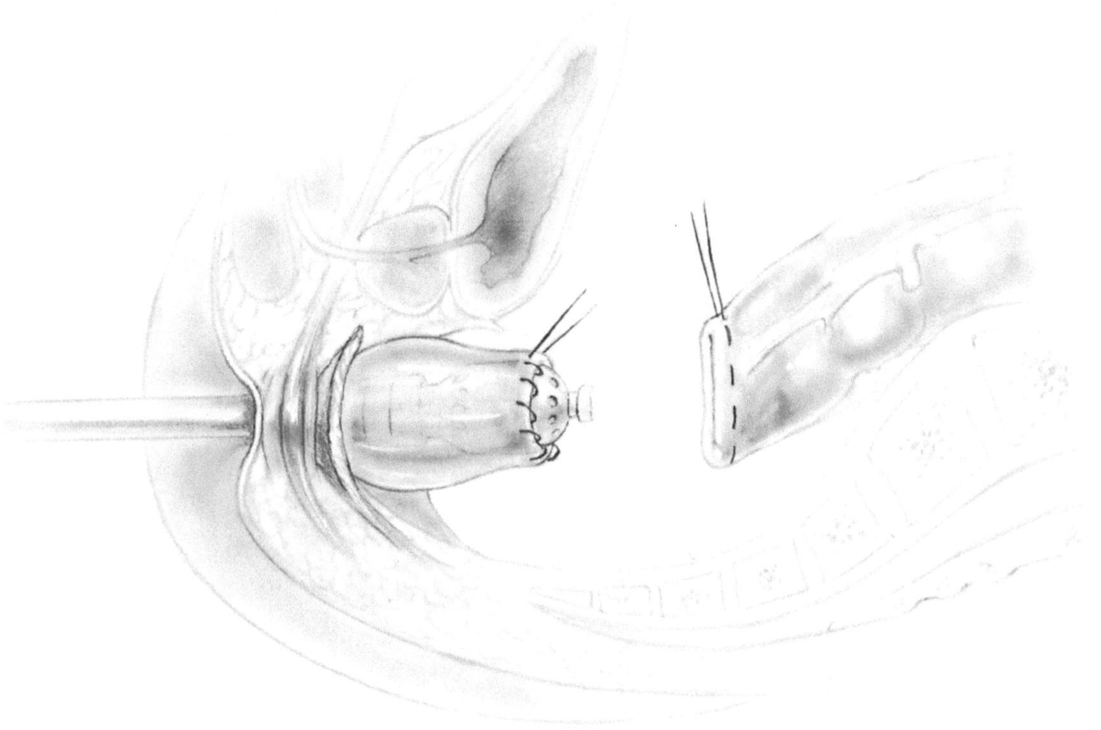

Fig. 6–27

areolar tissue. When the staples are fired, there should be no fat or mesentery between the muscular wall of the rectum and the seromuscular wall of the proximal colon. Grasp both ends of the Prolene purse-string suture in a hemostat. Irrigate the pelvis.

Now move to the perineal portion of the operative field. Check that the stapler is correctly assembled. Because devices from different manufacturers vary, it is crucial to be familiar with the circular stapling device in use. Lubricate the tip of the stapling device with sterile surgical jelly. Insert the device into the anal canal and the rectum with the trigger handles pointing anteriorly **(Fig. 6–27)**. Slowly push the anvil of the stapler through the lower rectal purse-string suture, then rotate the wing nut at the end counterclockwise until the device is wide open. Tie the rectal purse-string suture firmly around the shaft of the stapler **(Fig. 6–28)** and cut the tails 5 mm from the knot.

Apply three Allis clamps in triangular fashion to the cut end of the proximal colon, the lumen of which has been dilated so the colon may be brought over the cap of the circular stapler. When this has been accomplished, tie the colonic purse-string suture and cut its tails 5 mm from the knot **(Fig. 6–29)**. It is vital to observe the integrity of the two purse-string sutures, as any gap in the purse-string closures can cause a defect in the anastomosis.

Now *completely* close the circular stapler by rotating the wing nut in a clockwise fashion **(Fig. 6–30)**. Check the vernier marks to confirm complete closure.

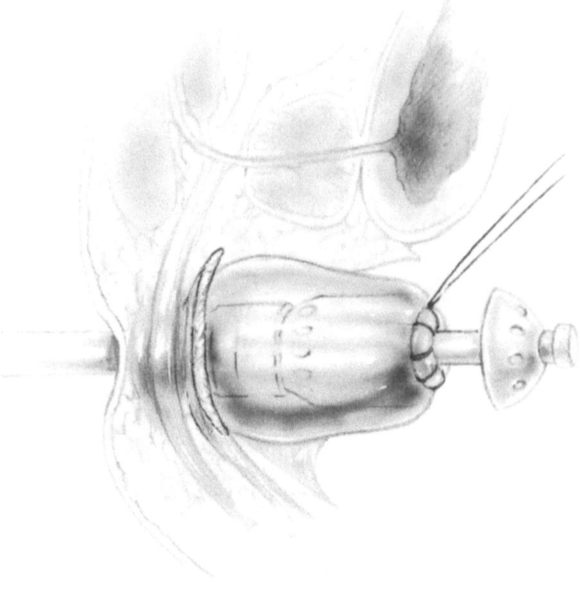

Fig. 6–28

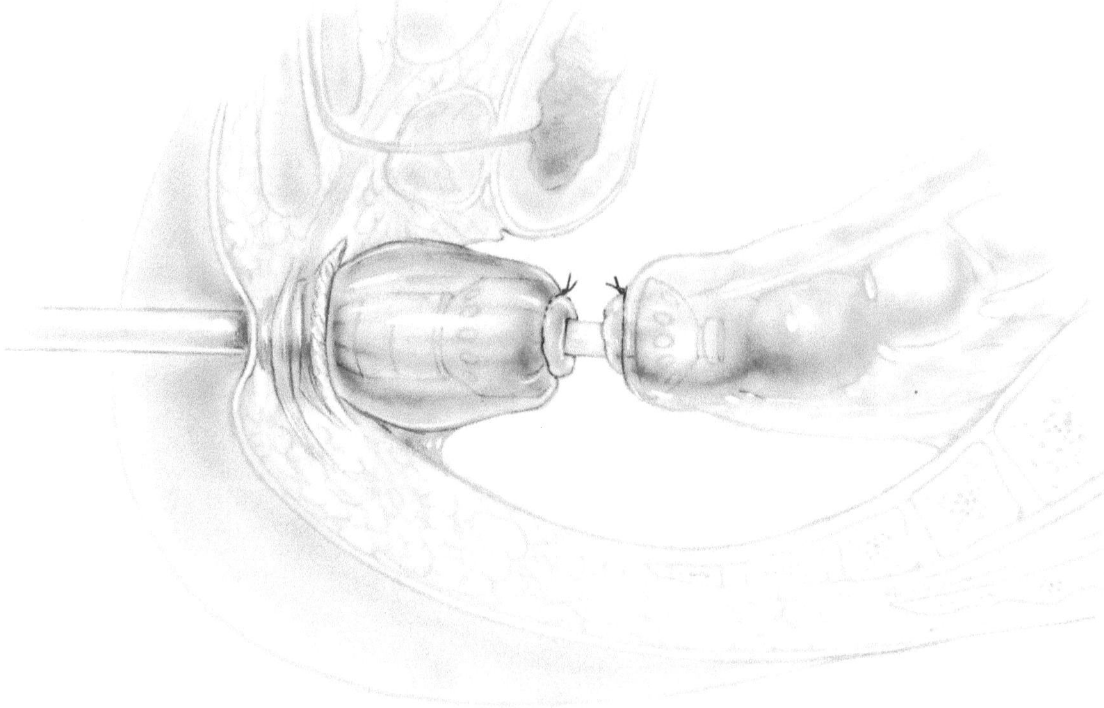

Fig. 6–29

This approximates the anvil to the staple cartridge. If closure is not complete, the staples are too far from the anvil and do not close to form the B shape. Be sure the vagina, bladder, and ureters are not grasped between the anvil and the cartridge during this step.

Unlock the trigger handles and then strongly compress them by applying a firm grip **(Fig. 6–31)**. Check the strength of the compression by observing if the black mark on the shaft of the instrument is in the proper location. If this step is done properly, two circular, concentric rows of staples are fired against

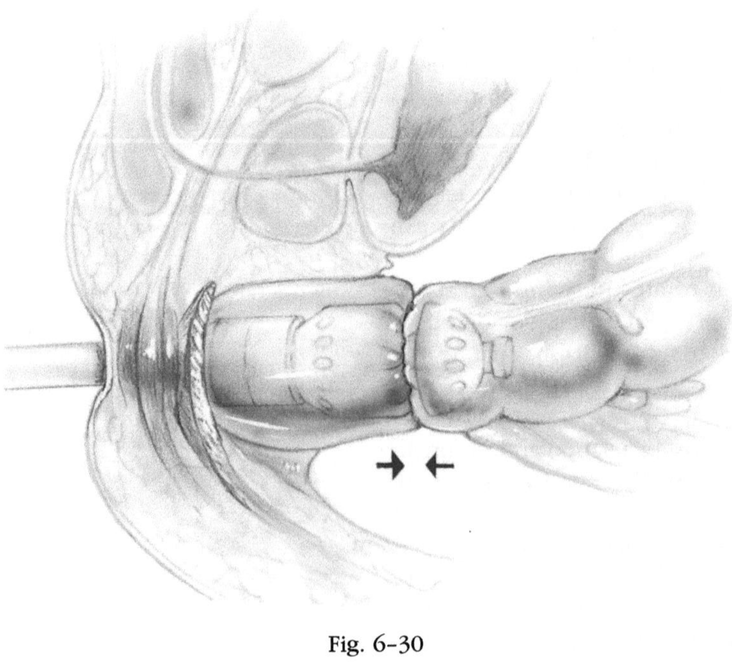

Fig. 6–30

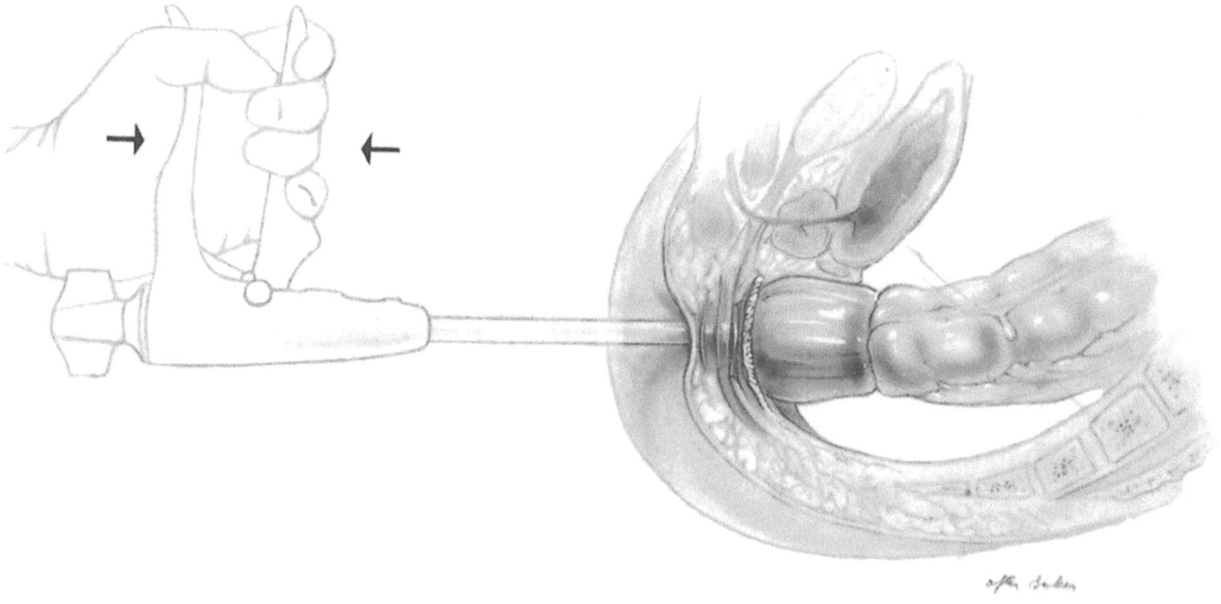

Fig. 6–31

an anvil, and a circular scalpel blade excises the tissues compressed by the two purse-string sutures in the rectum and colon, resulting in a circular stapled anastomosis.

Now rotate the wing nut counterclockwise the recommended number of turns to open the device and separate the anvil from the cartridge. Rotate the stapler at least 180° to the right and then to the left to free any adherent tissue. Remember that the anvil cap is larger than the inner diameter of the anastomosis. Extract the anvil by depressing the stapling device handle toward the floor, thereby elevating the anterior lip of the anvil. Extract this lip first; then deliver the posterior lip by elevating the handle. It is sometimes helpful if the assistant grasps the anterior rectal stump with a gauze pad or inserts a Lembert suture to stabilize the staple line while the anvil is being extracted **(Figs. 6–32, 6–33)**.

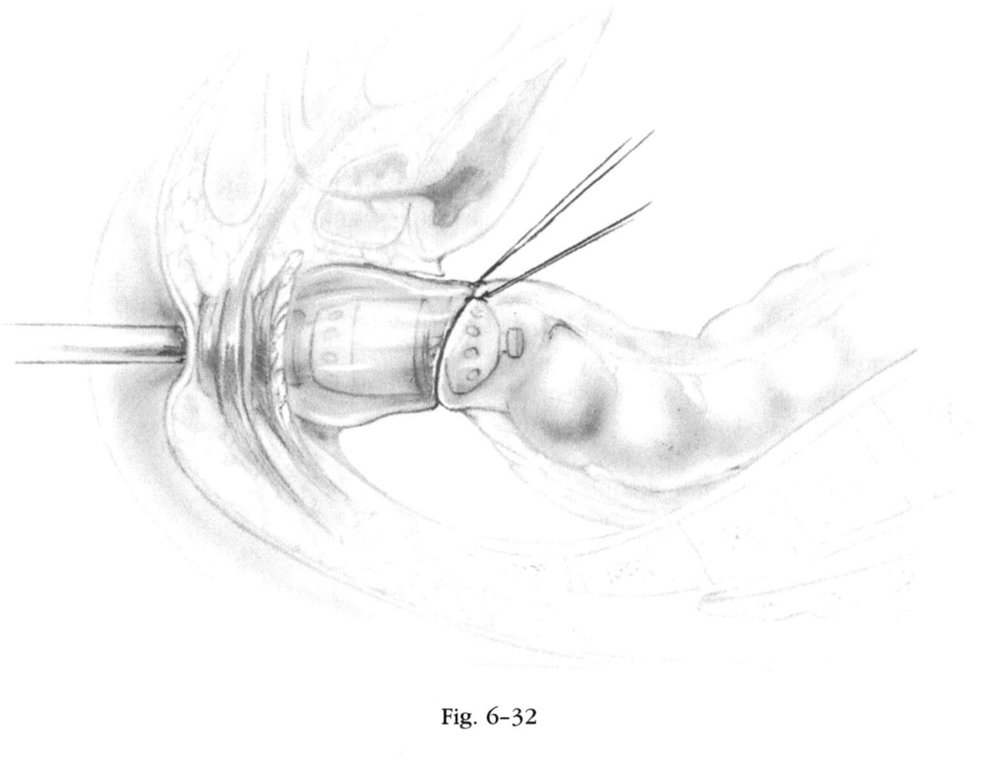

Fig. 6–32

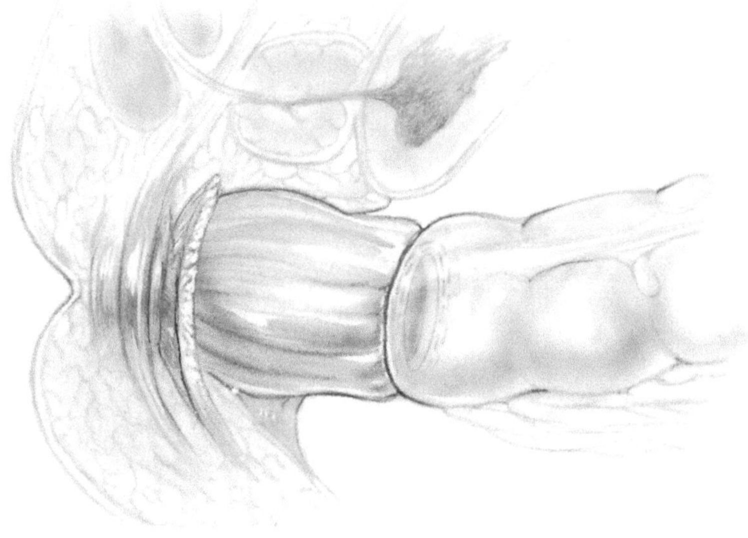

Fig. 6–33

After the instrument has been removed, turn the thumb screw on the cap of the staple cartridge counterclockwise and remove the cap containing the anvil to reveal the segments of rectum and colon that have been amputated. The cartridge should contain two complete circles, each resembling a small doughnut. One represents the proximal margin of the rectum and the other the distal margin of the proximal colon. Any gap in either of the two circles of bowel indicates a defect in the stapled anastomosis caused by the bowel pulling out of the purse-string suture before being stapled. Locate and repair any such defects. Consider a complementary colostomy or loop ileostomy.

Now check the integrity of the stapled anastomosis by digital examination. An additional test of integrity is to flood the pelvis with sterile saline. Wait until all air bubbles have disappeared and then apply an atraumatic Doyen clamp to the colon above the anastomosis. The assistant then inserts an Asepto-type syringe or a Foley catheter into the anus and pumps air into the rectum while the surgeon palpates the colon. When the colon is inflated with air under only a moderate degree of pressure, observe the pool of saline for air bubbles. The absence of air bubbles is fairly reliable evidence of an intact anastomosis. If air bubbles are detected, attempt to find the source of the leak and repair it with sutures. Create a transverse colostomy if the leak cannot be located or if the suture repair seems unreliable. Another method is to insert a Foley catheter into the rectum and, through it, instill a sterile solution of methylene blue dye. Inspect the anastomosis for leakage of the dye. Use a sterile angled dentist's mirror to help observe the posterior aspect of the anastomosis.

## *Double-Stapled Technique for Very Low Colorectal Stapled Anastomosis*

There are several situations in which the double-stapled method is advantageous. First, when the rectum is unusually thick or large, even the largest circular stapler cartridge is too small to accommodate the large bulk of tissue. Forcing this large bulk of tissue into the cartridge results in extruding some of the tissue between the colon and rectum being anastomosed **(Fig. 6–34)**. Because the tissue is devitalized, it may interfere with healing and cause leakage. When the rectum is bulky, instead of a purse-string suture apply the Roticulator-55 stapler and close the rectum with a line of staples. Then amputate the specimen. If a circular stapling device

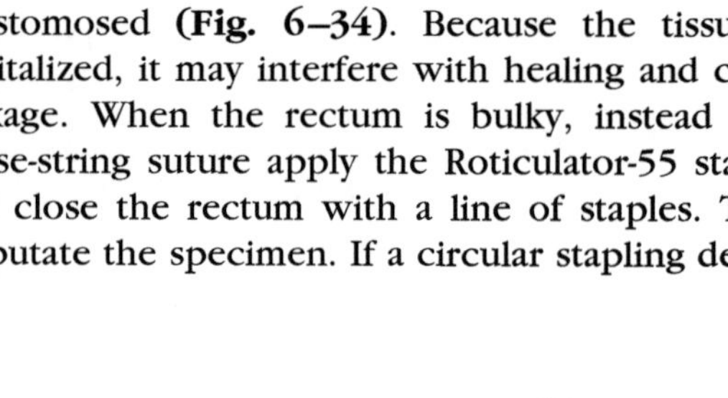

Fig. 6–34

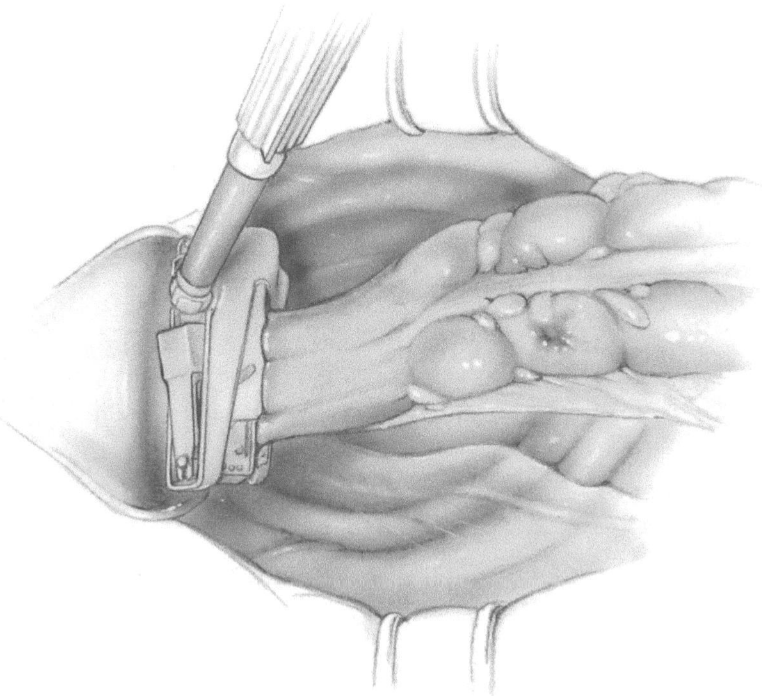

Fig. 6–35

is inserted into the rectum, the circular stapled colorectal anastomosis does not encompass a large bulk of rectum, only a relatively thin circle of rectum (Fig. 6–38). Second, it is possible to close the rectal stump at a significantly lower level, as it is much simpler to apply the stapler in this location than to insert a purse-string suture. Third, in patients who have undergone a Hartmann operation, when performing the colorectal anastomosis to the stump of rectum left behind after the Hartmann operation inserting the circular stapling device into the rectal stump makes reversal of the Hartmann operation much simpler than would construction of a sutured colorectal anastomosis.

Anterior resection of the rectum proceeds in the same manner as described above, except that the dissection generally continues farther into the pelvis than the average case, as the Roticulator-55 can be inserted closer to the anal canal than other methods of excising the rectum. After dissection is completed, using the usual retractors on the bladder or uterus, apply the Roticulator-55 to encompass the entire lower rectum and no adjacent pelvic tissues **(Fig. 6–35)**. Dissect the rectum down to the longitudinal muscle on all sides. After firing the stapler, apply a long-angled clamp to occlude the proximal rectum and then use the scalpel to divide the rectum flush with the proximal margin of the Roticulator device **(Fig. 6–36)**. Locate the upper end of the specimen. Divide the colon and remove the specimen. Insert a 2-0 Prolene purse-string suture close to the cut margin of the colon; then insert the detached anvil into the colon and tie the purse-string suture **(Fig. 6–37)**.

Insert the circular stapler cartridge, with the shaft containing the trocar recessed, through the anus into the rectum. Advance the instrument cautiously to the staple line of the closed rectal stump. Rotate the wing nut at the base of the stapler to advance the trocar through the rectal stump. Aim at a spot just anterior to the midpoint of the staple line. When the trocar has emerged through the rectal stump, remove the trocar (Fig. 6–37). Now engage the anvil shaft into the cartridge shaft. Under direct vision, slowly close the wing nut in such fashion that the anvil and the cartridge are properly approximated

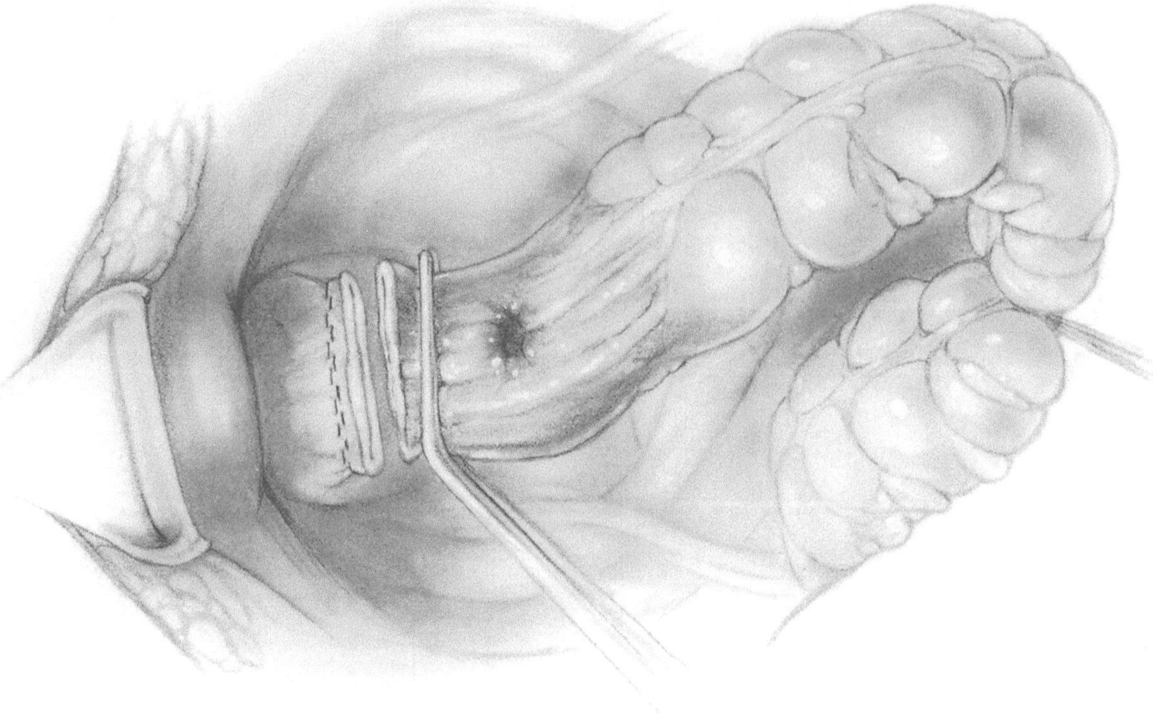

Fig. 6–36

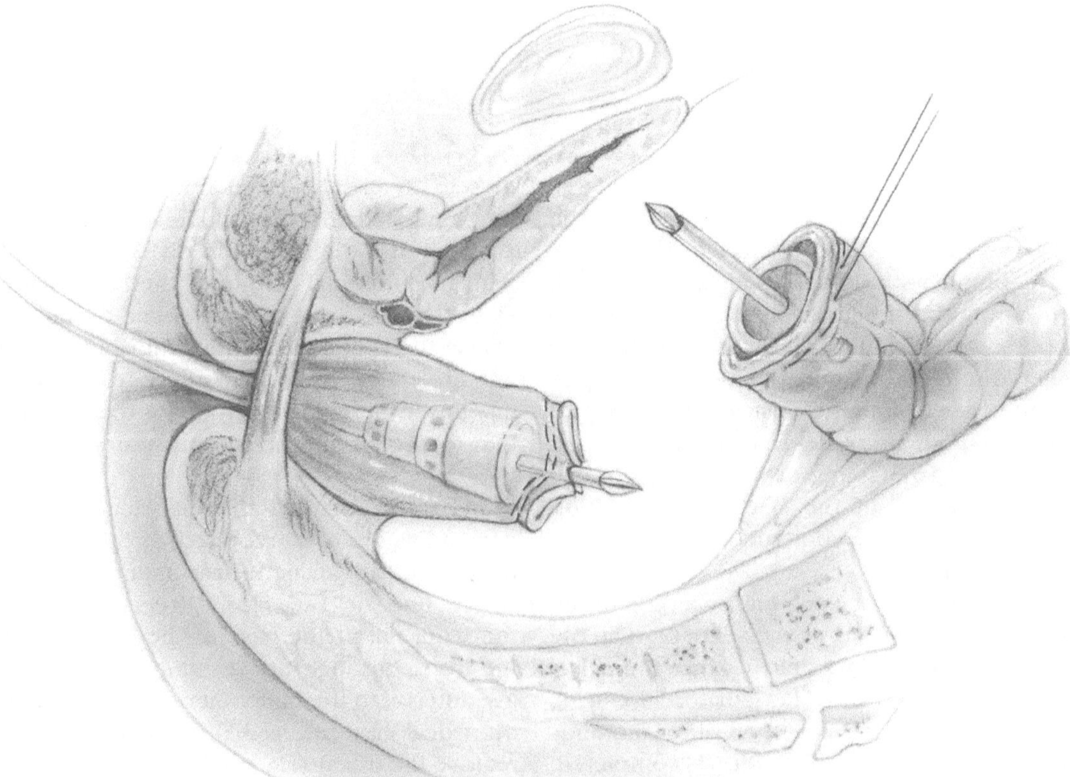

Fig. 6–37

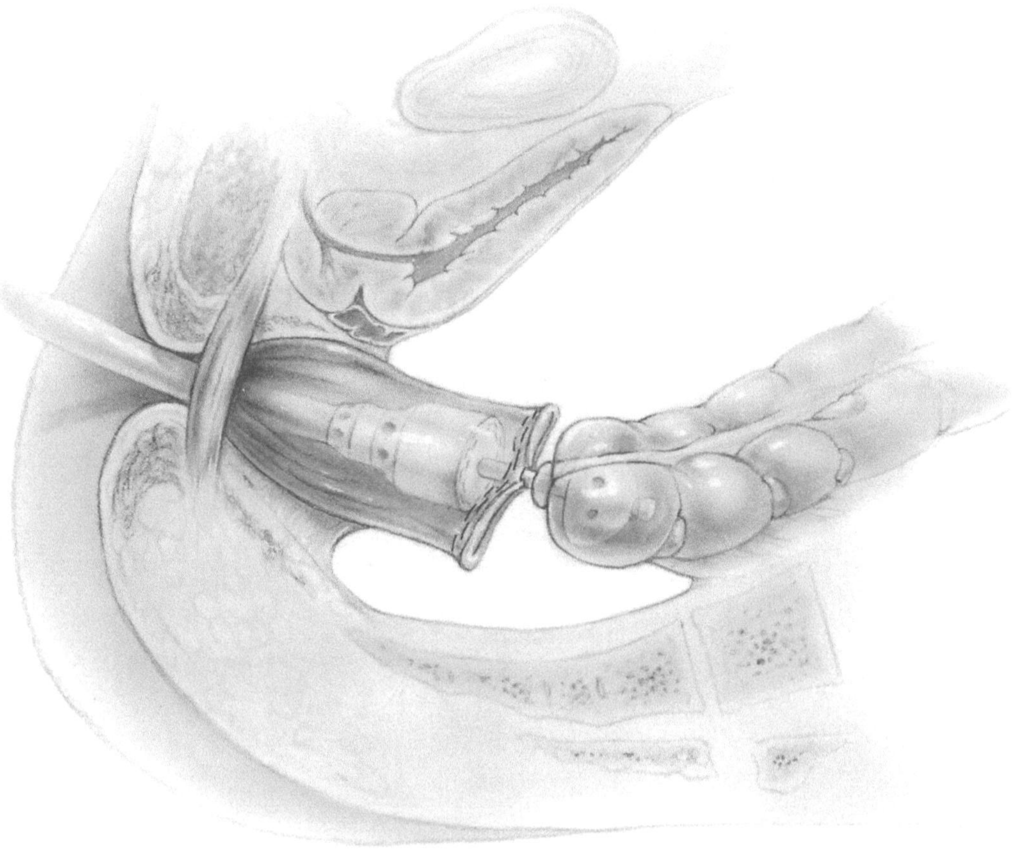

Fig. 6–38

**(Fig. 6–38)**. Then fire the stapler **(Fig. 6–39)**. Now open the stapler and remove it as previously described. Carefully check the anastomosis and both "doughnuts" as previously described.

## *Pitfalls and Danger Points of Circular Stapled Colorectal Anastomosis*

Most defects in the staple line are the result of an imperfect purse-string suture. If this suture does not hold the entire cut end of the bowel close to the shaft of the stapling instrument, the staples cannot catch the complete circumference of the colon or rectum, resulting in a defect and postoperative leakage. If complete doughnut-like circles of fullthickness rectum and colon can be identified after the device has been fired, it indicates that the staples have passed through complete circles of bowel and there should be no defect.

Low colorectal circular stapled anastomoses fail also when too much bowel is left beyond the purse-string sutures. When an excessive volume of tissue is admitted into the cartridge, the capacity of the cartridge is exceeded. This results in extrusion of tissue when the cartridge is compressed against the anvil. The devitalized extruded tissue may emerge between the two walls of stapled bowel and interfere with healing. It is also essential to remove fat from the two bowel walls in the area where the staples are to be inserted.

One important exception to use the whip-stitch is where the rectal diameter is large. When a whip-stitch is used to compress a large rectum, it is sometimes impossible to snug the entire diameter up close to the shaft of the stapling device. In this case close the rectum with a linear stapler and use the double-stapled method.

An additional pitfall should be noted. If the trigger handles of the instrument are not compressed fully, the circular scalpel blade fires incompletely. The staples may be driven home, but the redundant colon and rectum within the anvil *are not cut*. Forceful removal of the stapling device under these conditions disrupts the entire anastomosis.

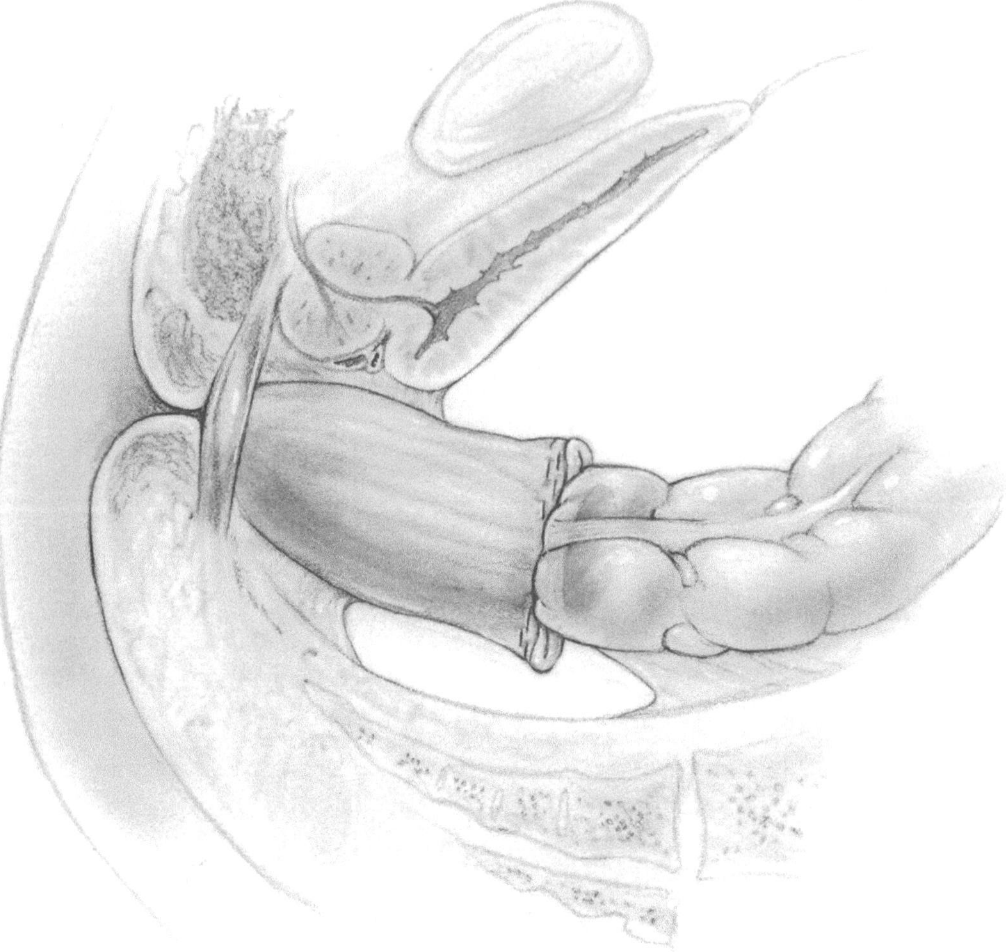

Fig. 6-39

When the anvil cannot be disengaged easily, do not use force. Rather, make a colotomy incision on the antimesenteric border of the upper colon 3–4 cm above the staple line. Then unscrew and remove the anvil through the colotomy. Extracting the stapler from the anus is now a simple matter. Inspect the interior of the anastomosis through the colotomy opening. If a septum of inverted bowel remains in the lumen inside the circle of staples, excise the septum using a Potts angled scissors. Close the colotomy with a 55 mm linear stapler.

An obvious cause of failure is the erroneous use of a cartridge or stapler that has been fired already. In this case the circular blade may function, but there are no staples; the surgeon is left with two cut ends of bowel, but no anastomosis. To avoid this error, before attaching the anvil look closely into the cartridge to be certain it is properly loaded with staples and a circular blade.

Unless the stapler is fully opened, it cannot be removed from the rectum after firing the staples. This mishap occurs because the anastomosed bowel is still being grasped between the staple cartridge and the anvil, and forceful attempts to dislodge the stapler disrupt the anastomosis.

As mentioned above, if the screw that caps the anvil is not screwed on tightly or if the wing nut near the handle is not completely closed before the staples are fired, the space between the staple cartridge and the anvil is excessive. It prevents proper closure of the legs of the staples, in which case the anastomosis may pull apart at the slightest stress. Never use hemostatic clips on any part of the colon or rectum that may be included in the stapled anastomosis because these metal clips prevent proper function of the staples and the stapler blade.

Intraluminal hemorrhage following a stapled anastomosis occurs if mesenteric blood vessels have been trapped in the staple line and are transected by the blade. Bleeding may be controlled by cautious electrocautery through a proctoscope or by inserting sutures through a proximal colotomy.

When the stapled anastomosis is situated at or above the cephalad margin of the anal sphincter muscles (i.e., at or above the puborectalis component of the levator muscle), fecal continence is not lost. However, because the proximal colon segment does not function as a reservoir, the patient defecates frequently during the first few months. Each peristaltic contraction results in evacuation of a small, formed stool; but there is no inadvertent loss of stool or liquid. On the other hand, if the anastomosis is at or below the dentate line, the loss of the internal sphincter results in some degree of fecal incontinence for 3–6 months and *sometimes permanently*.

Goligher (1979) described insertion of the purse-string suture into the rectal stump by a transanal approach after dilating the anus and inserting a self-retaining bivalve Parks rectal retractor. Goligher recommended this maneuver in cases where the purse-string suture cannot be inserted from the abdominal approach. Unfortunately, this technique results in excision of the internal sphincter muscle and produces some degree of fecal incontinence if the stapled anastomosis is placed at or below the dentate line. If the transanal approach is used, make every effort to insert the purse-string or whip-stitch into the rectal stump in the upper segment of the anal canal to ensure retention of the internal sphincter muscle. If the rectal stitch cannot be properly applied, one can perform a transanal end-to-end sutured anastomosis by the method of Parks, which makes a point of preserving the internal sphincter muscle. *A coloanal anastomosis may be constructed by a technique similar to that described in Chapter 48 for the ileoanal pouch.*

When the rectal stump is too short to insert a purse-string stitch from above, it is usually possible to use the Roticulator stapler instead (Fig. 6–35). We are enthusiastic about the double-staple technique for colorectal anastomoses that are so low it would be difficult to use sutures. We have resected tumors 6 cm from the anal verge using the stapler with a 2 cm margin of normal tissue, performing a successful stapled anastomosis flush with the upper margin of the anal canal.

Complementary colostomy and presacral drainage should be used following a stapled anastomosis under the same conditions that would lead the surgeon to use these modalities following a sutured colorectal anastomosis. We routinely employ closed-suction presacral drainage for low extraperitoneal anastomoses.

For stapled intraperitoneal anastomoses above the pelvis, we prefer a functional end-to-end anastomosis (see Figs. 6–35 through 6–38) rather than the circular stapled procedure. The latter often takes more time and is prone to more technical complications than the functional end-to-end method.

### Wound Closure and Drainage

Remove the wound protector drape. The surgical team should change its gloves and discard all contaminated instruments. Thoroughly irrigate the abdominal cavity and wound with an antibiotic solution. Close the incision in the usual fashion.

## POSTOPERATIVE CARE

Nasogastric suction for 3–5 days

No oral intake for the first 4–6 days

Continuation of perioperative antibiotics for 24 hours

Constant bladder drainage via Foley catheter for 6–7 days

Presacral suction catheters attached to closed suction drainage

Drainage catheter removed after 5 days unless there is significant drainage volume

Radiation therapy for selected patients, depending on the stage of disease

## COMPLICATIONS

*Bladder dysfunction* may follow low anterior resection, especially in men with prostatism, but it is much less common than after abdominoperineal proctectomy. Generally, function resumes after 6–7 days of bladder drainage.

*Pelvic sepsis* secondary to anastomotic leakage is the most common serious complication following low colorectal anastomosis. Any patient with fever, leukocytosis, and ileus following low anterior resection should be assumed to have a leaking anastomosis and a pelvic abscess. Clinical manifestations of this complication commonly occur between the sixth and ninth postoperative days. Cautious digital examination of the rectum by the surgeon may prove to be diagnostic if the finger discloses a defect in the suture line, generally on its posterior aspect. Careful proctoscopic examination may disclose evidence of a defect in the suture line.

The presence of pelvic sepsis can almost always be confirmed by pelvic CT and can often be treated by CT-guided percutaneous catheter drainage. A patient may have sustained a pelvic abscess even in the absence of a definite defect in the suture line. Consequently, a patient who is febrile and toxic should undergo drainage of any septic process if CT-guided percutaneous catheter drainage is not successful. In some cases the patient also requires fecal diversion by transverse colostomy or loop ileostomy.

Patients with mild systemic symptoms who are suspected of having a pelvic infection may be treated by food withdrawal, intravenous antibiotics, and hyperalimentation. Occasionally, a presacral abscess drains into the rectum through the anastomosis without making the patient seriously ill. It must be remembered, however, that anastomotic leakage and pelvis sepsis constitute potentially lethal complications that often require vigorous management.

*Sexual dysfunction* in men may follow low anterior resection, especially in patients with large tumors and who require extensive dissection of the presacral space, lateral ligaments, and prostatic area.

## REFERENCES

Baker JW. Low end to side rectosigmoidal anastomosis. Arch Surg 1950;61:143.

El Pakkastie T, Luukkonen PE, Jarvinen HJ. Anastomotic leakage after anterior resection of the rectum. Eur J Surg 1994;160:293.

Enker WE, Thaler HT, Cranor ML, Polyak T. Total mesorectal excision in the operative treatment of carcinoma of the rectum. J Am Coll Surg 1995;181:335.

Goligher JC. Surgery of the Anus, Rectum, and Colon, 3rd ed. London, Bailliere, 1975, p 662.

Goligher JC. Use of circular stapling gun with peranal insertion of anorectal purse-string suture for construction of very low colorectal or colo-anal anastomoses. Br J Surg 1979;66:501.

Longo WE, Milsom JW, Lavery IC, et al. Pelvic abscess after colon and rectal surgery: what is optimal management? Dis Colon Rectum 1993;36:936.

Nivatvongs S, Fang DT. The use of thumbtacks to stop massive presacral hemorrhage. Dis Colon Rectum 1986; 29:589.

Parks AG, Thomson JPS. Per-anal endorectal operative techniques. In Rob C, Smith R (eds) Operative Surgery, Colon, Rectum, and Anus, 3rd ed. London, Butterworths, 1997, 157.

Stolfi VM, Milson JW, Lavery IC, et al. Newly designed occluder pin for presacral hemorrhage. Dis Colon Rectum 1992;35:166.

Surtees P, Ritchie JK, Phillips RKS. High versus low ligation of the inferior mesenteric artery in rectal cancer. Br J Surg 1990;77:618.

Zu J, Lin J. Control of presacral hemorrhage with electrocautery through a muscle fragment pressed on the bleeding vein. J Am Coll Surg 1994;179:351.

# 7 Abdominoperineal Resection for Rectal Cancer

## INDICATIONS

Malignancy of distal rectum or anus not amenable to sphincter-preserving techniques

## PREOPERATIVE PREPARATION

Sigmoidoscopy and biopsy

Barium enema or colonoscopy

Computed tomography (CT) of abdomen and pelvis

Endorectal ultrasonography and other staging studies as indicated

Correction of anemia if necessary

Mechanical and antibiotic bowel preparation

Indwelling Foley catheter in bladder

Nasogastric tube

Perioperative antibiotics

## PITFALLS AND DANGER POINTS

Hemorrhage

- Presacral veins
- Left iliac vein
- Middle hemorrhoidal artery
- Hypogastric arterial branches
- Gastrointestinal vessels

Rupture of rectum during dissection

Colostomy ischemia, producing postoperative necrosis

Colostomy under excessive tension, leading to postoperative retraction and peritonitis

Separation of pelvic peritoneal suture line, causing herniation and obstruction of small intestine

Inadequate mobilization of pelvic peritoneum, resulting in failure of newly constructed pelvic floor to descend completely; resulting empty space encourages sepsis

Genitourinary

Ureteral trauma, especially during dissection in the vicinity of lateral ligaments of the rectum; inadvertent ureteral ligation; especially during reconstruction of pelvic floor

Urethral laceration during dissection of perineum in male patients

## OPERATIVE STRATEGY

### Abdominal Phase

The initial abdominal phase of the dissection is essentially identical to that performed for a low anterior resection. See Chapter 6 for a detailed discussion of the strategy relevant to this phase.

#### *Colostomy*

The colostomy may be brought out through the left lower quadrant musculature, the midline abdominal incision, or the belly of the left rectus muscle. If the colostomy is brought out laterally, the 3- to 5-cm gap between the colon and the lateral portion of the abdominal wall should be closed or a retroperitoneal colostomy performed; otherwise the small bowel may become incarcerated in the lateral space. On the other hand, if the colostomy is brought out somewhere near the midline of the abdomen, there is no need to close this space, which becomes so large that movement of small bowel can take place freely without complication.

Goligher (1958) reported a method of bringing the colostomy out through a retroperitoneal tunnel to the opening in the abdominal wall sited in the lateral third of the rectus muscle a few centimeters below the umbilicus. When the peritoneal pelvic floor is suitable for closure by suturing, this technique is another satisfactory method of creating the sigmoid colostomy (see Figs. 7-19 to 7-22).

To prevent necrosis of the colostomy, confirm that there is adequate arterial blood flow to the distal portion of the exteriorized colon, equivalent to that required if an anastomosis were made at this point. Even in the presence of adequate arterial flow, ischemia of the colostomy may occur if an obese mesentery is constricted by a tight colostomy orifice.

Postoperative retraction of the colostomy may result if abdominal distension causes the abdominal wall to move anteriorly. For this reason the limb of colon to be fashioned into a colostomy should protrude without tension for 5 cm beyond the level of the abdominal skin before any suturing takes place.

### *Pelvic Floor*

Because intestinal obstruction due to herniation of the ileum into a defect in the reconstructed pelvic floor is a serious complication, a number of surgeons now omit the step of resuturing the pelvic peritoneum. If no attempt is made to reperitonealize the pelvic floor, the small bowel descends to the level of the sutured levators or subcutaneous layers of the perineum. Intestinal obstruction during the immediate postoperative period does not appear to be common following this technique. However, if intestinal obstruction does occur at a later date, it becomes necessary to mobilize considerable small bowel, which is bound down by dense adhesions in the pelvis. It often results in damage to the intestine, requiring resection and anastomosis to repair it. Thus it appears logical to attempt primary closure of the pelvic peritoneum to prevent this complication, provided enough tissue is available for closure without undue tension. The peritoneal floor should be *sufficiently lax to descend to the level of the reconstructed perineum*. This eliminates the deadspace between the peritoneal floor and the other structures of the perineum. As total proctectomy is done primarily to remove lesions of the lower rectum, there is no need for radical resection of the perirectal peritoneum. One should conserve as much of this layer as possible. If it appears that a proper closure is not possible, it is preferable to leave the floor entirely open. Otherwise the deadspace between the peritoneal diaphragm and the perineal floor often leads to disruption of the peritoneal suture line and to bowel herniation. Creating a vascularized pedicle of omentum is a good way to fill the pelvic cavity with viable tissue and to prevent the descent of small bowel into the pelvis.

## Perineal Phase

### *Position*

Turning the patient to a prone position provides the best exposure for the surgeon but imposes a number of disadvantages on the patient. First, circulatory equilibrium may be disturbed by turning the patient who is under anesthesia. Also, changing positions prolongs the operative procedure, as it is not possible to have one member of the surgical team close the abdominal incision while the perineal phase is in process. Similar objections can be raised about the lateral Sims position.

For these reasons we favor the position described here. The patient lies supine, with the sacrum elevated on a folded sheet or sandbag and the lower extremities supported by Lloyd-Davies leg rests, causing the thighs to be widely abducted but flexed only slightly; the legs are supported and moderately flexed. This mild flexion of the thighs does not interfere in any way with the abdominal procedure, and the second assistant can stand comfortably between the patient's legs while retracting the bladder (see Figs. 6–3a, 6–3b).

Whether the abdominal and perineal phases are carried on synchronously by two operating teams or one team does the complete procedure, positioning the patient in this manner gives the surgeon the option of doing some portions of the procedure from below and then switching to the abdominal field in response to the exigencies of a particular step. It facilitates safe lateral dissection of large tumors and complete hemostasis in the pelvis. Some vessels may be easier to control from below, and others should be clamped from above. In addition, after the surgeon has completed suturing the pelvic peritoneum, suction can be applied from below to determine if there is a deadspace between the pelvic floor and the perineal closure. After removing the specimen it is fairly simple to have closure of both the abdomen and perineum proceed simultaneously.

### *Closure of Perineum*

Primary closure of the perineum is now routine, particularly if there has been no fecal spillage in the pelvis during the course of resection, and good hemostasis has been accomplished. Primary healing has been obtained in most of our patients operated on for malignancy when the perineum is closed per primam with insertion of a closed-suction drainage catheter. Suction applied to the catheter draws the reconstructed peritoneal pelvic floor downward to eliminate any empty space.

In patients with major presacral hemorrhage, tamponade the area with a sheet of topical hemostatic agent covered by a large gauze pack, which is brought out through the perineum. Remove the gauze in the operating room on the first or second postoperative day after correcting any coagulopathy and achieving full resuscitation.

In patients who have experienced major pelvic contamination during the operation, the perineum should be closed only partially and drained with both latex and sump drains. In female patients, management of the perineum depends on whether one has elected to remove the posterior vagina. For small anterior malignancies, the adjacent portion of the posterior vagina may be removed with the specimen, leaving sufficient vagina for primary closure with PG. When the entire posterior vaginal wall has been removed along with large anterior lesions, the perineum should be closed with sutures to the levator muscles, subcutaneous fat, and skin. This leaves a defect at the site of the vaginal excision through which loose gauze packing should be inserted. If there is primary healing of the perineal floor, granulation fills this cavity and vaginal epithelium regenerates in 1–3 months. Vaginal resection need not be done for tumors confined to the posterior portion of the rectum.

### *Dissection of Perineum*

The most serious pitfall during perineal dissection is inadvertent transection of the male urethra. This can be avoided if the anterior part of the dissection is delayed until the levator muscles have been divided throughout the remainder of the circumference of the pelvis and the prostate identified. It is important not to divide the rectourethralis muscle at a point more cephalad than the plane of the posterior wall of the prostate (see Fig. 7–11). Alternatively, one should identify the transverse perineal muscles. If the dissection is kept on a plane posterior to these muscles, the urethra is out of harm's way.

## Hemostasis

All bleeding during the perineal dissection can be controlled by accurate application of electrocautery. Here, as elsewhere during abdominal surgery, if electrocautery is applied to a vessel that is well isolated from surrounding fat, ligature is not necessary. Whether electrocautery is applied directly to a bleeding point or to forceps or a hemostat depends on the preference of the surgeon. With the cautery device it is possible to obtain complete control of bleeding in this area without undue loss of blood or time.

# OPERATIVE TECHNIQUE

## Position

Place the patient in the supine position, with the sacrum elevated on several folded sheets or a sandbag and the thighs flexed only slightly but abducted sufficiently to allow adequate exposure of the perineum. The legs should be flexed slightly and the calves padded with foam rubber and supported in Lloyd-Davies leg rests (see Figs. 6–3a, 6–3b). If the thighs are not flexed excessively, there is no interference with performance of the abdominal phase of the operation. The second assistant should stand between the patient's legs during the abdominal phase. Bring the indwelling Foley catheter over the patient's groin and attach it to a plastic tube for gravity drainage into a bag calibrated to facilitate measurement of hourly urine volume. In men, fix the scrotum to the groin with a suture. Close the anal canal with a heavy purse-string suture.

Carry out routine skin preparation of the abdomen, perineum, and buttocks. Drape the entire area with sterile sheets. After these steps have been completed, the operation can be performed with two teams working synchronously or by one team alternating between the abdomen and the perineum.

## Incision and Exploration: Operability

Make a midline incision beginning at a point above the umbilicus and continuing to the pubis (see Fig. 6–3a). Separate the pyramidalis muscles as the pubis is approached because getting an extra 1–2 cm closer to the pubis improves the exposure significantly. Open the peritoneum and carry out a general exploration.

In most cases the resectability of a rectal carcinoma cannot generally be determined until a later step in the operation, when the presacral space is open. Accurate preoperative staging has eliminated most of these intraoperative dilemmas. When a tumor invades the sacrum posteriorly or the prostate anteriorly, attempting to core out the rectum by forcing a plane through the tumor is a fruitless and sometimes dangerous endeavor. If much tumor is left behind in the presacral space, the palliation attained is negligible because if it invades the presacral nerves it produces the most distressing of all symptoms in this disease, extreme perineal pain. On the other hand, many tumors are firmly adherent to the sacrum without having invaded it. These lesions should be resected. Cases of borderline resectability may benefit from preoperative neoadjuvant therapy. Local invasion of the ureter does not contraindicate resection, as the divided ureter at this low level can be implanted into the bladder.

## Mobilization of Sigmoid, Lymphovascular Dissection, and Presacral Dissection

The abdominal phase of this operation proceeds down to the levator diaphragm, as previously outlined (see Figs. 6–4 through 6–11).

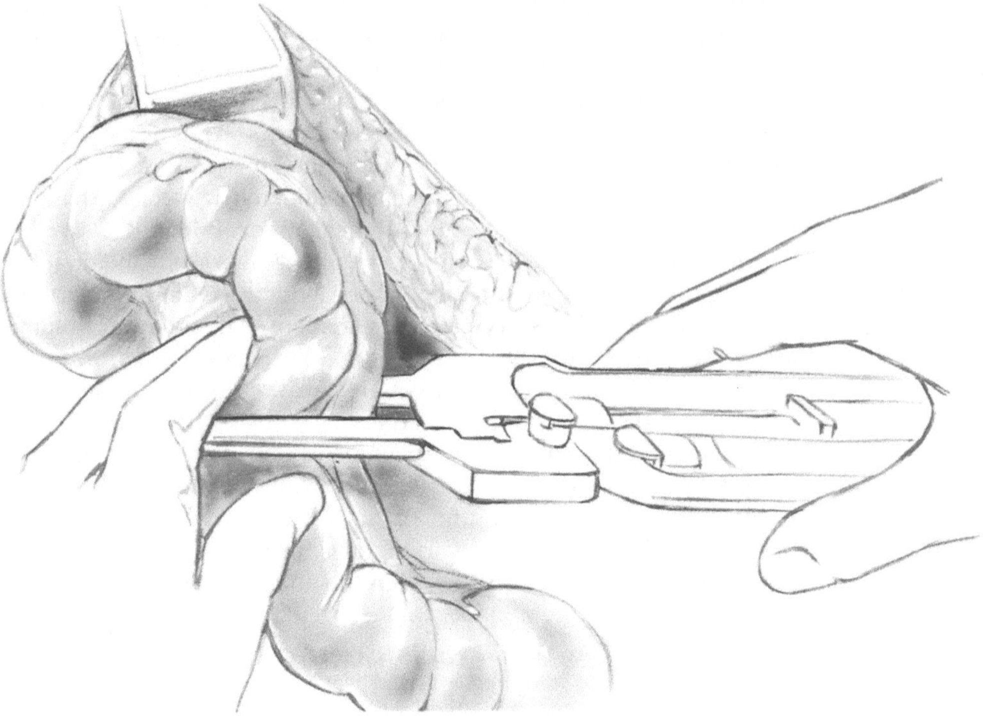

Fig. 7-1a

The last step in the abdominal portion of the procedure is to divide the sigmoid colon at a point that permits the proximal colon to be brought out of the abdominal incision with at least 5 cm of slack to form an end-colostomy. Use the GIA stapling device, which simultaneously applies staples and divides the colon **(Figs. 7–1a, 7–1b)**. Tie a rubber glove over the end of the distal sigmoid to preserve sterility (see Figs. 6-14a, 6-14b). After this step abandon the abdominal dissection temporarily and initiate the perineal stage.

## Pelvic Hemostasis

Obtain pelvic hemostasis as previously described (see Chapter 6). Sometimes bleeding is more easily controlled after the perineal phase is completed. If massive hemorrhage is encountered and cannot be controlled, place gauze packs in the pelvis and remove them in 24-48 hours through the perineum.

## Perineal Dissection

The anus is already closed by a heavy, silk pursestring suture. In male patients make an elliptical incision in the skin beginning at a point 3-4 cm anterior to the anal orifice and terminating at the tip of the coccyx **(Fig. 7–2)**. In female patients with small posterior lesions make the incision from a point just behind the vaginal introitus to the tip of the coccyx. For anterior lesions in women, leave a patch of posterior vagina, including the posterior portion of the vaginal introitus, attached to the rectum in the region of the tumor **(Figs. 7–3, 7–4)**.

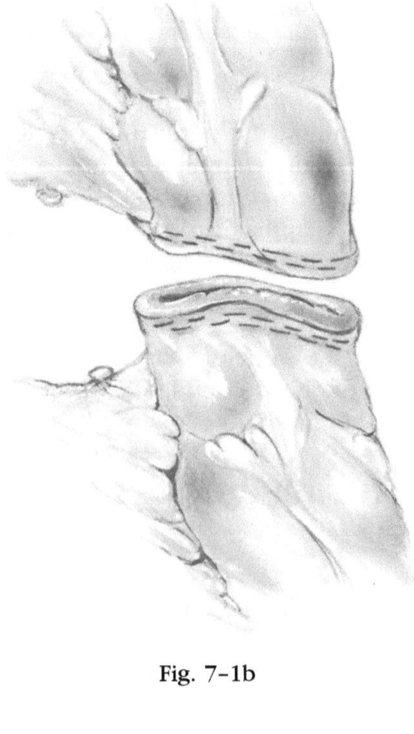

Fig. 7-1b

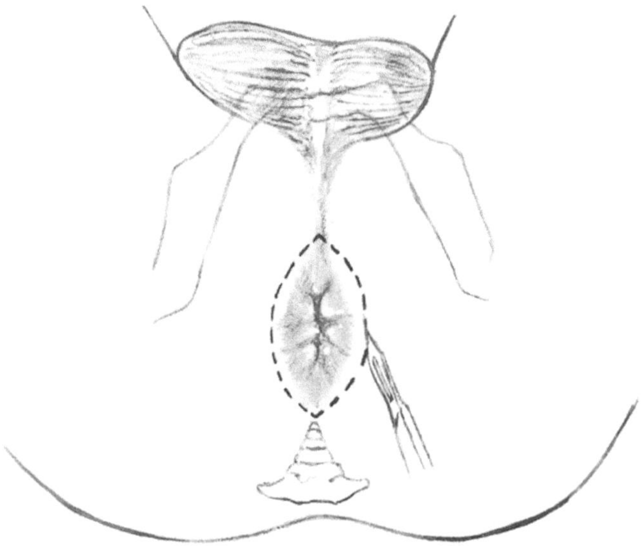

Fig. 7-2

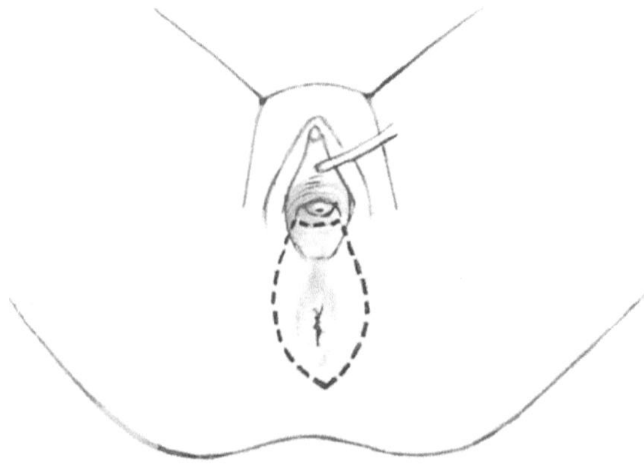

Fig. 7-3

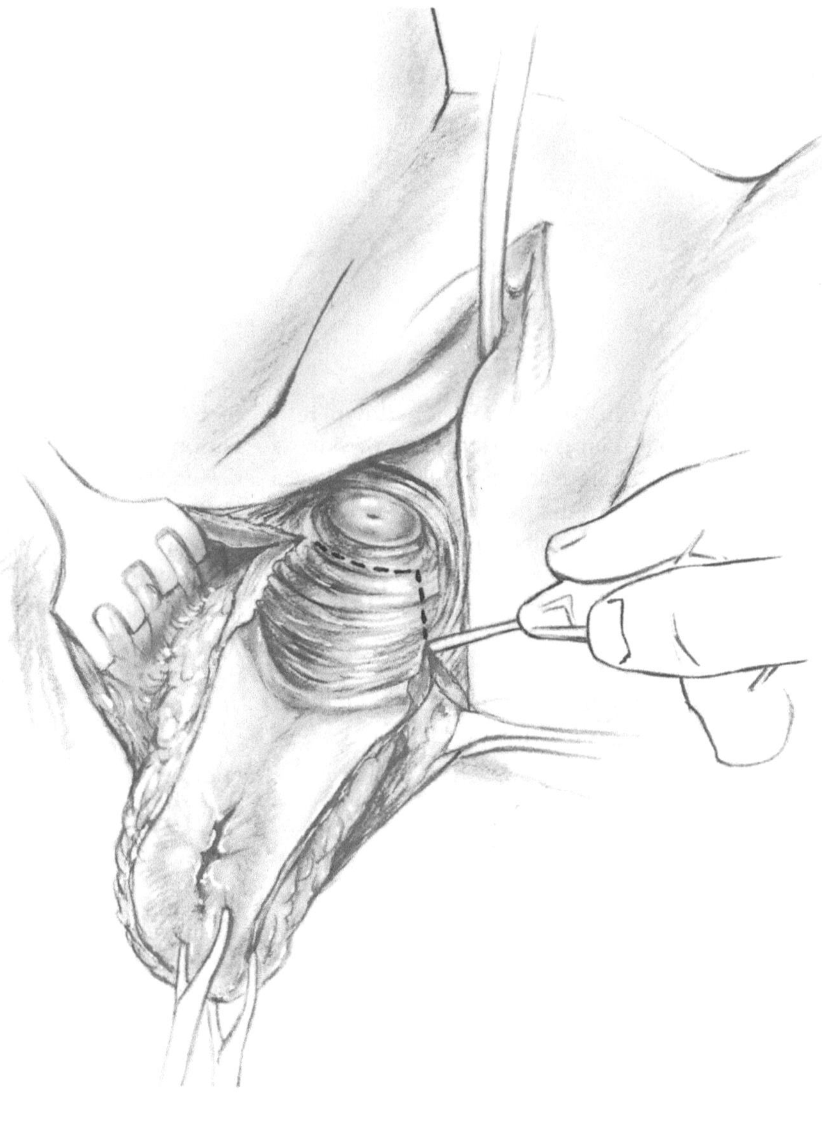

Fig. 7-4

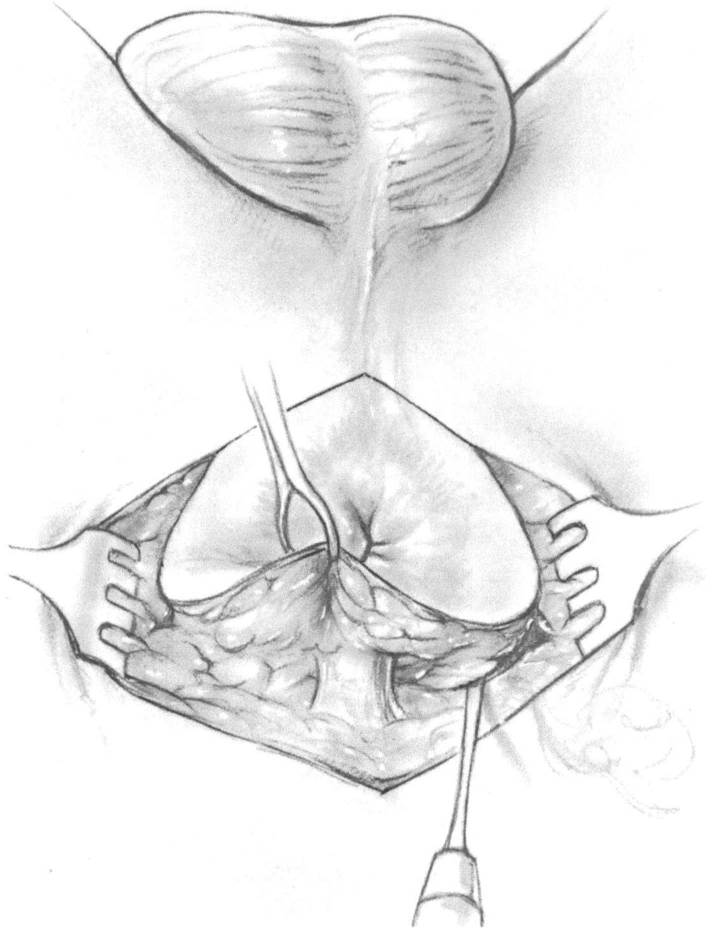

Fig. 7-5

In all cases carry the scalpel incision down into the perirectal fat and then grasp the ellipse of skin to be removed in three Allis clamps. While the anus is retracted to the patient's right, have the assistant insert a rake retractor to draw the skin of the perineum to the patient's left. Then incise the perirectal fat down to the levator diaphragm **(Fig. 7–5)**. Generally, two branches of the inferior hemorrhoidal vessels appear in the perirectal fat just superficial to the levators. Each may be secured by electrocautery. Accomplish the identical procedure on the right side of the perineum.

After identifying the anococcygeal ligament at the tip of the coccyx, use electrocautery to divide this ligament transversely from its attachment to the tip of the coccyx **(Figs. 7–6, 7–7)**. Note at this point that if the surgeon's index finger is inserted anterior to the tip of the coccyx it may be unable to enter the presacral space. A dense condensation of fascia (Waldeyer's fascia) attaches the posterior rectum to the presacral and precoccygeal area. If this fascia is torn off the sacrum by blunt technique, the presacral venous plexus may be entered, producing hemorrhage. Therefore Waldeyer's fascia must be incised at the termination of the abdominal portion of the presacral dissection or at the present stage during perineal dissection. From the perineal aspect this is a simple maneuver, as it requires only sharp division of the fascia with a scalpel or electrocautery in the plane just deep to the anococcygeal ligament. As soon as this is

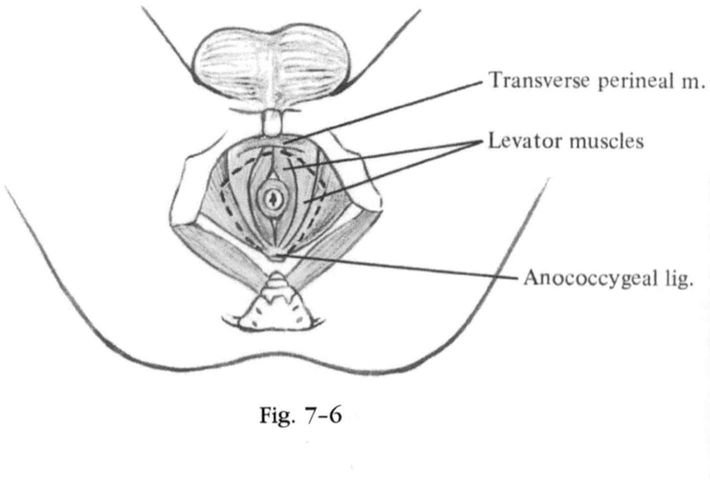


Fig. 7-6

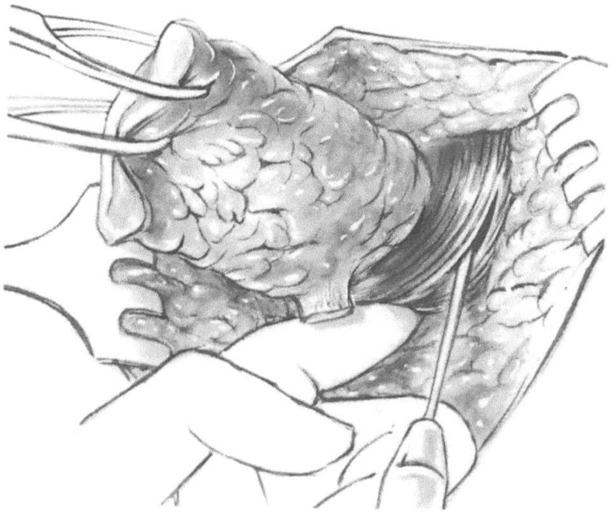

Fig. 7-7

accomplished it becomes evident that the abdominal and perineal phases of the dissection have joined.

The surgeon should then insert the left index finger underneath the left side of the levator diaphragm and, with the coagulating current, transect the levator muscles upward beginning from below, leaving a portion of the diaphragm attached to the specimen (Fig. 7-7). Continue this incision in the muscular diaphragm up to the region of the puborectalis sling on the anterior aspect of the perineum but not through it.

Use the identical procedure to divide the right-hand portion of the levator diaphragm. Because the greatest danger of the perineal dissection in men is the risk of traumatizing the urethra, delay the anterior portion of the dissection until all the other landmarks in this area have been delineated. To facilitate this delineation, the transected rectosigmoid specimen may be delivered through the opening in the posterior perineum at this time **(Fig. 7–8)**. Insert an

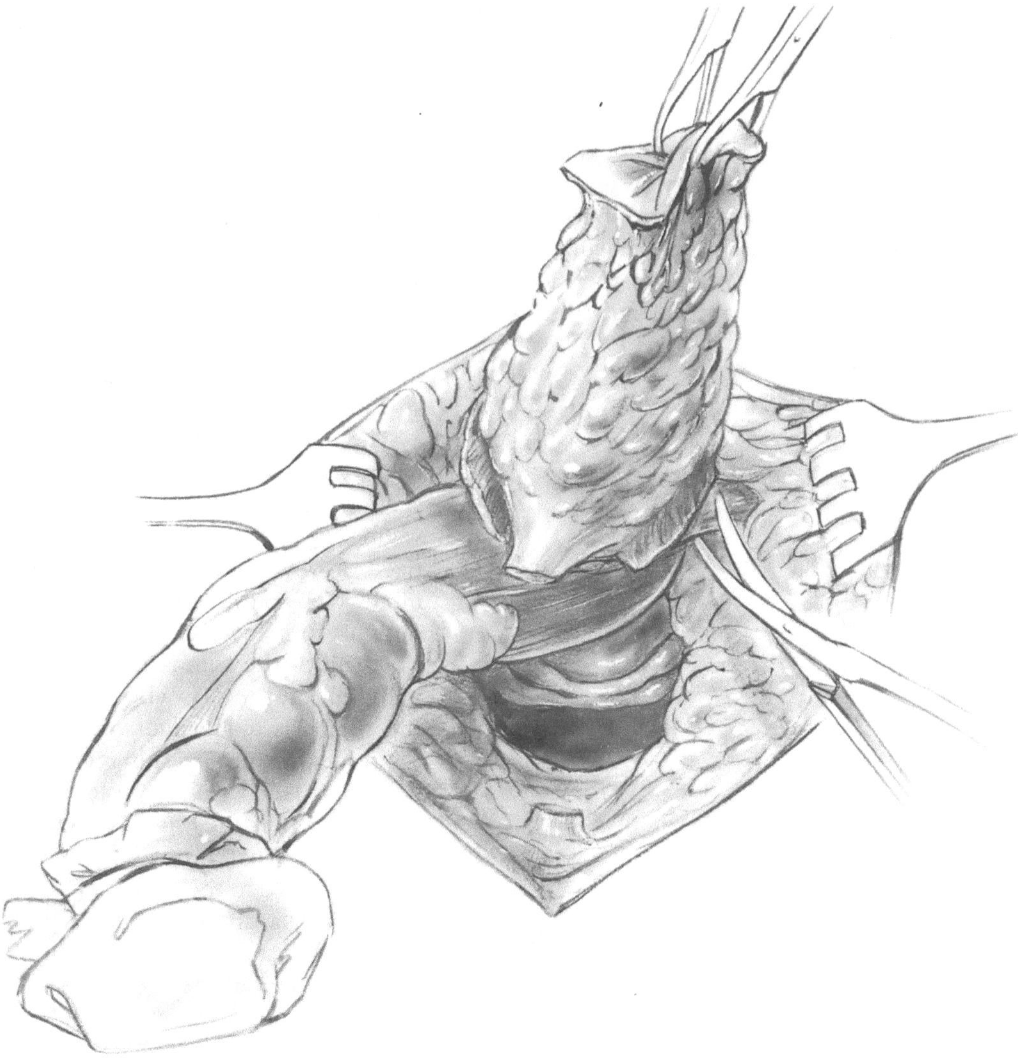

Fig. 7-8

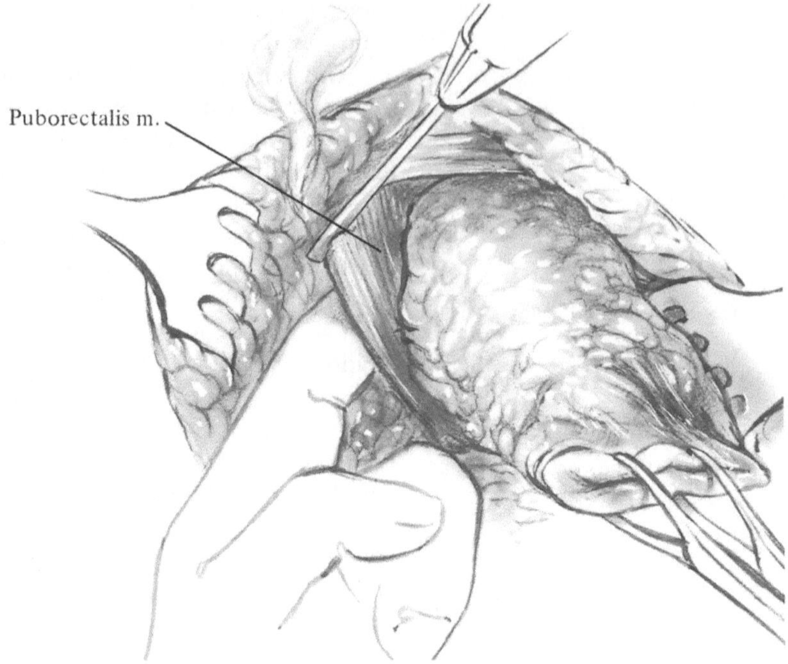


Fig. 7-9

index finger underneath the puborectalis muscle and transect it with electrocautery **(Figs.** 7-8, **7–9)**. The prostate was exposed during the abdominal dissection; at this time palpate it and visualize it from below. Make a projection of the plane along the posterior aspect of the prostate gland **(Fig. 7–10)**.

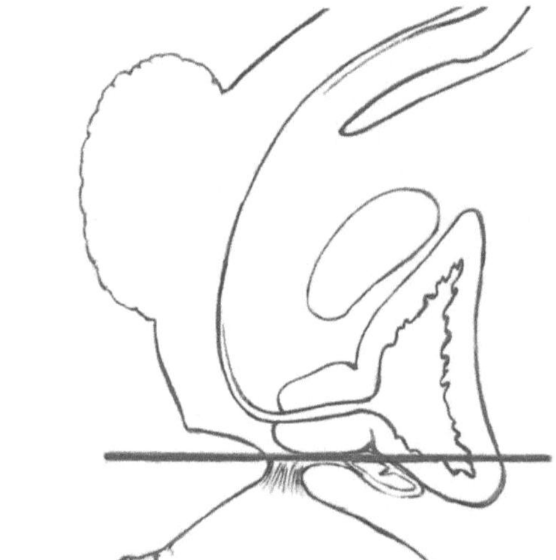

Fig. 7-10

Where this plane crosses the rectourethralis muscle, the muscle may be transected safely and the specimen removed **(Fig. 7–11)**. Another landmark, sometimes difficult to identify in obese patients, is the superficial transverse perineal muscles. The anterior plane of dissection should be posterior to these muscles. Finally, divide the remaining attachments to the prostate **(Fig. 7–12)** and remove the specimen.

The above precautions do not apply in women. If the vagina is to be preserved, the anterior dissection should follow a plane just posterior to the vagina. The wall of the vagina should not be traumatized or devascularized during this dissection, as it might well lead to a perineovaginal fistula, which is difficult to manage. It is better to excise the posterior wall of the vagina than to devascularize it partially during the dissection. If the posterior wall of the vagina is to be removed, use electrocautery to continue the perineal skin incision across the vaginal introitus (Fig. 7-4). Complete hemostasis is easily attained when the vagina is incised by electrocautery. Leave a patch of vagina of appropriate dimensions attached to the specimen. Irrigate the presacral space with a dilute antibiotic solution. Hemostasis should be absolute and complete and is easily accomplished using electrocautery and ligatures as one assistant works from above and the surgeon works from below.

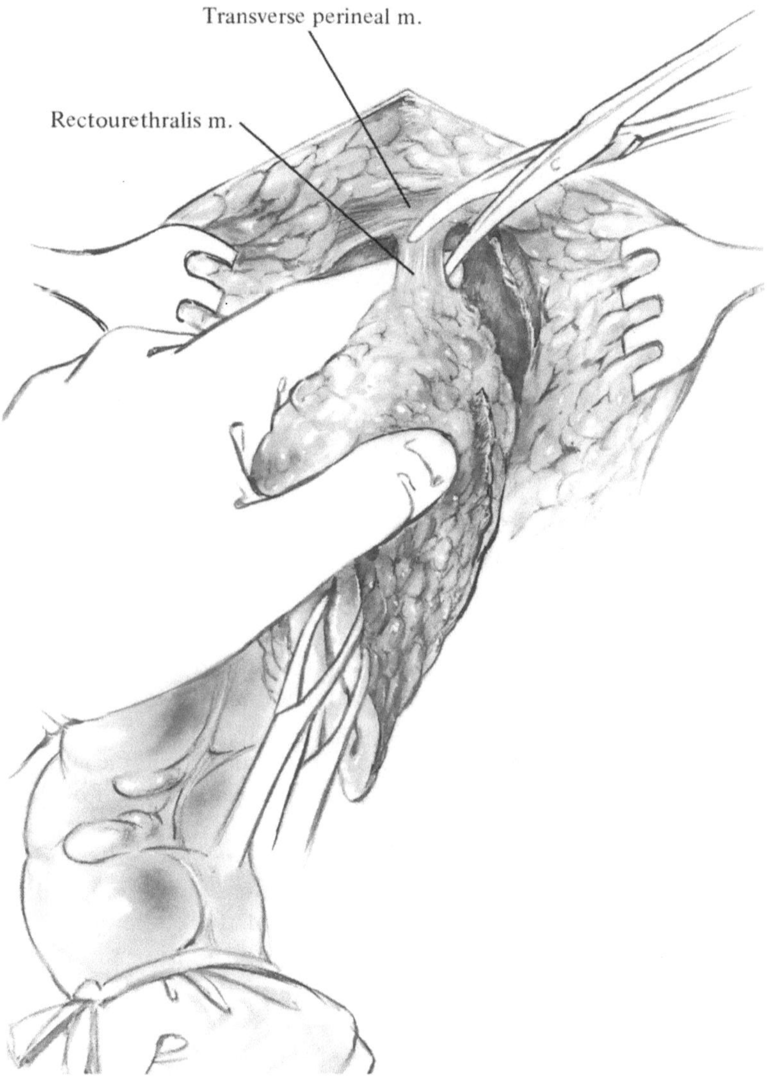


Fig. 7-11

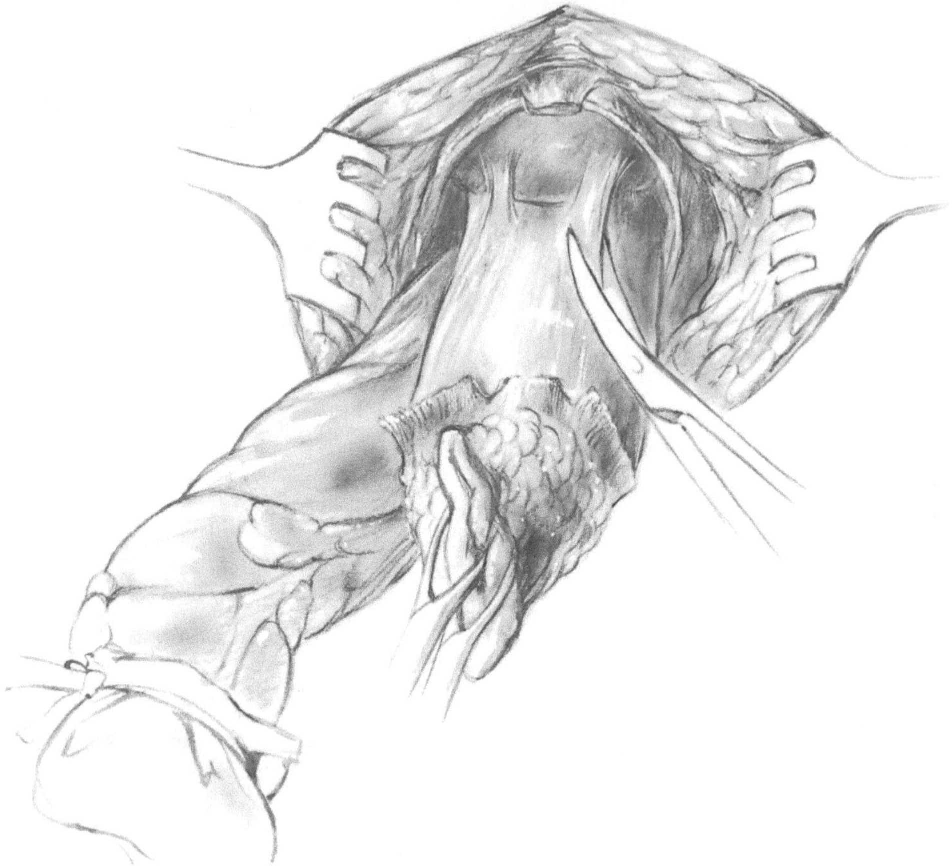

Fig. 7-12

## Management of Pelvic Floor

In women whose posterior vaginal wall remains intact and in all men, the perineum may be closed per primam if there has been no fecal contamination and if hemostasis is excellent. First, accomplish presacral drainage by inserting one or two closed-suction drainage catheters, each 6 mm in diameter. Introduce one catheter through a puncture wound of the skin in the posterior portion of the perineum about 4 cm to the left of the coccyx and a second through a similar point at the right. Suture each catheter to the skin surrounding its exit wound **(Fig. 7–13)**. Place the tips of the catheters in the presacral space. In some cases the posterior levator diaphragm may be partially reconstructed using 2-0 PG sutures. Accomplish the remainder of the perineal closure with one or two layers of interrupted PG to the subcutaneous fat and a subcuticular suture of 4-0 PG to close the skin. As soon as the abdominal surgeon has closed the pelvic peritoneum, apply continuous suction to the two drainage catheters to draw the peritoneum down to the newly reconstructed pelvic floor. The surgeon's aim must be to *eliminate any possible deadspace* between the peritoneal closure and the pelvic floor. These closed suction drains may also be brought out via a stab wound in the lower abdominal wall.

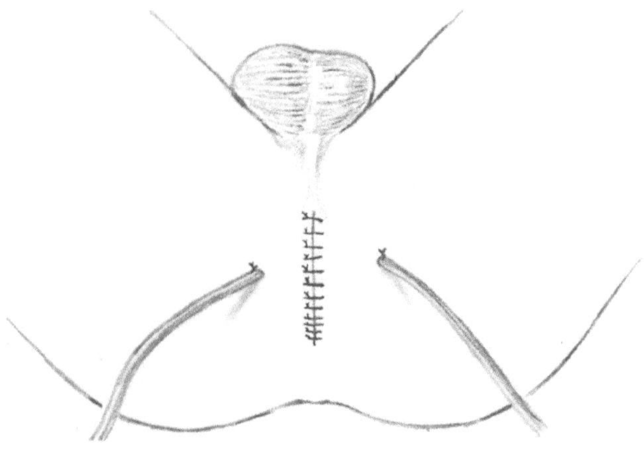

Fig. 7-13

When the posterior vaginal wall and the specimen have been excised, attempt to fabricate a substitute

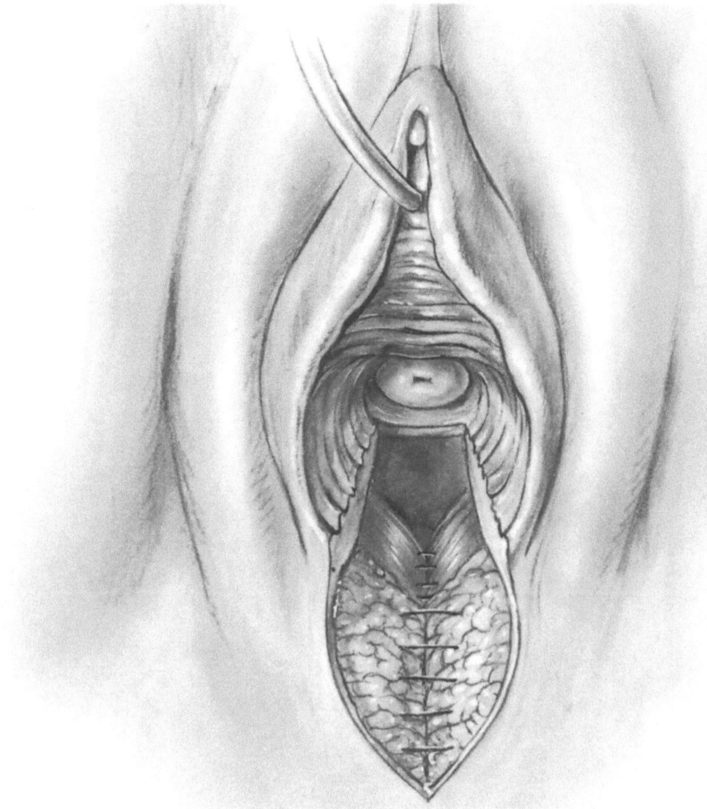

Fig. 7-14

posterior wall with interrupted PG sutures to the perineal fat and to the residual levator muscle **(Fig. 7–14)**. If this can be accomplished, within a few months after the operation the vaginal mucosa grows over this newly constructed pelvic floor, restoring the vaginal tube. Pack the posterior defect loosely with sterile gauze. Bring the gauze out through the newly reconstructed vaginal introitus after the remainder of the perineal fat and skin have been closed, as described above **(Fig. 7–15)**. If it is deemed desirable, a sump catheter can be brought out from the presacral space through the same defect, but it is not done routinely.

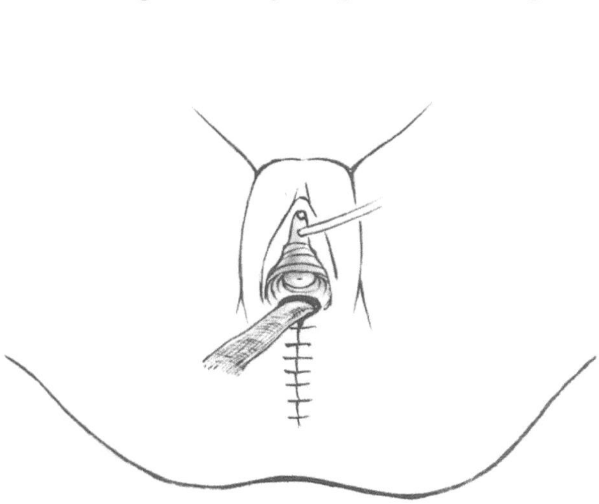

Fig. 7-15

While the assistant is closing the perineum, the surgeon should return to the abdominal approach to dissect the pelvic peritoneum free from its surrounding attachments to the lateral pelvic walls and bladder. This enables the peritoneum to be closed without tension **(Fig. 7–16)**. Use a continuous atraumatic suture of 2-0 PG. If there is insufficient peritoneum to permit the peritoneal diaphragm to descend to the level of the newly constructed perineal floor, leave the peritoneum completely unsutured.

## Colostomy

The colostomy may be brought out through the upper portion of the midline incision, in which case it is not necessary to close the intraperitoneal gap lateral to the colostomy. Through the midline incision, at a point where 5 cm protrudes from the

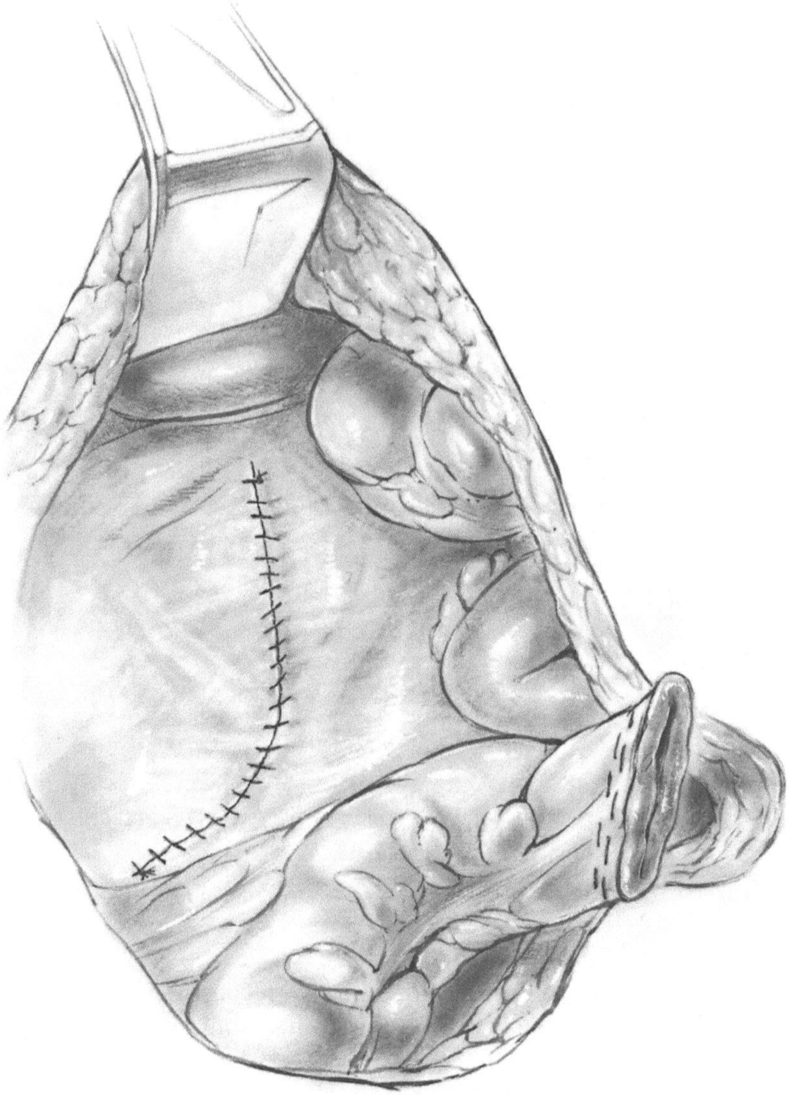

Fig. 7-16

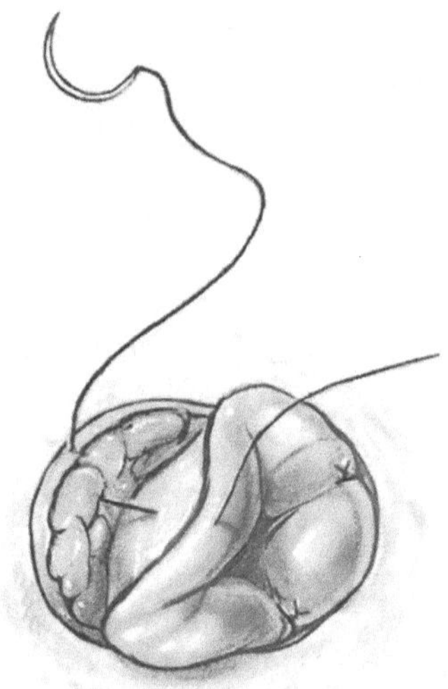

Fig. 7-17

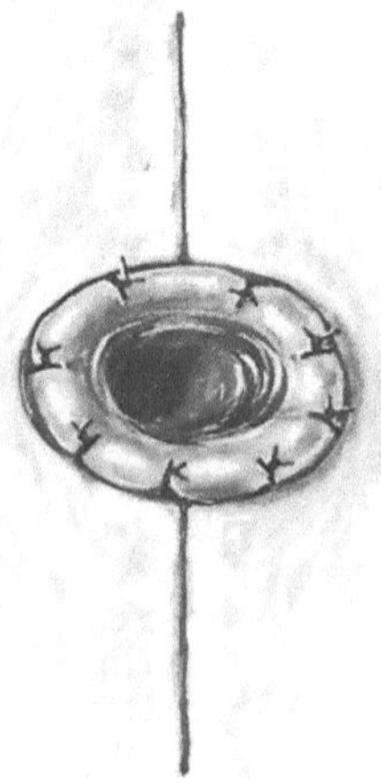

Fig. 7-18

anterior abdominal skin surface without tension, bring out the segment of colon previously selected to form the colostomy. If this point is near the umbilicus, excise the umbilicus for more postoperative cleanliness. Close the abdominal wall with one layer of monofilament 1-0 PDS; an index finger should fit without tension between the colostomy and the next adjoining suture. Close the skin above and below the colostomy with a continuous subcuticular suture of 4-0 PG. Before closing the skin, irrigate with a dilute antibiotic solution.

After these steps have been completed, excise the line of staples previously used to occlude the colon. Immediately mature the colostomy, using interrupted or continuous sutures of 4-0 PG to attach the full thickness of the colon to the subcuticular plane of the skin **(Figs. 7–17, 7–18)**. No additional sutures are necessary to attach the colon to the fascia or to any other layer of the abdominal wall.

When the peritoneal pelvic floor is suitable for reconstruction by suturing, the retroperitoneal type of colostomy may be performed. Elevate the previously incised peritoneum of the left paracolic gutter from the lateral abdominal wall by finger dissection. Continue until a hand is freely admitted up to the point in the lateral portion of the rectus muscle that has been previously selected for the colostomy **(Figs. 7–19, 7–20)**, generally about 4 cm below the level of the umbilicus.

Excise a circle of skin about the size of a nickel and expose the fascia of the left rectus muscle. Make cruciate incisions in the anterior rectus fascia, separate the rectus muscle fibers bluntly, and incise the underlying posterior rectus sheath and peritoneum. The aperture in the abdominal wall should be large enough to admit two fingers.

Bring the colon through the retroperitoneal tunnel and out the opening made for the colostomy **(Fig. 7–21)**. Begin the suture line that closes the pelvic peritoneum near the bladder. Continue this suture of 2-0 atraumatic PG in a cephalad direction, closing the entire defect by suturing the free edge of the peritoneum to the anterior seromuscular wall of the sigmoid colon as it enters the retroperitoneal tunnel to become a colostomy **(Fig. 7–22)**. Then close the abdominal incision. Mature the colostomy by a mucocutaneous suture as described above. Attach a temporary colostomy bag to the

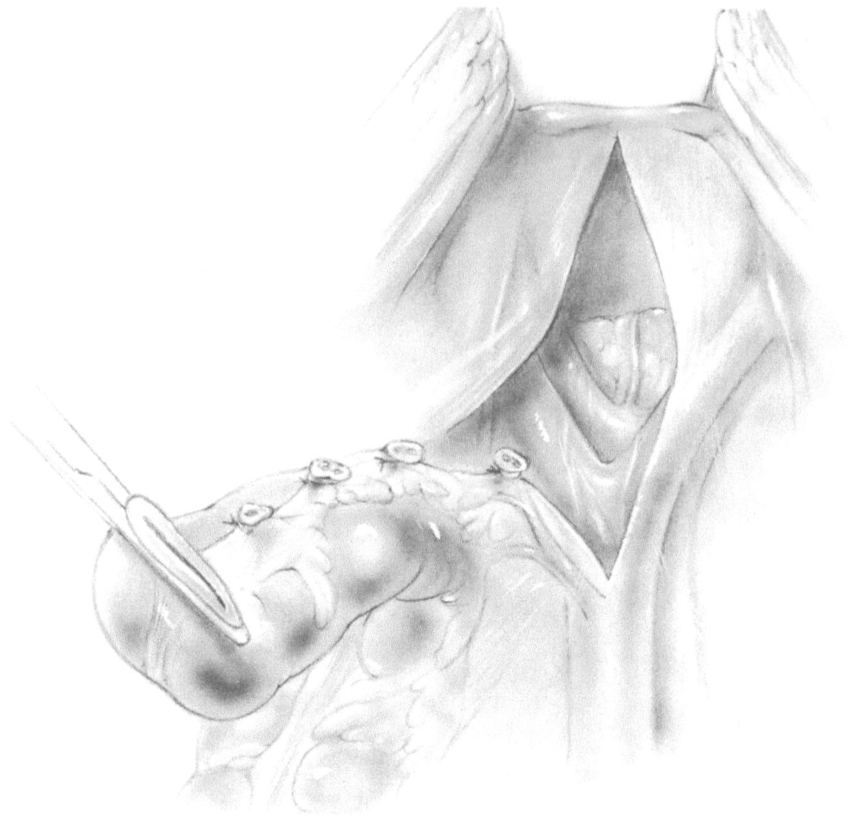

Fig. 7-19

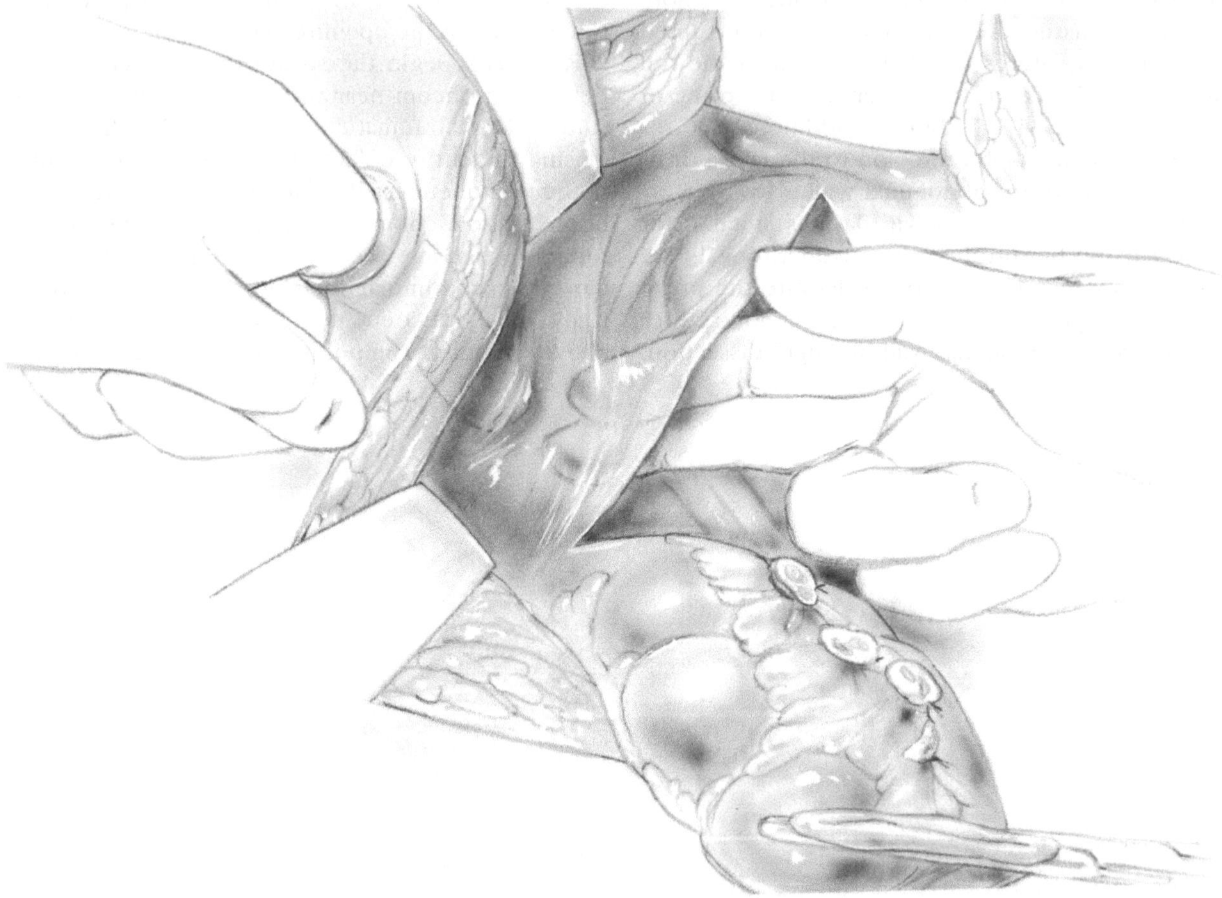

Fig. 7–20

Fig. 7–21

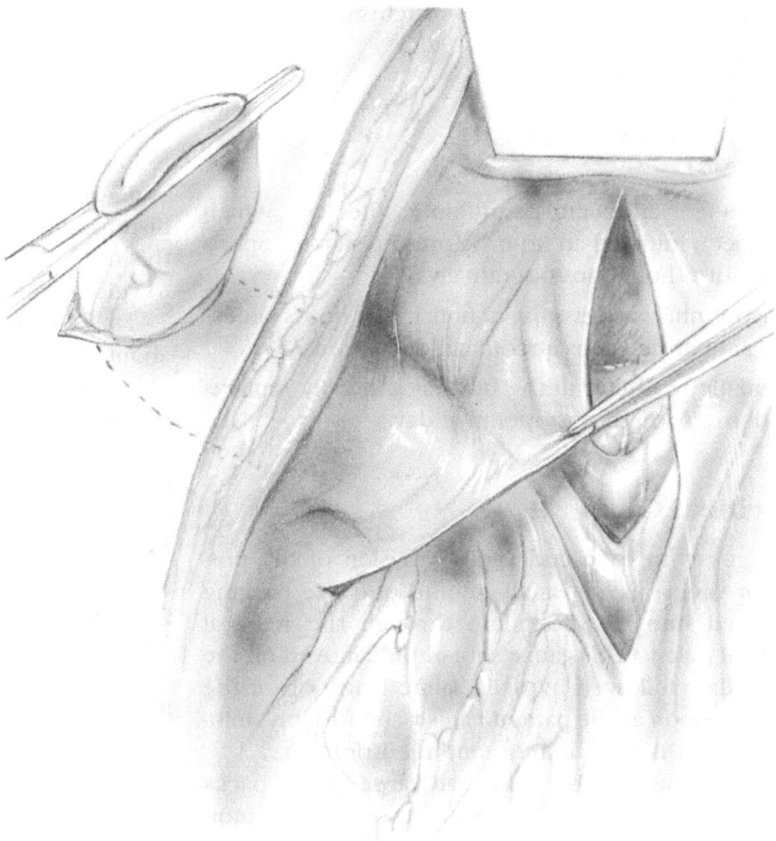

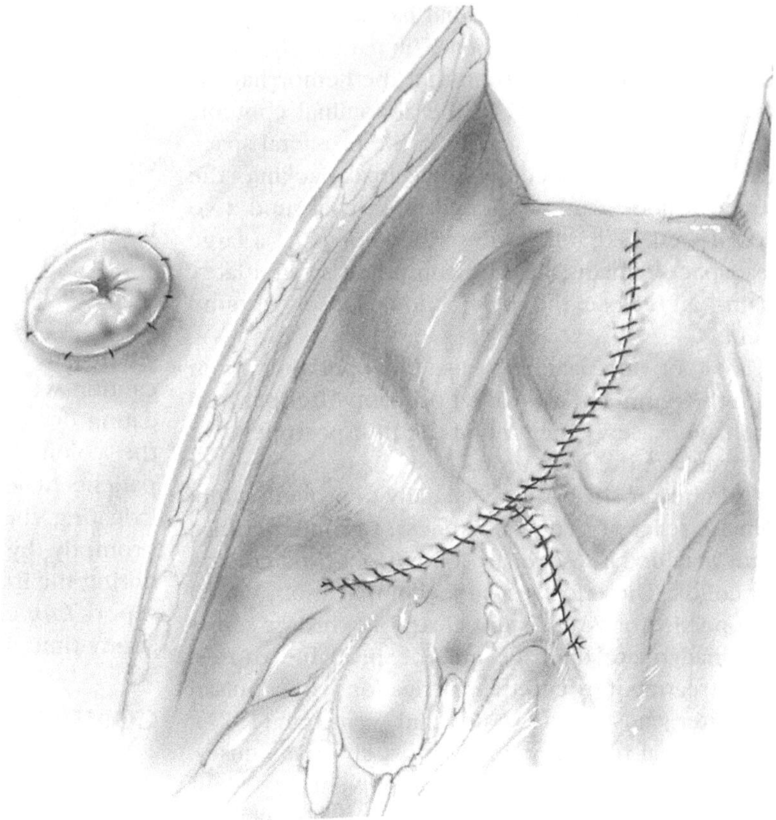

Fig. 7–22

abdominal wall at the conclusion of the operation.

## POSTOPERATIVE CARE

Continue perioperative antibiotic therapy, which had been initiated an hour before the start of operation, for 6 hours postoperatively.

Discontinue nasogastric suction in 24 hours unless the patient develops abdominal distension.

The Foley catheter in the bladder generally remains until the seventh postoperative day.

### Perineal Care

Patients who have undergone excision of the posterior vagina have a small amount of gauze packing inserted into the perineum through the residual vaginal defect. This gauze should be removed on the third day, followed by daily saline irrigation of the area. As soon as the patient can sit comfortably, initiate sitz baths daily and discontinue irrigation.

The patients who have had large gauze packs inserted in the presacral region to control hemorrhage should be brought back to the operating room on the first or second postoperative day so the pack can be removed under general anesthesia. The sheet of topical hemostatic agent that had been applied to the sacrum is left undisturbed. The patient should be observed briefly to ascertain that the hemorrhage is under complete control. If the abdominal contents descend to occupy the cavity in the presacral space that had been created by the gauze packing, the perineal floor can be closed tightly around two closed-suction drains, as described above. If a large deadspace remains, insert a sump and several latex drains and close the pelvic floor loosely around them.

Most of our patients leave the operating room with the perineum closed per primam. After perineal drainage ceases, generally on the fifth postoperative day, remove the catheters.

Administer sitz baths twice daily to provide symptomatic relief of perineal soreness. Chronic perineal sinus may occur, especially following a proctectomy for colitis. The etiology of this complication, which may persist for years, is not clear, but chronic sepsis and inadequate drainage are the probable causes. Local treatment by curettage, irrigation with a pulsating water jet as noted by Sohn and Weinstein (1977), and perineal hygiene remedy most chronic sinuses. Frequent shaving is necessary to prevent loose hair from entering deep into the sinus and producing a foreign-body granuloma.

### Colostomy Care

Observe the colostomy daily through the transparent bag to detect signs of possible necrosis. That the colostomy does not function during the first 6–7 days following the operation need not be a cause for concern if the patient does not develop abdominal distension or cramps. If there is no function beyond this date, abdominal radiography must be performed to rule out an obstruction of the small bowel.

The patient should begin receiving instructions about daily colostomy irrigation during the second week of hospitalization. No patient should leave the hospital before acquiring the skills necessary to perform the irrigation effectively. It is important to understand that the aim of colostomy irrigation is not simply to wash out the distal few inches of colon. Patients sometimes insert a catheter a few inches into the colon, and when the water runs into the colon they permit it promptly to run out alongside the catheter. This is ineffective. Water is instilled into the distal colon for the purpose of dilating the area sufficiently to produce a reflex peristaltic contraction that evacuates the entire distal colon. For many patients this requires injection of more than 1 liter of water before they begin to feel "crampy" discomfort. At this point the catheter should be removed and the patient encouraged to keep the colostomy orifice occluded for a few more minutes, until peristalsis is well underway.

Some patients use a cone-shaped device through which the fluid channel passes, to occlude the lumen. In other cases the patient is able to occlude the lumen by lightly grasping and manually compressing the abdominal wall around the inflow catheter or cone. There are many variations in devices and techniques for colostomy management: When one fails, however, it usually is because the patient has not retained the injected fluid long enough for distension of the distal colon to occur. Without such distension there can be no reflex peristaltic contraction.

All patients must be urged to exercise extreme caution when passing the catheter or any other irrigating device to avoid the possibility of perforating the colon. This complication may occur even in patients who have had 15–20 years of experience irrigating their colostomy. It is generally heralded promptly by the onset of severe abdominal pain during the irrigation. The patient should be urged to report *immediately* for examination if pain occurs at any time during irrigation.

## COMPLICATIONS

*Acute intestinal obstruction.* The small intestine may become obstructed by adhesion to the pelvic suture line or herniation through a defect in the pelvic floor. Adhesions elsewhere in the abdomen, which may occur after any abdominal procedure, can also cause obstruction. If colostomy function has not begun by the sixth or seventh postoperative day, radiographs of the abdomen should be obtained. If small bowel obstruction appears to have occurred and there is no evidence of strangulation, a *brief* trial of a long intestinal tube may be initiated. If this is not promptly successful (3–4 days), secondary laparotomy for relief of the obstruction is indicated.

*Hemorrhage*. Hemorrhage is rare in properly managed cases. If there is evidence of significant bleeding (by vital signs and laboratory tests or by visible bleeding from the perineal drains), prompt reoperation is preferable to expectant management.

*Sepsis*. Sepsis that occurs following primary closure of the perineal wound is generally not difficult to detect. It is accompanied by fever, local pain, and purulent drainage through the suction catheters. Under these conditions the perineal incision should be opened sufficiently to insert two fingers, a sump, and several latex or Penrose drains. If this measure does not relieve the infection quickly, the entire wound may be reopened and a gauze pack inserted. The gauze should be changed at least once daily.

*Bladder obstruction*. Because many men who undergo proctocolectomy for carcinoma are at an age when prostatic hypertrophy is common, this factor combined with the loss of bladder support in the absence of the rectum and some degree of nerve injury leads to a high incidence of urinary tract obstruction. If the obstruction cannot be managed by conservative means, urologic consultation and prostatectomy may be necessary.

*Sexual impotence*. Some studies have indicated that virtually all operations for radical removal of malignancies in the middle and lower rectum of men have been followed by sexual impotence, although Goligher's (1958) findings were not as bleak. This complication has been rare after operations for benign disease when special precautions are observed (see Chapter 49).

*Colostomy complications*. Ischemia, retraction, or prolapse of the colostomy may occur if the colostomy is not properly constructed. Parastomal hernia is an occasional late complication.

*Chronic perineal sinus*. Although a persistent sinus is rare after a properly managed resection for carcinoma, it appears to be common following operations for inflammatory bowel disease. If all the local measures fail and the sinus persists for several years, Silen and Glotzer (1974) recommended a saucerization procedure that consisted of excising the coccyx and the chronically infected wall of the sinus down to its apex. After saucerization, persistent attention to encouraging healing from the bottom has proved successful. Another technique is insertion of a perforated split-thickness skin graft following local débridement and cleansing.

## REFERENCES


Anderson R, Turnbull RB Jr. Grafting the unhealed perineal wound after coloproctectomy for Crohn's disease. Arch Surg 1976;111:335.

Goligher JC. Extraperitoneal colostomy or ileostomy. Br J Surg 1958;46:97.

Lechner P, Cesnik H. Abdominopelvic omentopexy: preparatory procedure for radiotherapy in rectal cancer. Dis Colon Rectum 1992;35:1157.

Meade PG, Blatchford GJ, Thorson AG, Christensen MA, Tement CA. Preoperative chemoradiation downstages locally advanced ultrasound-staged rectal cancer. Am J Surg 1995;170:609.

Niles B, Sugarbaker PH. Use of the bladder as an abdominopelvic partition. Am Surg 1989;55:533.

Nivatvongs S, Fang DT. The use of thumbtacks to stop massive presacral hemorrhage. Dis Colon Rectum 1986;29:589.

Silen W, Glotzer DJ. The prevention and treatment of the persistent perineal sinus. Surgery 1974;75:535.

Sohn N, Weinstein MA. Unhealed perineal wound lavage with a pulsating water jet. Am J Surg 1977;134:426.

Weiss EG, Wexner SD. Laparoscopic segmental colectomies, anterior resection, and abdominoperineal resection. In Scott-Conner CEH (ed) The SAGES Manual: Fundamentals of Laparoscopy and GI Endoscopy. New York, Springer-Verlag, 1999, pp 286–299.

# 8 Laparoscopic Abdominoperineal Resection and Total Proctocolectomy with End Ileostomy

Steven D. Wexner
Giovanna M. DaSilva

## ABDOMINOPERINEAL RESECTION

## INDICATIONS

Low rectal cancer (within 5 cm from the anal verge) without invasion of adjacent organs

## PREOPERATIVE PREPARATION

The preoperative management is exactly the same as that for laparotomy. On the day before surgery, the patients are instructed to eat a light meal at lunch, have only clear liquids after lunch, and refrain from having anything to eat or drink after midnight. Bowel preparation is undertaken using a mechanical cathartic and both oral and parenteral antibiotics. The stoma site is preoperatively marked by an enterostomal therapist and heparin or low molecular weight heparin and sequential compression stockings are utilized for venous thrombosis prevention.

## PITFALLS AND DANGER POINTS

Damage to the epigastric vessels during port placement

Damage to the ureters during colon mobilization

Injury to the spleen during mobilization of the splenic flexure (if performed)

Injury to the autonomic nerves during dissection near the aorta and in the pelvis

Injury to major vessels

Injury to the presacral vessels

Bleeding from the stapler line

## OPERATIVE TECHNIQUE

### Room Setup and Trocar Placement

With the patient under general anesthesia, a Foley catheter is placed into the bladder and a nasogastric tube is inserted into the stomach. Ureteric stents may be indicated in selected cases (previous surgery, pelvic phlegmon, large tumor, prior radiation therapy) to facilitate intraoperative identification. The patient is positioned in a modified lithotomy position using Allen stirrups (Allen Medical, Bedford Heights, OH). Both arms are tucked at the patient's sides and the hips and legs are only minimally elevated and flexed to avoid interference with handling of the laparoscopic instruments. Care should be taken to firmly secure the patient to the table as a considerable amount of Trendelenburg and tilting of the table is used during the operation. As with open procedures, the anus is closed with a double purse string suture to prevent leakage of stool during the perineal dissection.

**Figure 8–1** shows the positioning of monitor and surgical team. The surgeon and second assistant (cameraoperator) stand at the right side of the patient while the first assistant and the nurse are at the patient's left side or between the legs. Two monitors are used; one on either side of the patient.

Three ports are normally used for this procedure (Fig. 8-1). We prefer 10–12 mm ports which allow flexibility for the camera and all instruments. The camera port is placed in an infra- or supraumbilical position using a Veress needle or an open Hasson technique and the two remaining ports are placed under direct vision, on the right side, one in the iliac fossa and one in the right paraumbilical region. Care is taken to visualize the epigastric vessels before port placement. An optional additional fourth 10–12 mm port can be placed at the site of the preoperatively marked colostomy.

### Exploration of the Abdominal Cavity

A 15 mm Hg of carbon dioxide ($CO_2$) pneumoperitoneum is established and a 30 degree camera is used to inspect the peritoneal cavity and liver for metas-

Fig. 8-1a

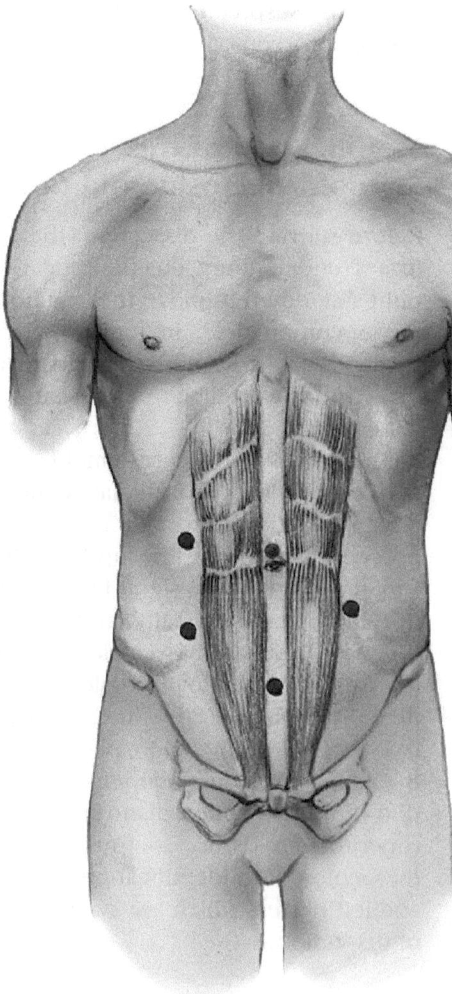

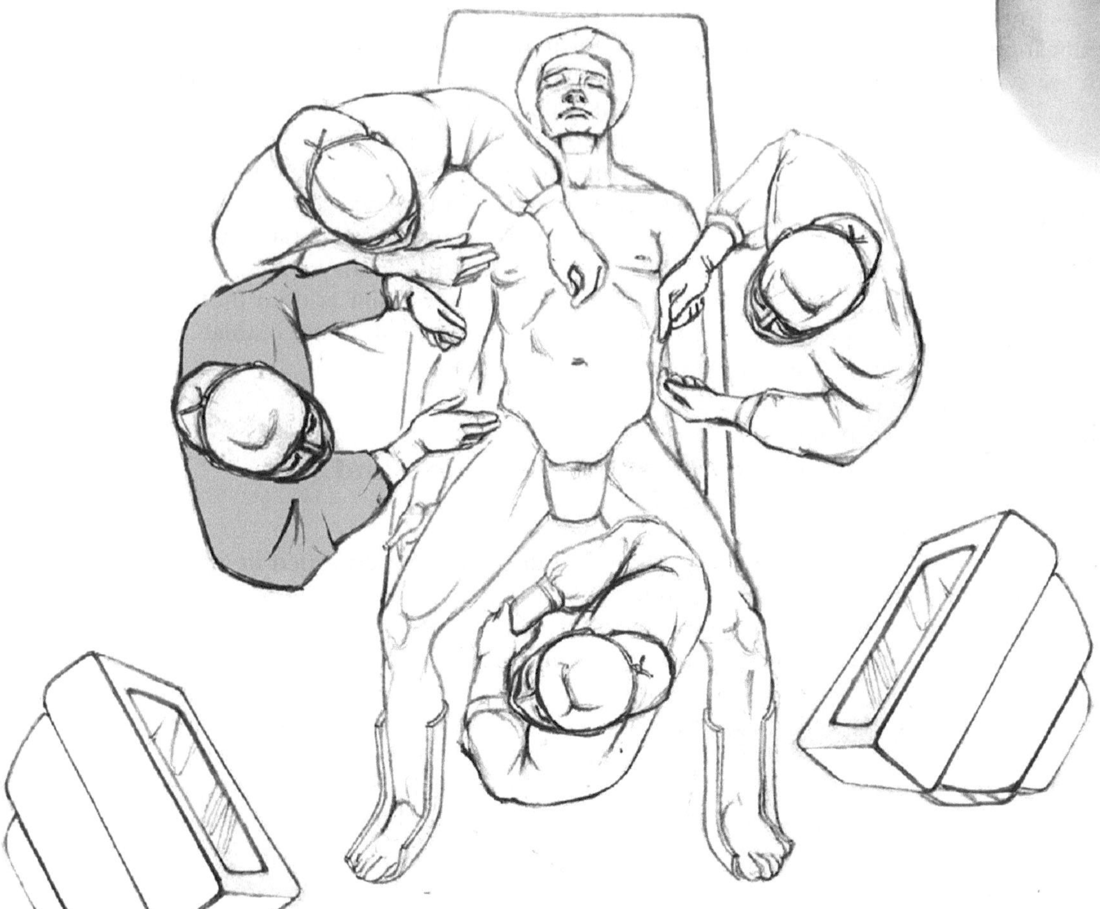

Fig. 8-1b

tases. Any suspicious lesions are biopsied with laparoscopic forceps.

## Mobilization of the Sigmoid/Rectosigmoid Colon

Before starting the dissection, the patient is placed in a Trendelenburg position and the table is titled right-side down to move the small bowel away from the operating field. In females, the uterus can be suspended with a suture through the anterior abdominal wall to facilitate visualization during pelvic dissection.

Dissection of the rectosigmoid can follow a medial-to-lateral or lateral-to medial sequence. Our preference is to utilize the same technique as is the open procedure. By using the upper right side port, the surgeon retracts the sigmoid colon with a Babcock to the right and cranially stretching the lateral peritoneum. Dissection is carried out along the white line of Toldt, up to the splenic flexure, using the harmonic scalpel (Ethicon Endosurgery Inc, Cincinnati, Ohio) introduced through the lower port **(Fig. 8–2)**. The harmonic scalpel provides good visualization of the dissection plane and hemostasis. The retroperitoneal tissue is thus dissected from the mesocolon with identification of the gonadal vessels and left ureter, which are swept away from the area of dissection.

## Division of the Inferior Mesenteric Vessels

Identification and preparation for ligation and division of the inferior mesenteric vessels is best accomplished by retracting the sigmoid anteriorly and to the left, and then scoring the medial aspect of the peritoneum extending the incision down into the pelvis and cephalad towards the mesenteric pedicle near its origin. A window is created anterior to the aorta and at the right of the mesenteric vessels. The hypogastric nerves can be generally identified and posteriorly reflected at this point. The inferior mesenteric artery and vein are separately divided using the Ligasure, clips or a 30 mm linear vascular stapler. We prefer to use the endoscopic stapler for the mesenteric vessels and either clips or the harmonic scalpel for any smaller branches. A good maneuver prior to vascular division is to pass the endoscopic stapler through the closed window before ligation in order to ensure easy passage when opened **(Fig. 8–3)**. Care is taken to visualize the ureter prior to ligation and division of the mesenteric vessels. Bleeding from the stapler line can usually be controlled by the use of clips.

## Division of the Sigmoid/Descending Colon

After ligation of the inferior mesenteric vessels, the mesosigmoid is divided towards the sigmoid colon. The colon is then transected at a suitable point with an endo GIA Stapler introduced through the right lower quadrant port. The position of the stapler tip should be checked to ensure no other structure has been inadvertently grasped by the stapler **(Fig. 8–4)**.

## Rectal Mobilization

The peritoneum is incised along both sides of the rectum down to the peritoneal reflection. Rectal dissection is initiated posteriorly by dissecting the mesorectum from the Waldeyer's fascia in an avascular plane as low as possible down into the pelvis while the rectum is retracted cranially and anteriorly with a Babcock placed in its upper part. At the level of aortic bifurcation, the superior hypogastric plexus nerves can be identified and the right and left trunks along the pelvic side wall **(Fig. 8–5)**. The surgeon then performs lateral rectal mobilization, while the rectum is retracted to the sides. The "lateral ligaments" and medial arteries are divided with the harmonic scalpel. Care is taken to preserve the inferior hypogastric plexus located at the level of the ligaments. The rectum is then mobilized in its anterior aspect facilitated by cranial traction **(Fig. 8–6)**.

## Perineal Dissection and Specimen Removal

The perineal dissection is performed in an identical manner to the open procedure. The specimen is retrieved through the perineal wound and the pneumoperitoneum is deflated. The perineal wound is then closed in layers and pneumoperitoneum is recreated. The abdominal cavity is rinsed with warm saline solution and checked for hemostasis. The proximal colon is brought out through the left port with Babcock forceps and the terminal colostomy is fashioned **(Fig. 8–7)**; a drain is placed in the pelvis through the right lower port.

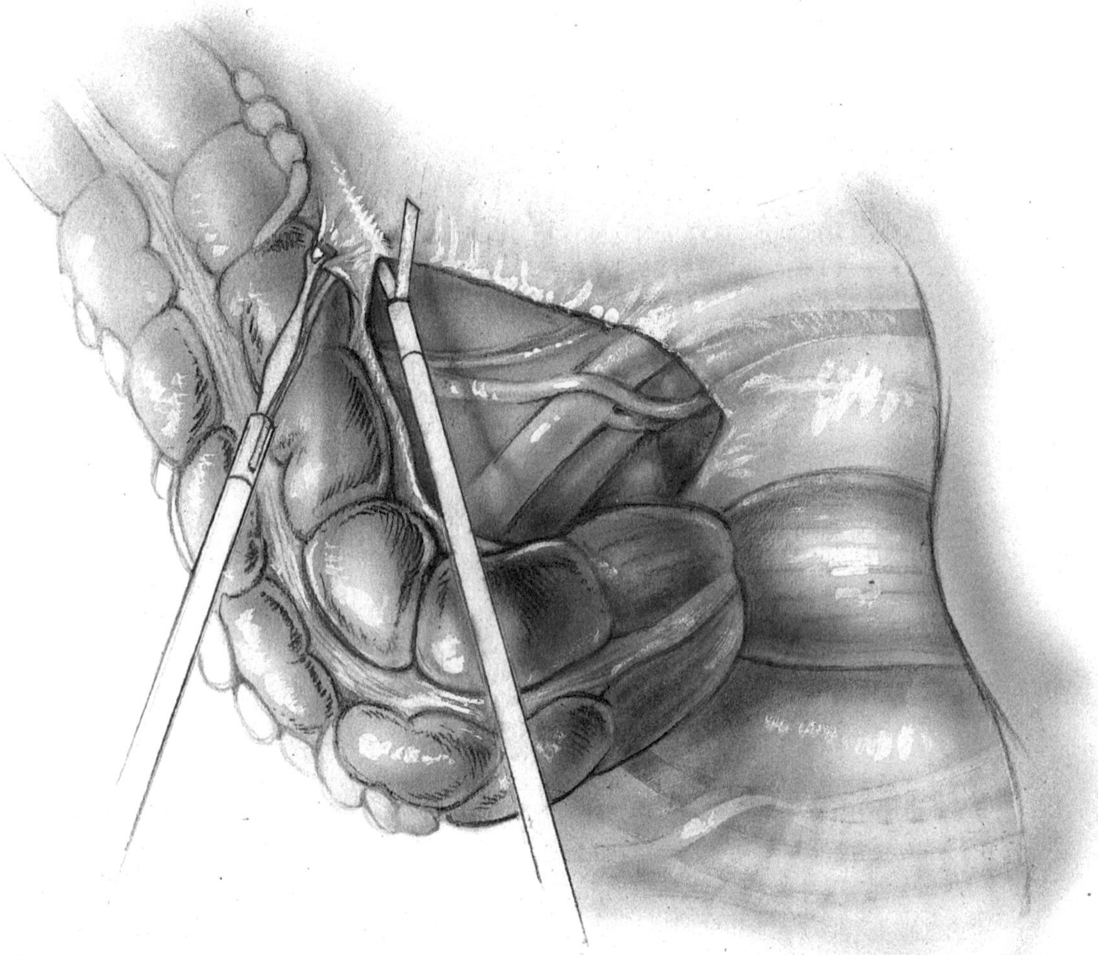

Fig. 8–2

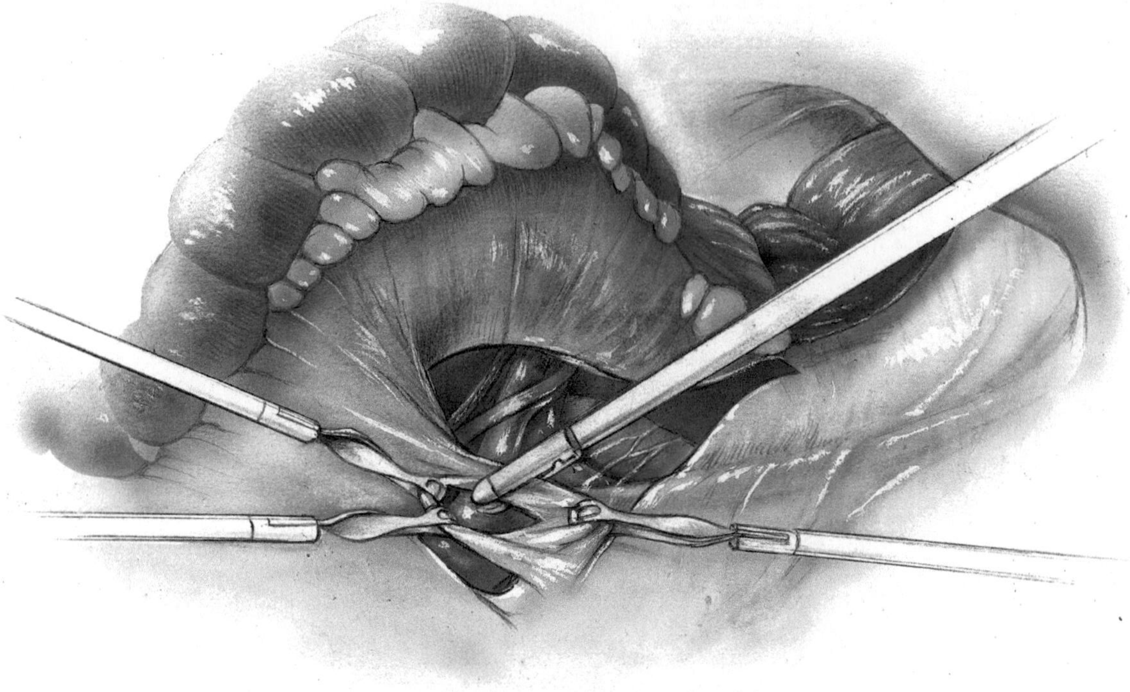

Fig. 8-3

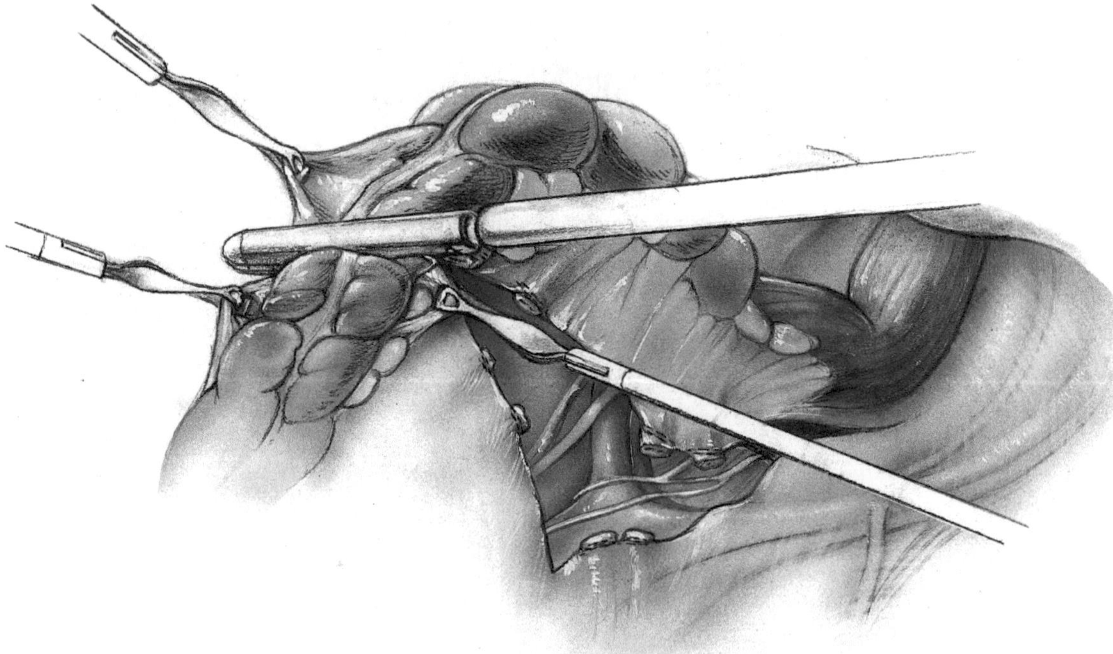

Fig. 8-4

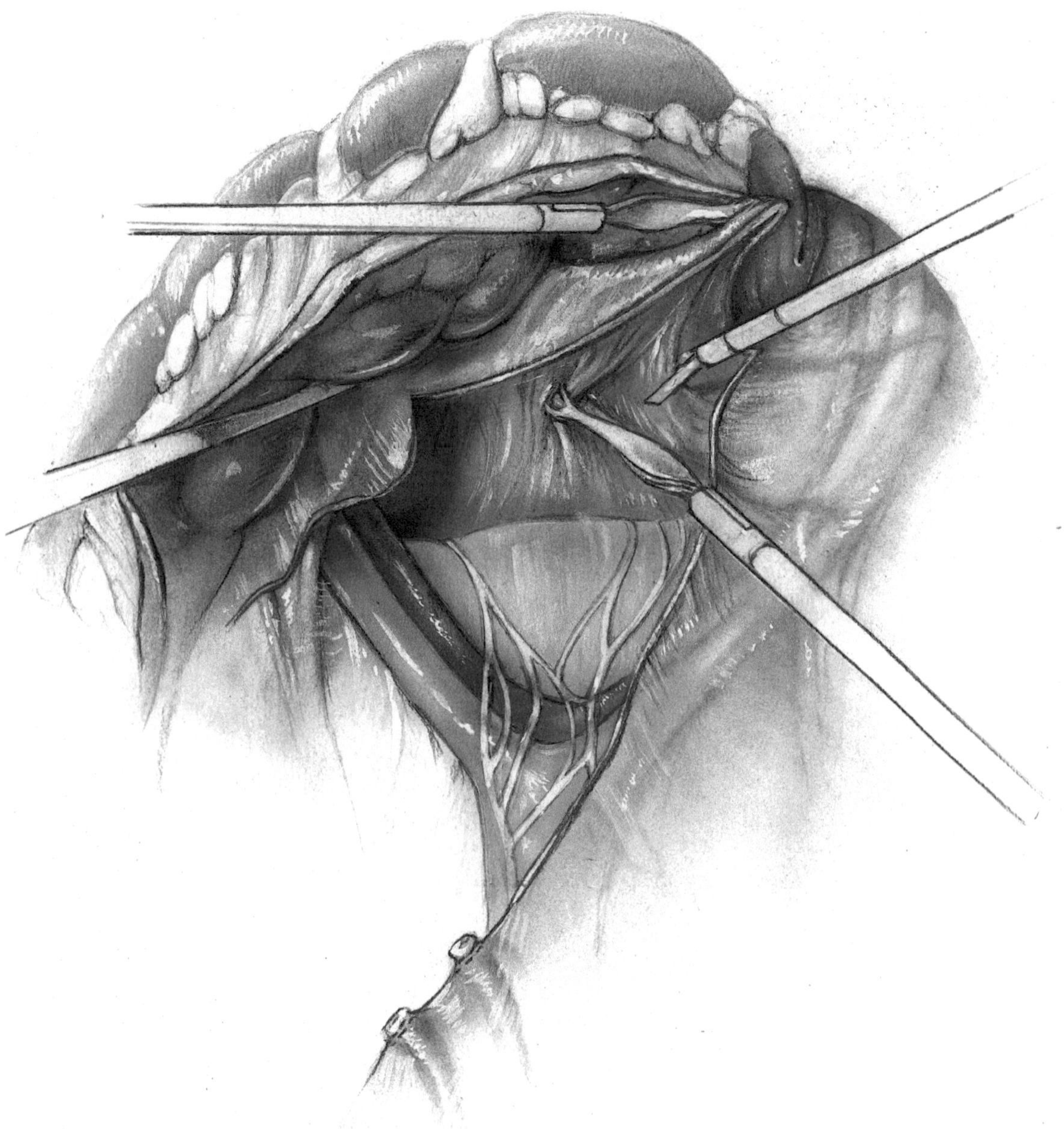

Fig. 8–5

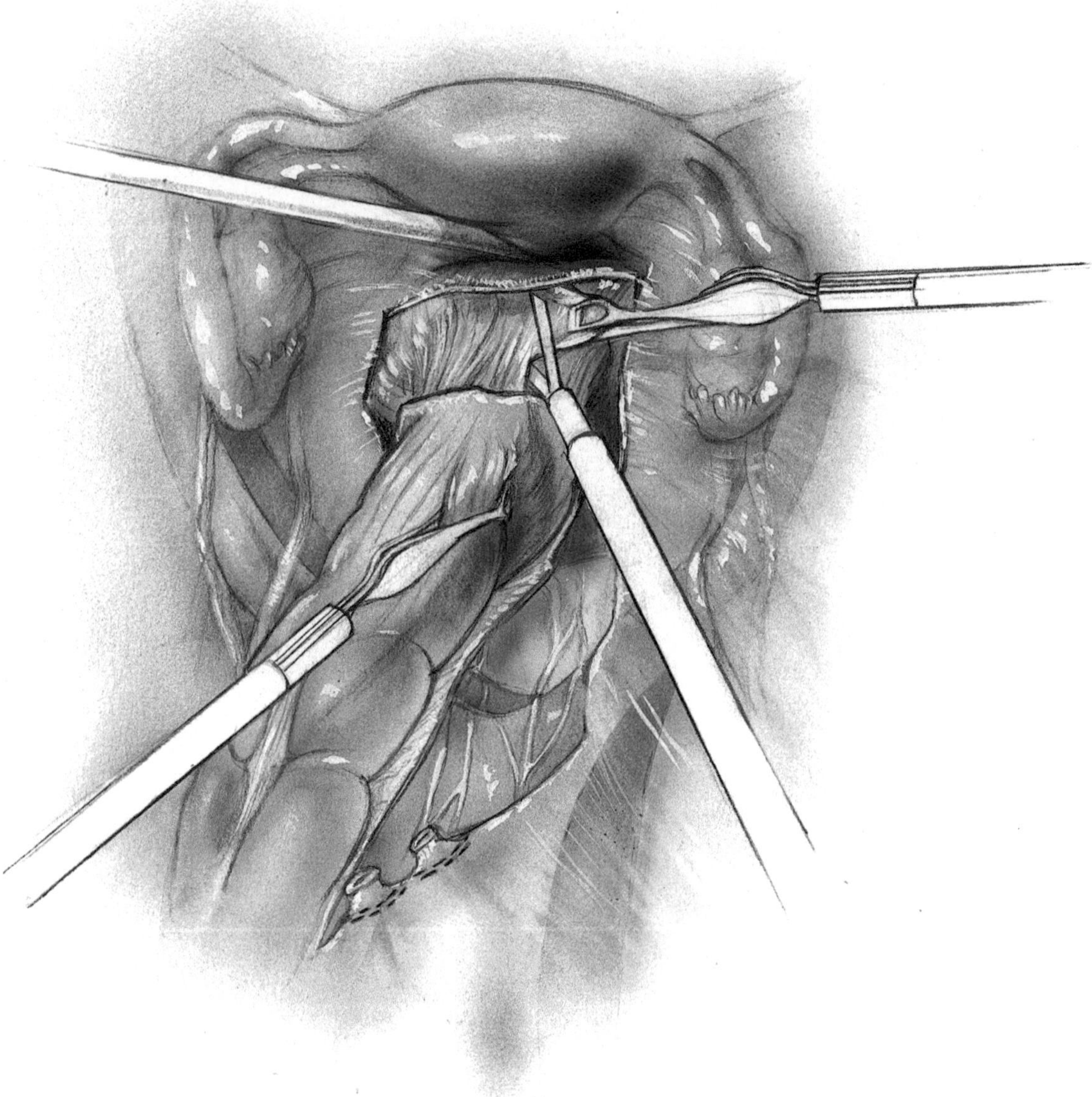

Fig. 8-6

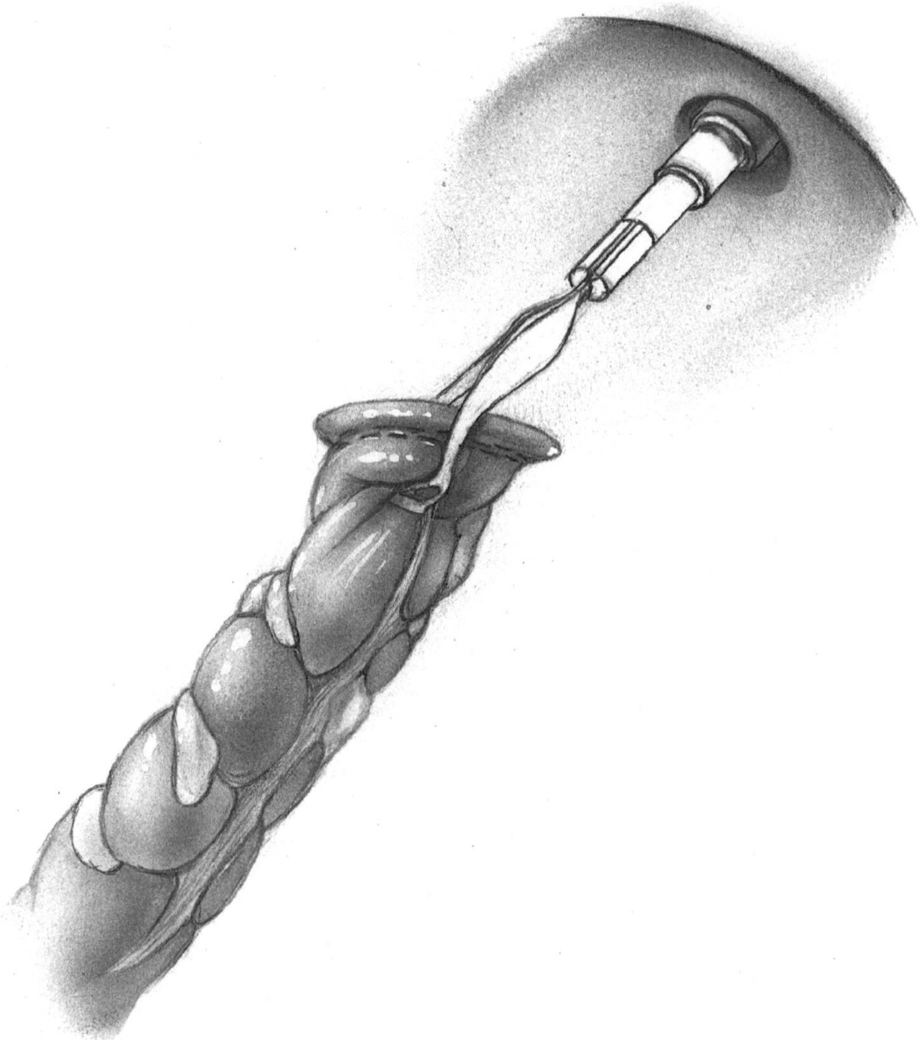

Fig. 8–7

## TOTAL PROCTOCOLECTOMY WITH END ILEOSTOMY

### INDICATIONS

Patients with Crohn's disease of the rectum

### PREOPERATIVE PREPARATION

The preoperative preparation is the same as for abdominoperineal resection.

### PITFALLS AND DANGER POINTS

Pitfalls are similar to those for abdominoperineal resection. In addition, duodenal injury may occur during right colon mobilization.

### OPERATIVE TECHNIQUE

#### Room Setup and Trocar Placement

The room is set up in a similar fashion as for abdominoperineal resection. After insertion of the camera port, four additional ports are generally required for the procedure, two on each on the left and right side **(Fig. 8–8)**. Similar to abdominoperineal resection, the lower ports should be placed at the proposed ileostomy and potential drain sites. The position of surgical team varies according to localization of the dissection. The surgeon stands on the opposite side of the colon being mobilized or between the patient's legs.

After placement of the ports, the small bowel is careful examined for evidence of Crohn's disease using two laparoscopic Babcock clamps. Dissection can start from any segment of the colon. Some sur-

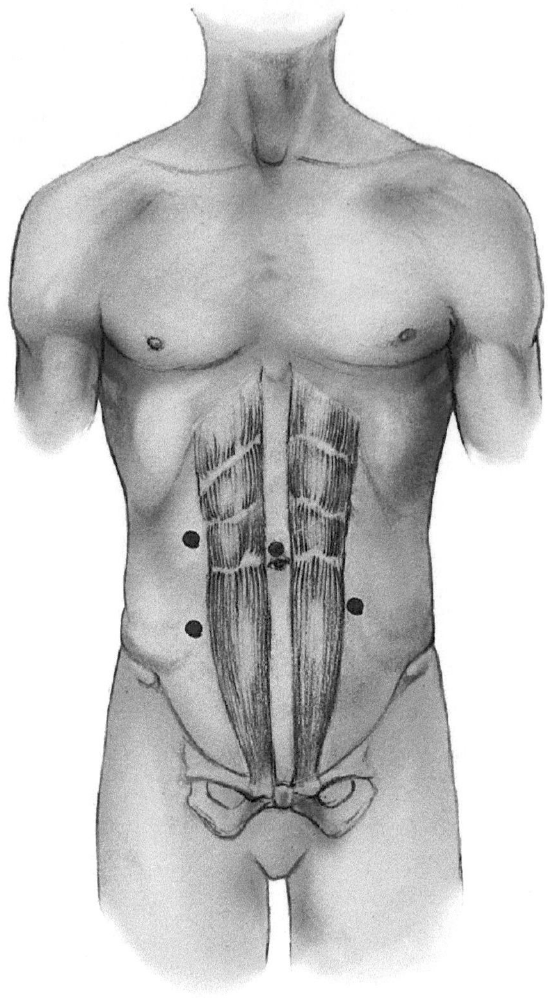

Fig. 8–8a

geons prefer to mobilize the sigmoid and rectum as far as possible prior to the ascending, transverse, and descending colon to avoid difficult retraction of these structures from the pelvis once they are mobilized. We usually start the dissection from the ileocecal valve and ascending colon as in the open procedure. The colon is retracted toward the midline and the lateral peritoneum is divided along the white line of Toldt, extending towards the hepatic flexure. During mobilization, the spermatic vessels, the right ureter and the duodenum are identified **(Fig. 8–9)**. The left colon is mobilized with identification of the left ureter followed by mobilization of the splenic flexure with division of the phrenocolic, splenocolic and renocolic ligaments **(Fig. 8–10)**. The transverse colon is then separated from the greater omentum by either dividing the avascular plane along the omentocolic junction or, alternatively, by transecting the omentum **(Fig. 8–11)**. At this point, if the procedure is continued totally laparoscopically, the rectum is dissected as described for abdominoperineal resection and the vessels are ligated intracorporeally. After the terminal ileum is divided with an endoscopic linear cutter, the entire specimen is then extracted through a standard perineal wound. Unlike peripheral excision for malignancy, the proctectomy is performed in an intersphincteric plane. The ileum is divided externally and the remainder of the operation proceeds as described

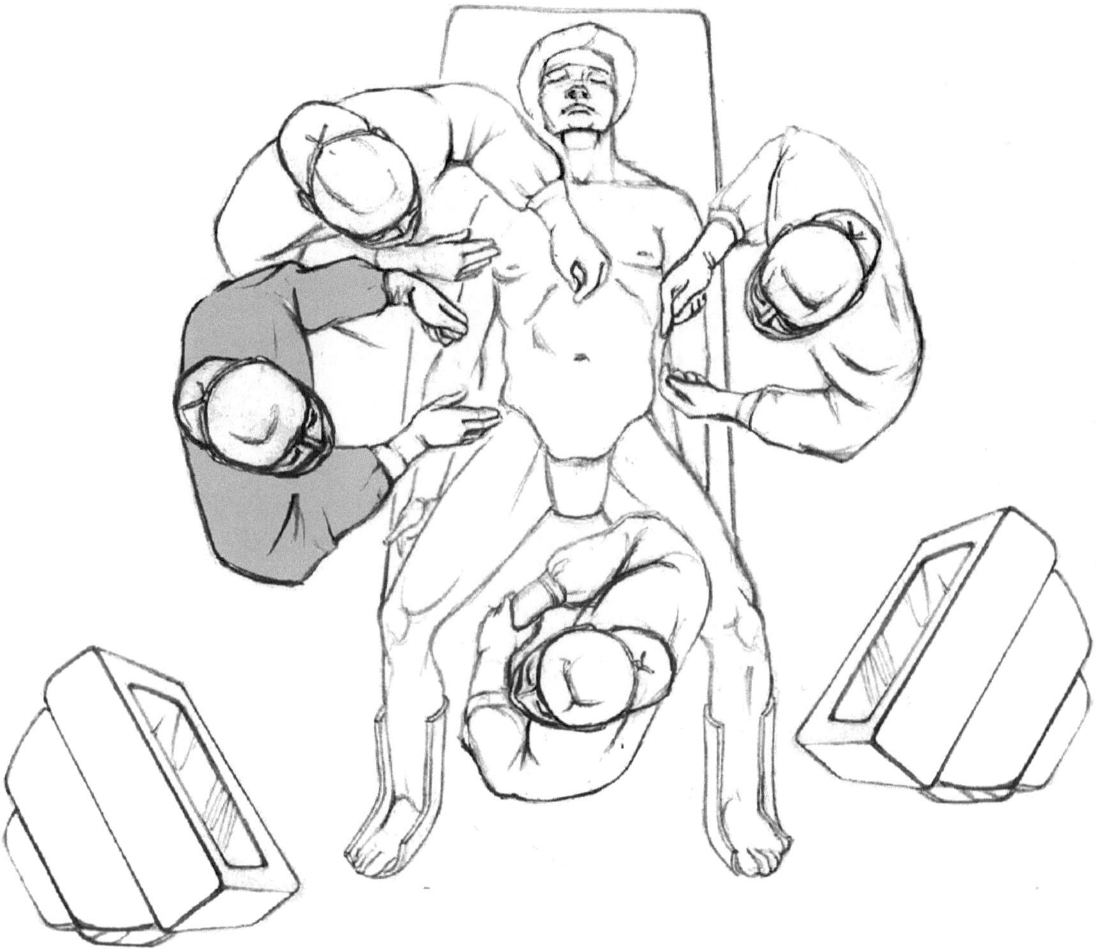

Fig. 8-8b

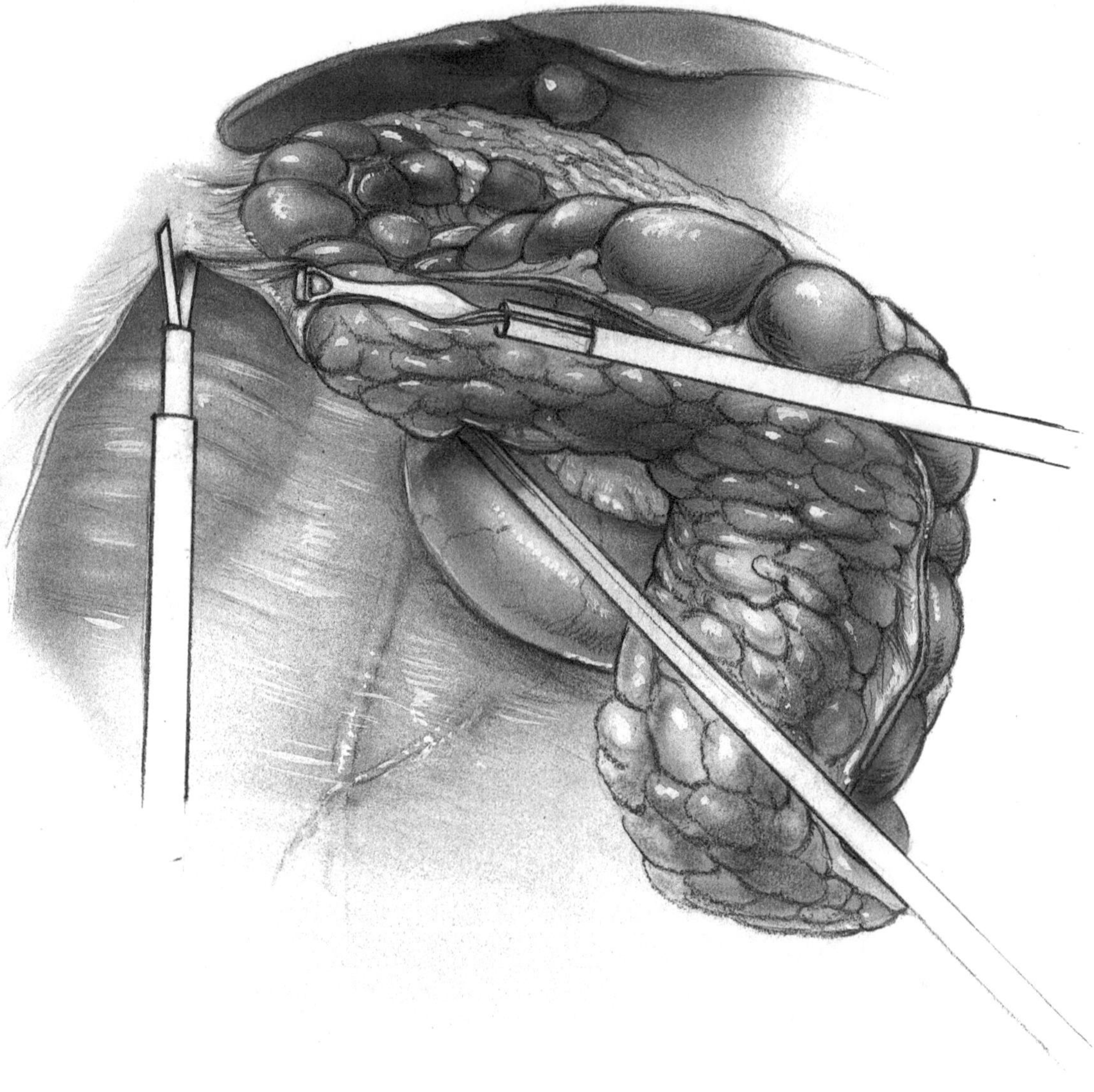

Fig. 8-9

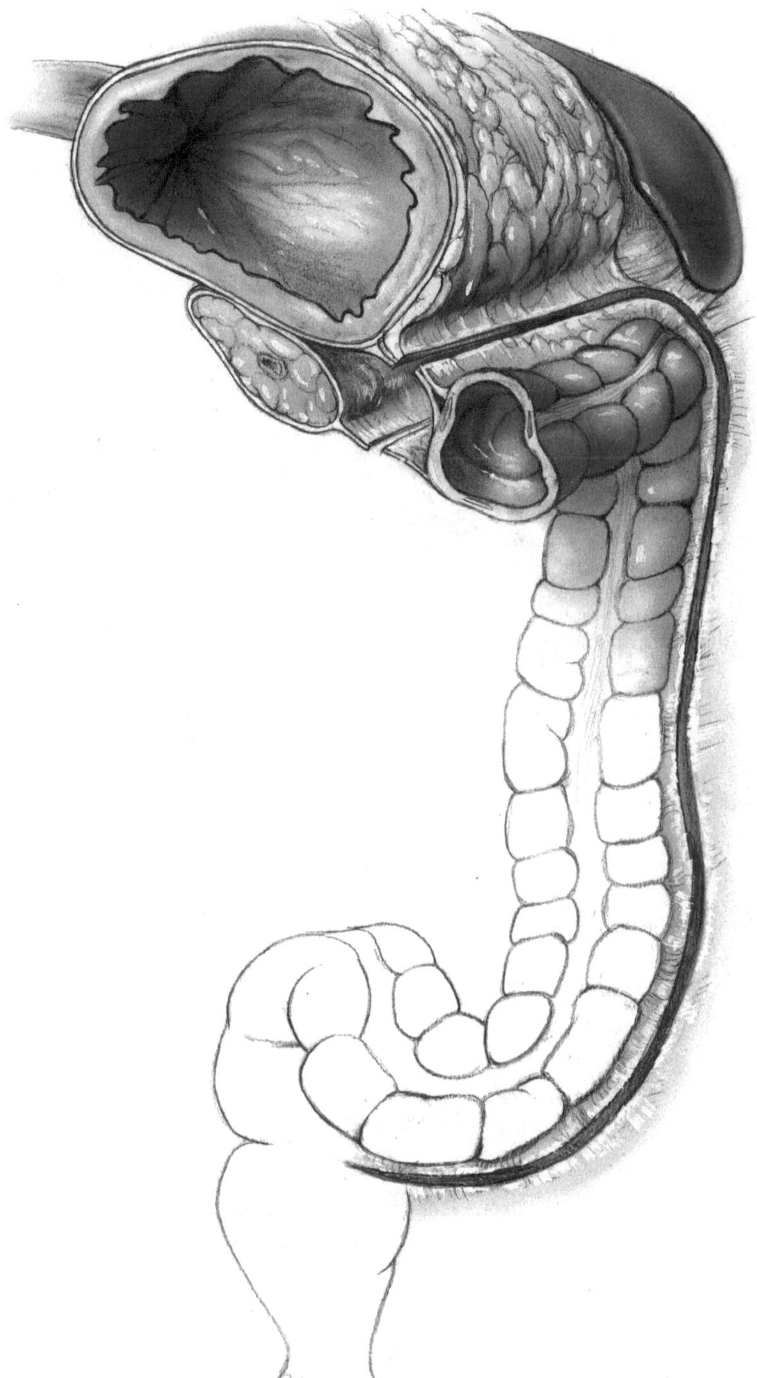

Fig. 8–10

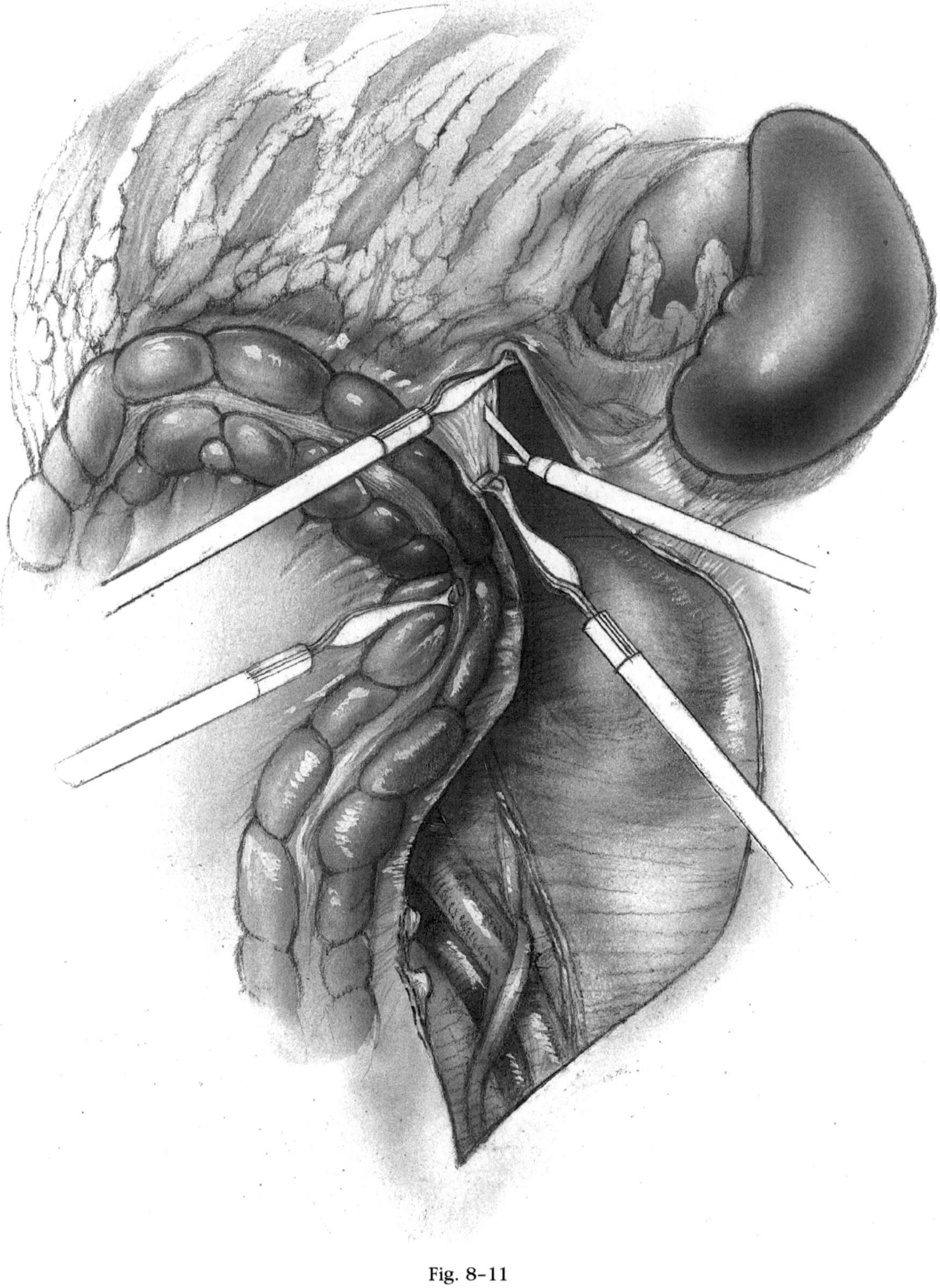

Fig. 8-11

for abdominoperineal resection. Alternatively, once the colon has been mobilized, a small Pfannenstiel incision is performed and rectal dissection is completed as in the open procedure. The colon is exteriorized and the ileum and mesenteric vessels are extracorporeally divided.

## COMPLICATIONS

Stoma-related complications (retraction, stenosis, prolapse, dehydration)

Postoperative small bowel obstruction

Nonhealing perineal wound

## POSTOPERATIVE CARE

Postoperatively, the nasogastric tube is removed in the operating room. A clear liquid diet is initiated immediately after surgery, as tolerated, and advanced to a regular diet once there is passage of flatus or bowel movement through the stoma. Patients can often be discharged home after 3 to 4 days.

# 9 Subtotal Colectomy with Ileoproctostomy or Ileostomy and Sigmoid Mucous Fistula

## INDICATIONS

See Chapter 1 for discussion of issues related to the choice of operative procedure.

Familial polyposis

Chronic ulcerative colitis

Crohn's colitis

## PREOPERATIVE PREPARATION

Patients with cachexia may require nutritional support.

Adrenal suppression may be present in patients who have been on steroids for a long time.

For *emergency* colectomy, restitution with blood and electrolytes should be accomplished.

Perioperative antibiotics are prescribed.

## PITFALLS AND DANGER POINTS

Operative contamination of the peritoneal cavity with colonic contents, leading to sepsis (with toxic megacolon)

Improper construction of ileostomy

## OPERATIVE STRATEGY

When choosing an emergency operative procedure for the patient with complications of inflammatory bowel disease (hemorrhage, perforation, toxic megacolon), consider both the immediate problem and the long-term result. Remember that sphincterspar-ing procedures are now available for most of these patients, even when the rectum is involved by disease. Whenever possible retain the rectosigmoid, as it allows restorative proctocolectomy (see Chapter 10) to be performed at a later date.

Sepsis is not uncommon following an emergency colectomy for inflammatory bowel disease and its complications. In Crohn's disease one often finds a fistula to the adjacent bowel or to the skin. In some cases paracolic abscesses are encountered, making gross contamination of the peritoneal cavity inevitable.

When resecting a toxic megacolon, the surgeon should be aware that the colon, especially the distal transverse colon and splenic flexure, may have the consistency of wet tissue paper and can be ruptured by even minimal manipulation. This causes massive, sometimes fatal contamination of the abdominal cavity, and it must be avoided. Make no attempt to dissect the omentum off the transverse colon, as it may unseal a perforation. Elevation of the left costal margin by a Thompson retractor generally provides good exposure of the splenic flexure.

Intraoperative tube decompression may decrease the risk of perforating the colon. Divide the mesentery at a point of convenience nearer to the colon, rather than performing extensive mesenteric excision (as is done for malignancy). Minimize postoperative ileostomy problems by constructing an ileostomy that protrudes permanently from the abdominal wall, like a cervix, for 2 cm. This helps prevent the contents of the small bowel from leaking between the appliance and the peristomal skin. It also greatly simplifies the patient's task of placing the appliance accurately. Finally, close the gap between the cut edge of ileal mesentery and the lateral abdominal wall to avoid internal herniation.

## OPERATIVE TECHNIQUE

### Placement of Ileostomy

On the day before the operation the surgeon should obtain a face-plate from an ileostomy appliance, or some facsimile, and apply it tentatively to the patient's abdominal wall. Test proper placement with the patient sitting erect. In some patients, if the appliance is not properly placed the rim strikes the costal margin or the anterior spine of the ilium. Generally, the proper location is somewhere near the outer margin of the right rectus muscle, about 5 cm lateral to the midline and 4 cm below the umbilicus. In this position the face-plate generally does not impinge on the midline scar, the umbilicus, the anterior superior spine, or the costal margin no matter what position the patient assumes. If the wafer covers the incision, we prefer a subcuticular skin closure for better skin approximation. The stoma should also be sited so the patient can see it when he or she is erect.

## Operative Position

If there is a possibility that the colectomy and total proctectomy will be performed in one stage, position the patient in Lloyd-Davies leg rests (see Figs. 6-3a, 6-3b). Otherwise, the usual supine position is satisfactory.

## Incision

We prefer a midline incision because it does not interfere with the ileostomy appliance. It also leaves the entire left lower quadrant free of scar in case ileostomy revision and reimplantation become necessary in the future. On the other hand, many surgeons use a left paramedian incision to permit a wider margin between the ileostomy and the scar. The incision should extend from the upper epigastrium down to the pubis **(Fig. 9–1)**. Because the splenic flexure is foreshortened in many cases of ulcerative colitis and toxic megacolon, exposure for this area is often good, with the Thompson retractor applied to the left costal margin.

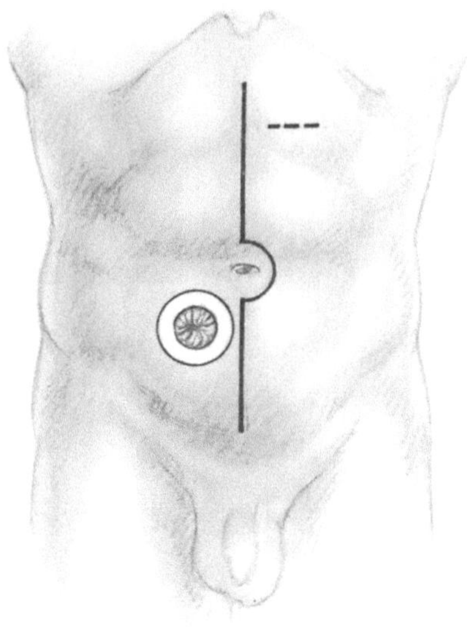

Fig. 9-1

## Evacuation of Stool

For patients undergoing an operation for acute toxic megacolon, insert a heavy purse-string suture on the anterior surface of the terminal ileum. Make a small enterotomy in the center of the purse-string suture and pass a suction catheter through it, threading the catheter across the ileocecal valve into the cecum. After decompressing the colon, remove the tube and tie the purse-string suture.

## Dissection of Right Colon and Omentum

Make an incision in the right paracolic peritoneum lateral to the cecum and insert the left index finger to elevate the avascular peritoneum, which should be divided by scissors in a cephalad direction **(Fig. 9–2)**. If local inflammation has produced increased vascularity in this layer, use electrocautery to carry out the division. Throughout the dissection keep manipulation of the colon to a minimum. Continue the paracolic incision around the hepatic flexure, exposing the anterior wall of the duodenum.

For emergency operations for toxic megacolon, divide the omentum between Kelly hemostats 5 cm above its line of attachment to the transverse colon. If the omentum is fused to the transverse mesocolon, it may be divided simultaneously with the mesocolon in one layer. In most *elective* operations, the omentum can be dissected off the transverse colon through the usual avascular plane **(Fig. 9–3)**.

## Dissection of Left Colon

Remain at the patient's right side and make an incision in the peritoneum of the left paracolic gutter in the line of Toldt, beginning at the sigmoid. With the aid of the left hand elevate the avascular peritoneum and divide it in a cephalad direction with Metzenbaum scissors. Carry this incision up to and around the splenic flexure **(Fig. 9–4)**. Mobilize the splenic flexure as described in Chapter 44 (see Figs. 4-5 through 4-8). In patients who suffer from toxic megacolon, perform this dissection with extreme caution so as not to perforate the colon.

## Division of Mesocolon

Turn now to the ileocecal region. If the terminal ileum is not involved in the disease process, preserve

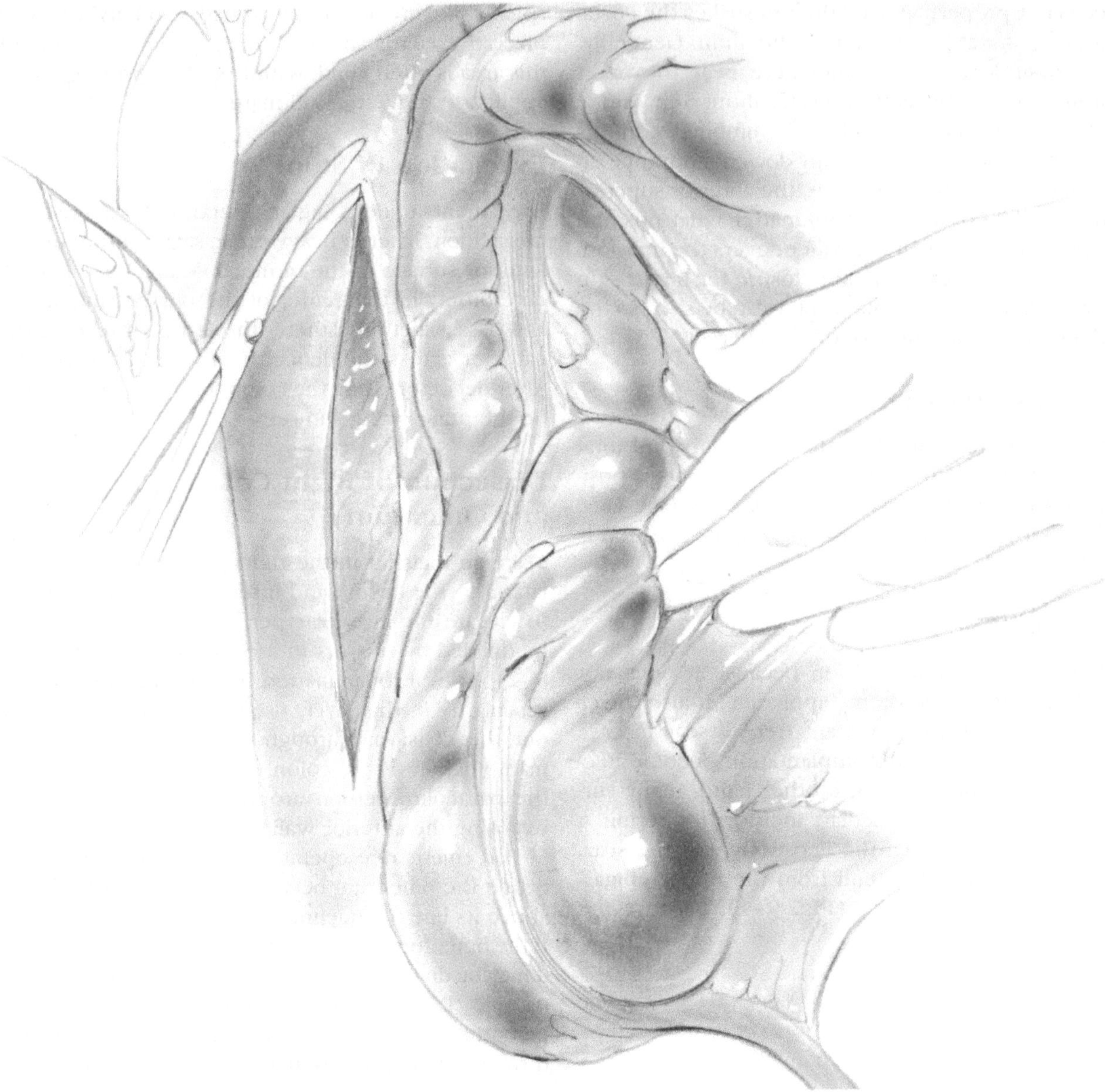

Fig. 9–2

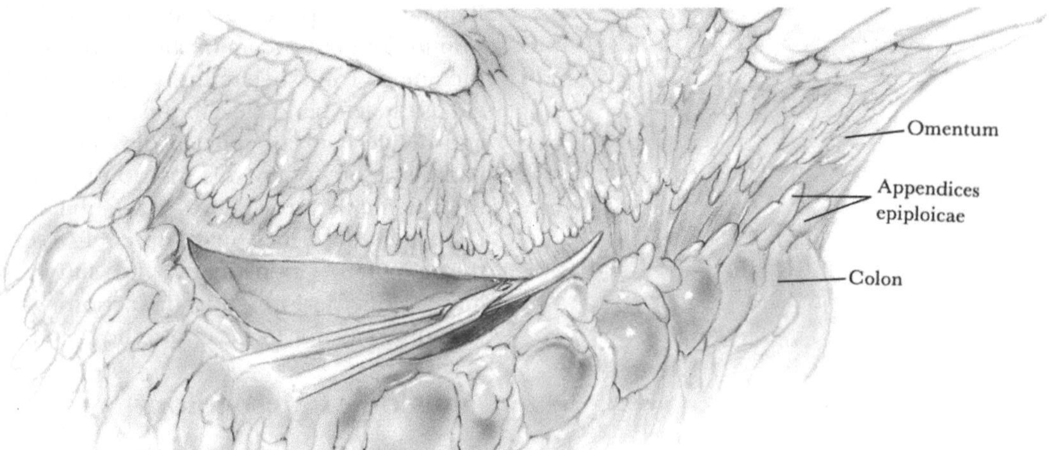


Fig. 9–3

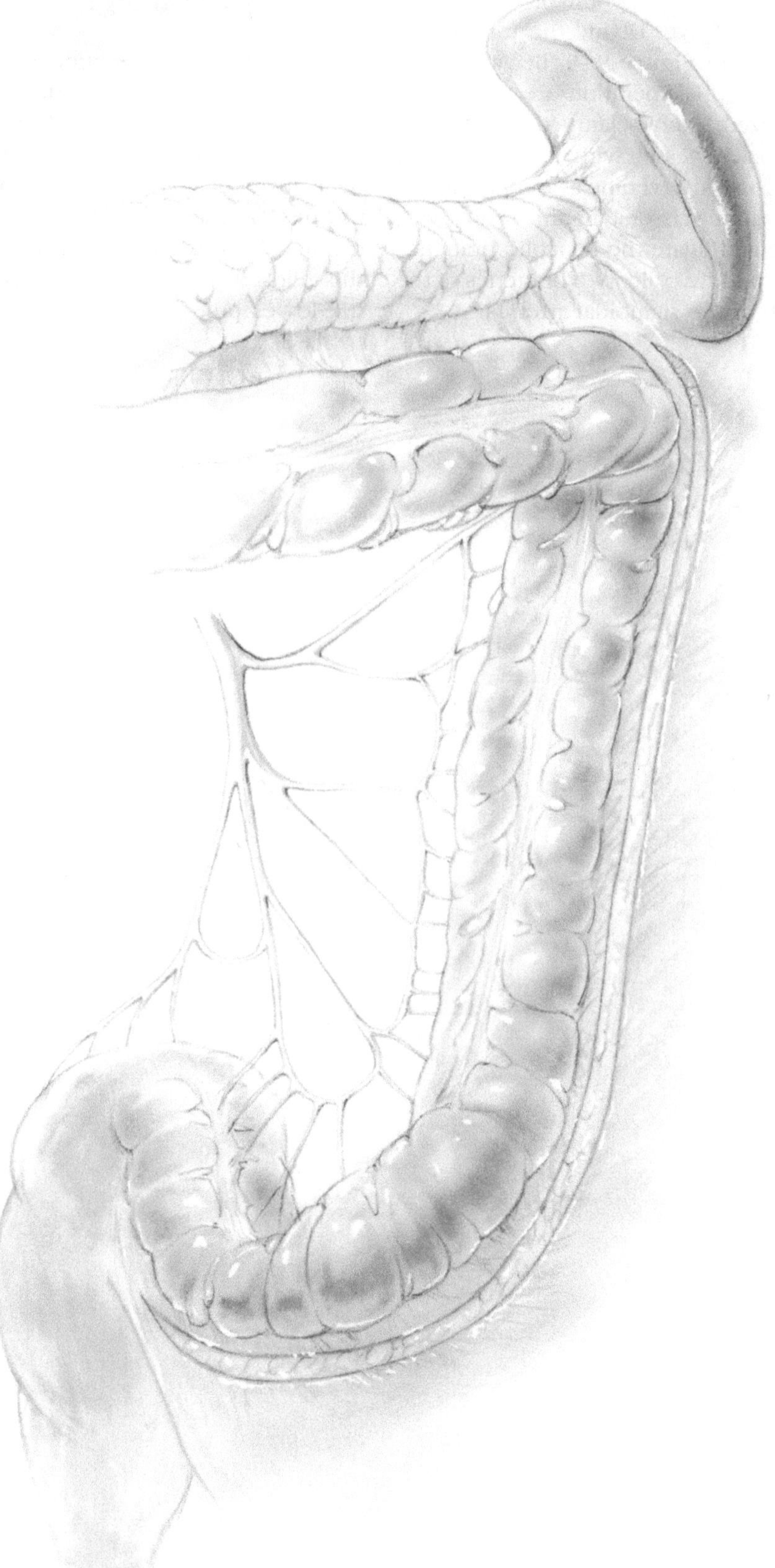

Fig. 9-4

its blood supply and select a point of transection close to the ileocecal valve. Divide the mesocolon along a line indicated in **Figure 9–5**. Because most patients who require this operation are thin, each vessel can be visualized, double-clamped, and divided accurately. Ligate each vessel with 2-0 PG or silk ligatures and divide the intervening avascular mesentery with Metzenbaum scissors. In the same way, sequentially divide and ligate the ileocolic branches and the right colic, middle colic, two branches of the left colic, and each of the sigmoidal arteries.

## Ileostomy and Sigmoid Mucous Fistula

The technique of fashioning a permanent ileostomy, including suturing the cut edge of the ileal mesentery to the right abdominal wall, is depicted in Figures 12-1 through 12-9. After the sigmoid mesentery has been divided up to a suitable point on the wall of the distal sigmoid, divide the colon with De-Martel clamps (as shown) or a linear cutting stapler. Bring this closed stump of the rectosigmoid through the lower pole of the incision **(Fig. 9–6)**. Fix the

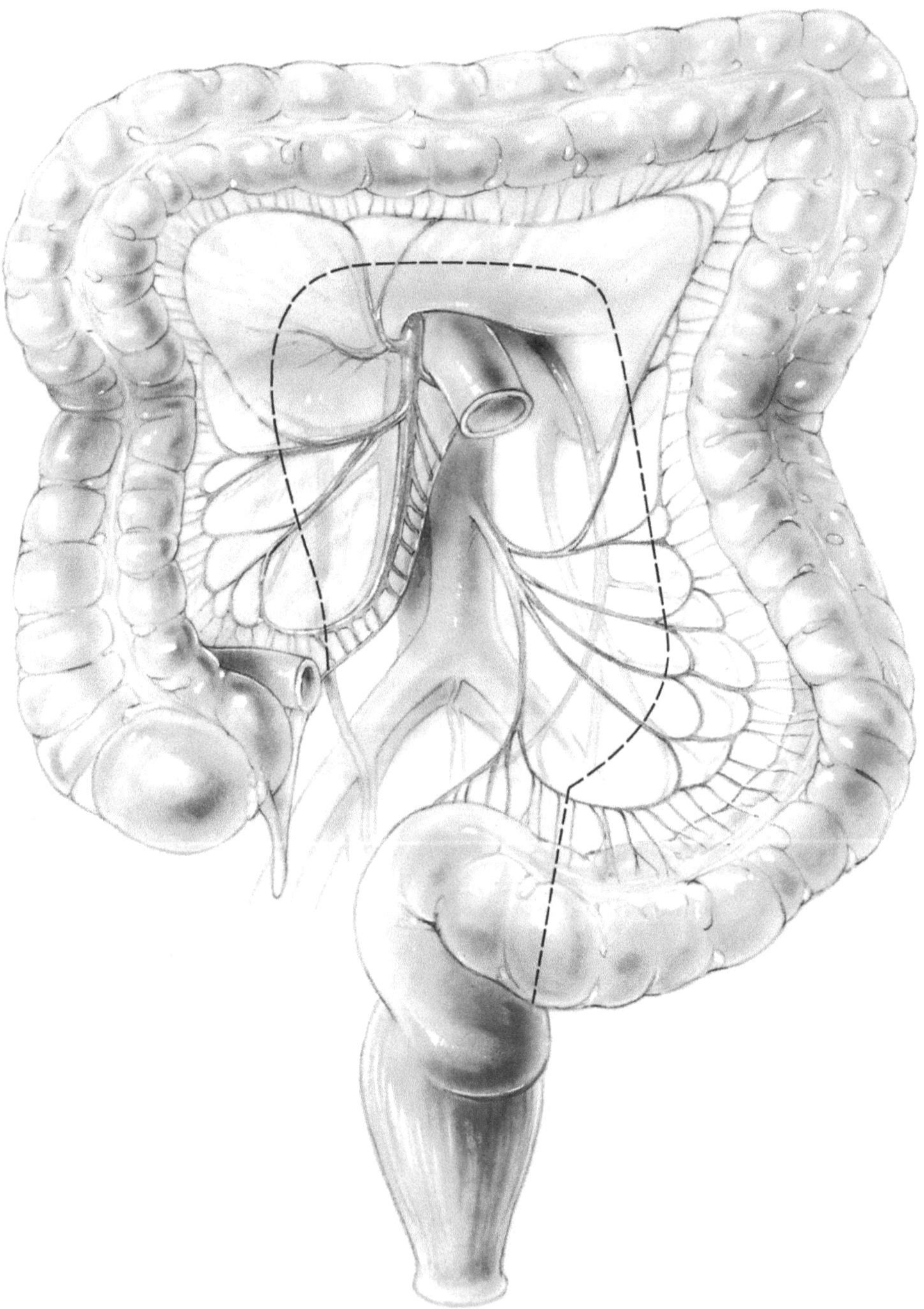

Fig. 9–5

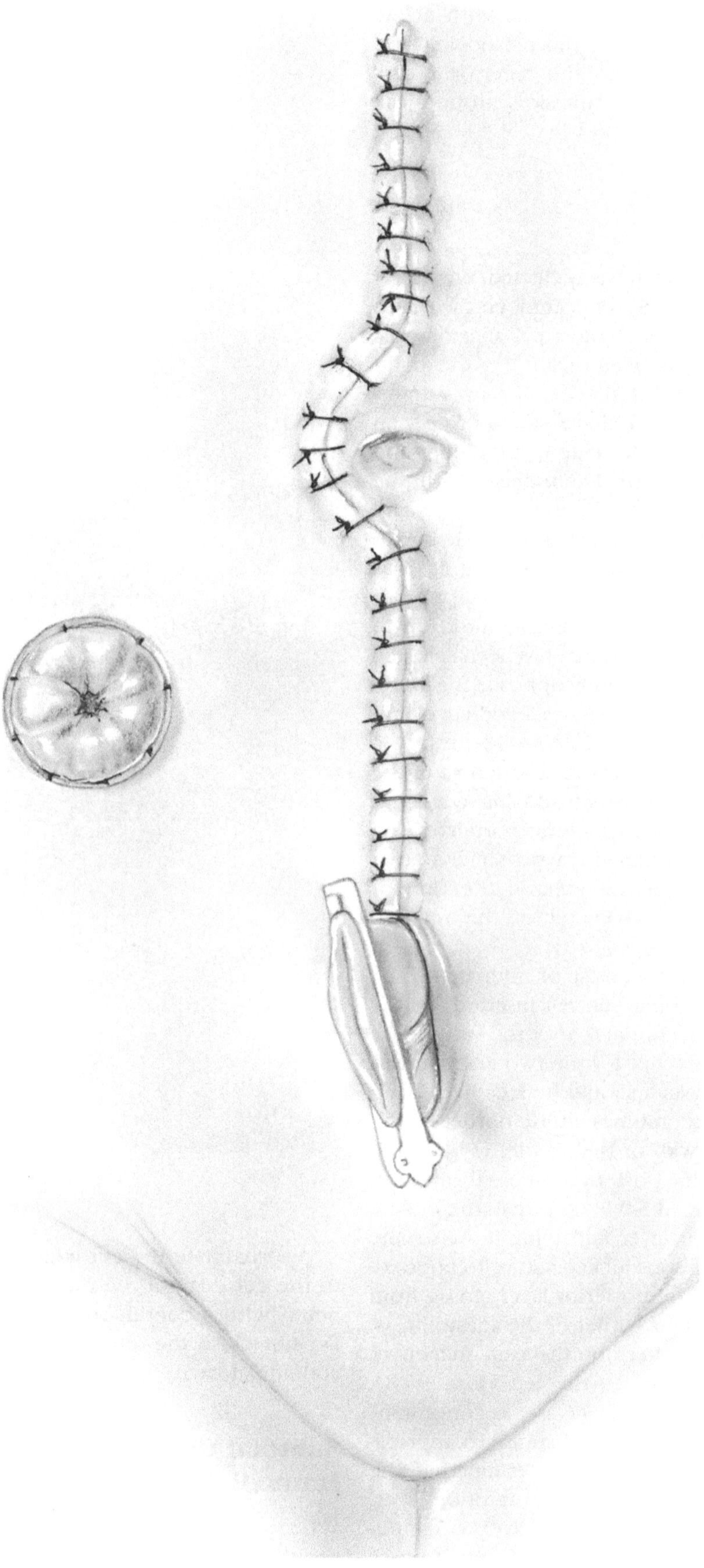

Fig. 9–6

rectosigmoid stump to the lower pole with a few 3-0 PG sutures, approximating the mesocolon and the appendices epiploicae to the anterior rectus fascia. Close the abdominal incision around the mucous fistula.

## Ileoproctostomy

When an ileorectal anastomosis is elected, we prefer the side-to-end modified Baker technique (see Figs. 6–12 through 6–23) for the colorectal anastomosis. After the mesentery has been cleared at the point selected for transection of the ileum, apply transversely and fire a 55/3.5 mm linear stapler. Apply an Allen clamp to the specimen side of the ileum and with a scalpel transect the ileum flush with the stapler. Lightly cauterize the everted mucosa and remove the stapling device. Inspect the staple line to ensure that proper B formation of the staples has occurred.

Divide the mesentery of the rectosigmoid up to the point on the upper rectum that has been selected for transection, which is generally opposite the sacral promontory. Apply a right-angle renal pedicle clamp to the colon to exclude colonic contents from the field. Dissect fat and mesentery off the serosa of the rectum at the site to be anastomosed. Make a linear scratch mark on the antimesenteric border of the ileum beginning at a point 1 cm proximal to the staple line and continuing in a cephalad direction for a distance equal to the diameter of the rectum, usually 4–5 cm.

The first layer should consist of interrupted 4-0 silk seromuscular Cushing sutures inserted by the successive bisection technique. After the sutures are tied, cut all the tails except for the two end sutures, to which small hemostats should be attached. Then make incisions on the antimesenteric border of the ileum and the back wall of the rectum **(Fig. 9–7)**. Initiate closure of the posterior mucosal layer by inserting a double-armed 5-0 PG suture in the middle point of the posterior layer and tying it. With one needle insert a continuous locked suture to approximate all the coats of the posterior layer, going from the midpoint to the right corner of the anastomosis. Use the other needle to perform the same maneuver going from the midpoint to the left **(Fig. 9–8)**. Amputate the specimen. Then use a continuous Cushing, Connell, or seromucosal suture to approximate the anterior mucosal layer, terminating the suture line at the midpoint of the anterior layer. Close the final anterior seromuscular layer with interrupted 4-0 silk Cushing sutures **(Fig. 9–9)**. If possible, cover the anastomosis with omentum.

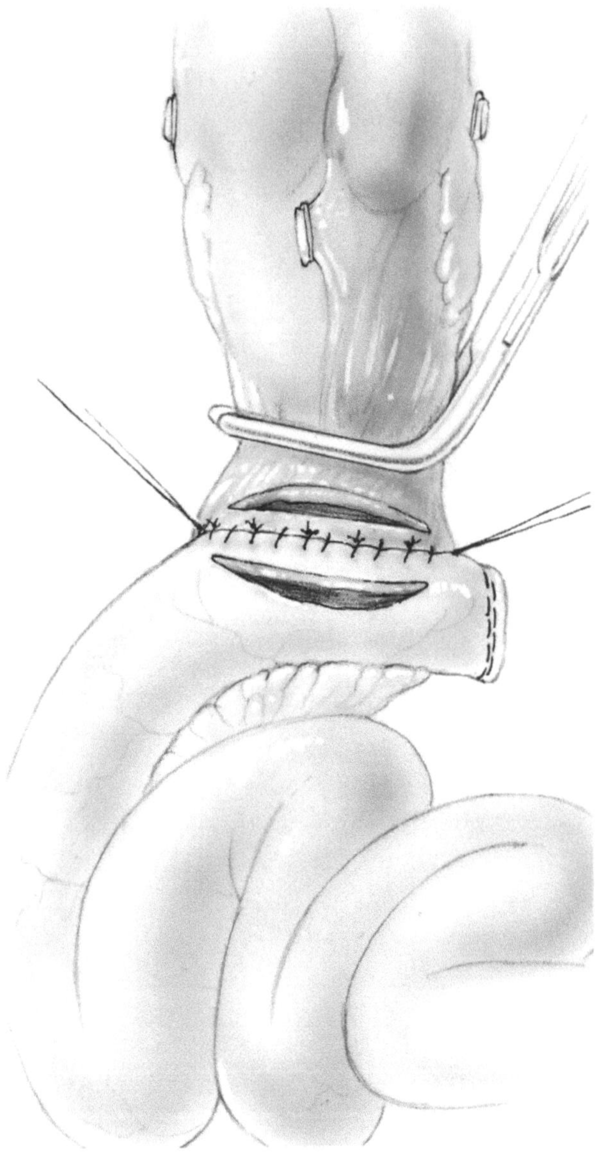

Fig. 9–7

Approximate the cut edge of the ileal mesentery to the cut edge of the right lateral paracolic peritoneum with a continuous 2-0 atraumatic PG suture. Do not close the left paracolic gutter. Irrigate the abdominal cavity.

## Subtotal Colectomy Combined with Immediate Total Proctectomy

When a proctectomy is performed at the same stage as a subtotal colectomy, occlude the rectosigmoid by a layer of TA-55 staples. Apply an Allen clamp to the

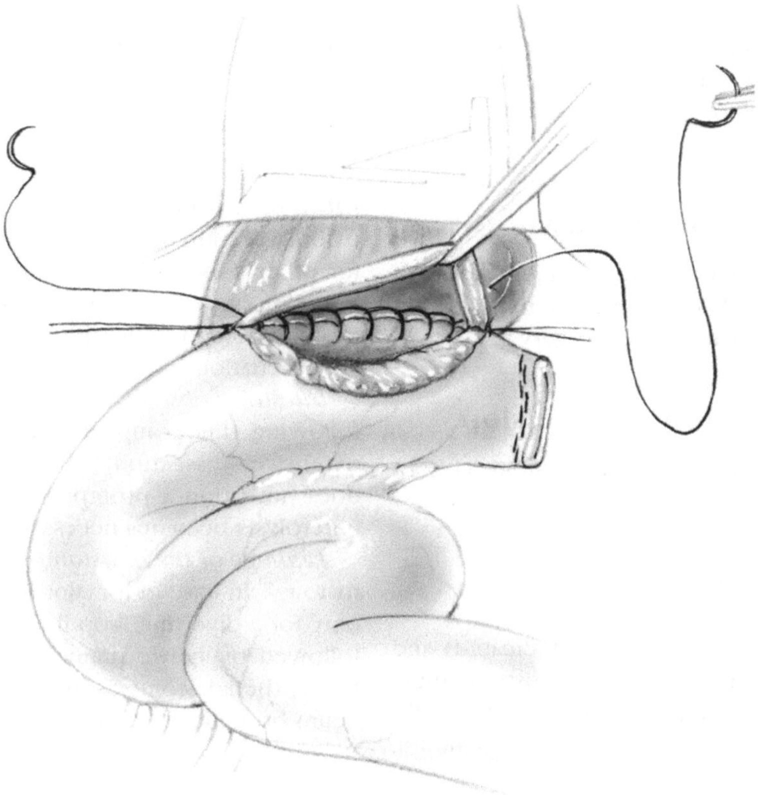

Fig. 9-8

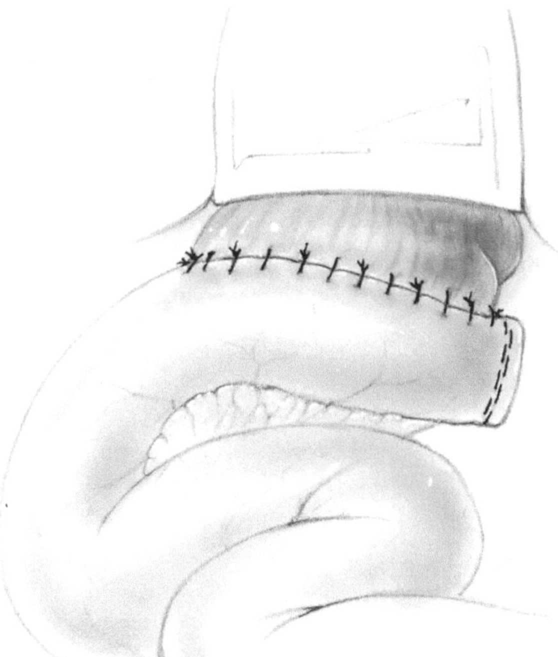

Fig. 9-9

specimen side of the colon, which should be transected with removal of the specimen. Construct the ileostomy as depicted in Figures 12-1 through 12-9. Then perform abdominoperineal proctectomy by the technique described in Chapter 11.

### Needle-Catheter Jejunostomy

Consider performing needle-catheter jejunostomy in any patient suffering from malnutrition to permit enteral feeding immediately after surgery.

### Closure of the Abdominal Incision

Close the abdominal wall in routine fashion without drains.

## POSTOPERATIVE CARE

Continue nasogastric suction (when indicated) and intravenous fluids until there is good ileostomy function. If there was no operative contamination, discontinue the operative antibiotics within 6 hours. Otherwise, continue antibiotics, modifying as indicated by the operative findings and the postoperative course.

In the operating room apply a Stomahesive disk to the ileostomy after cutting a properly sized opening. Over the disk place a temporary ileostomy bag. Instruct the patient in the details of ileostomy management and encourage him or her to join one of the organizations of ileostomates, where considerable emotional support can be derived by meeting patients who have been successfully rehabilitated.

## COMPLICATIONS

*Intraabdominal abscess* is more common after colon resection for inflammatory bowel disease than for other conditions. When signs of intraabdominal infection appear, prompt laparotomy or percutaneous computed tomography-guided catheter drainage for evacuation of the abscess is indicated.

*Intestinal obstruction* due to adhesions is not rare following this group of operations because of the extensive dissection. If nonoperative treatment does not bring a prompt response, laparotomy for enterolysis becomes necessary.

*Leakage of the anastomosis* may follow ileoproctostomy. In case of a major leak, immediate laparotomy for a diverting loop ileostomy (see Chapter 13) followed by pelvic drainage is mandatory. Alternatively, the anastomosis may be taken down and the ileum brought out as a terminal ileostomy.

## REFERENCES

Chevalier JM, Jones DJ, Ratelle R, et al. Colectomy and ileorectal anastomosis in patients with Crohn's disease. Br J Surg 1994;81:1379.

Longo WE, Oakley JR, Lavery IC, Church MJ, Fazio VW. Outcome of ileorectal anastomosis for Crohn's colitis. Dis Colon Rectum 1992;35:1066.

# 10 Ileoanal Anastomosis with Ileal Reservoir Following Total Colectomy and Mucosal Proctectomy

## INDICATIONS

Selected patients requiring proctocolectomy for ulcerative colitis, in whom preservation of continence is desired

Familial polyposis

## CONTRAINDICATIONS

Cohn's disease

Perianal fistulas

Rectal muscular cuff that is strictured and fibrotic, not soft and compliant

## PREOPERATIVE PREPARATION

Treat inflammation and ulcerations of the lower rectum preoperatively. If the patient has had a subtotal colectomy and ileostomy, it may be necessary to treat the rectum with steroid enemas or free fatty acid enemas.

Nutritional rehabilitation is applied when necessary.

Perioperative antibiotics as prescribed.

Nasogastric tube is inserted.

Foley catheter is placed in the bladder.

Endoscopy of ileum via the ileostomy is undertaken when Crohn's disease is suspected after subtotal colectomy.

If one-stage colectomy with reconstruction is anticipated, appropriate mechanical and antibiotic bowel preparation is indicated.

## PITFALLS AND DANGER POINTS

Performing an inadequate mucosectomy, which may produce a cuff abscess and possibly lead later to carcinoma

Establishing inadequate pelvic, reservoir, or anastomotic hemostasis, which may result in postoperative hemorrhage or hematoma

Injuring the nervi erigentes or the hypogastric nerves so sexual impotence or retrograde ejaculation results

Failing to diagnose Crohn's disease, resulting in Crohn's ileitis in the reservoir

Using improper technique when closing the temporary loop ileostomy, which leads to postoperative leakage or obstruction

## OPERATIVE STRATEGY

Multiple techniques have been described for restorative proctocolectomy. The method described here has served well and accomplishes maximum ablation of the abnormal mucosa. An alternative technique avoids the mucosal proctectomy altogether and creates the anastomosis between the anus and the perineal pouch by means of a double stapling technique. A roticulating linear stapler and circular stapler are used in a manner analogous to that described in Chapter 6. The anastomosis is constructed 1–2 cm above the dentate line, leaving some transitional zone epithelium behind. References at the end of the chapter detail operative results with various techniques and give additional technical details for other methods.

### Mucosectomy

The mucosectomy is performed most easily with the patient in the prone jacknife position. The dissection is expedited by injecting a solution of epinephrine (1:200,000) into the submucosal plane. It is performed as the first stage in the procedure; if the rectum is so badly diseased that mucosectomy cannot be reasonably accomplished, the operative plan must be modified. Generally, proctocolectomy is then required.

Good fecal continence can be maintained if the mucosa is dissected away from the rectum up to a point no more than 1–2 cm above the puborectalis, the upper end of the anal canal. This amount of dissection can generally be accomplished transanally with less difficulty in the adult patient than occurs when using the abdominal approach. There must be complete hemostasis in the region of the retained rectum. Generally, careful electrocoagulation can accomplish this end.

Some surgeons advocate the use of a Cavitron ultrasonic aspirator (CUSA) to facilitate the mucosal proctectomy. Frozen-section histologic examination of the excised mucosa may be helpful for ruling out Crohn's disease.

## Abdominal Dissection

When performing the colectomy, transect the ileum just proximal to its junction with the ileocecal valve to preserve the reabsorptive functions of the distal ileum. If a previous ileostomy is being taken down, again preserve as much terminal ileum as possible.

## Rectal Dissection

When dissecting the rectum away from the sacrum, keep the dissection immediately adjacent to the rectal wall. Divide the mesenteric vessels near the point where they enter the rectum and leave the major portion of the "mesentery" behind. In this way the hypogastric nerves are preserved.

Similarly, when the lateral ligaments are divided, make the point of division as close to the rectum as possible to avoid dividing the parasympathetic nerves essential for normal male sexual function. Anteriorly, the dissection proceeds close to the rectal wall posterior to the seminal vesicles and Denonvilliers' fascia down to the distal end of the prostate.

## Division of Waldeyer's Fascia

In the adult patient it is not possible to expose the levator diaphragm unless the fascia of Waldeyer is divided by sharp dissection. This layer of dense fascia is attached to the anterior surface of the sacrum and coccyx and attaches to the posterior wall of the rectum. Unless it is divided just anterior to the tip of the coccyx, it is not possible to expose the lower rectum down to the level of the puborectalis muscle.

## Temporary Loop Ileostomy and Ileostomy Closure

The loop ileostomy (see Chapter 13) completely diverts the fecal stream, yet is simple to close. It should be used whenever there is the slightest doubt as to the integrity of the anastomoses in the pelvis.

## Ileoanostomy

To facilitate anastomosing the ileum or the ileal reservoir to the anus, it is helpful to flex the thighs on the abdomen to a greater extent than is usually the case when the patient is placed in the lithotomy position for a two-team abdominoperineal operation. Be certain the rectal mucosa has been divided close to the dentate line. Otherwise, it will be necessary to insert sutures high up in the anal canal where transanal manipulation of the needle is extremely difficult. Also, it is important to remove all of the diseased mucosa in this operation to eliminate the possibility of the patient developing a rectal carcinoma at a later date.

One method of achieving exposure with this anastomosis is to insert the bivalve Parks retractor with large blades into the rectum. Then draw the ileum down, between the open blades of the retractor, to the dentate line. Insert two sutures between the ileum and the anterior wall of the anus. Insert two more sutures between the ileum and the posterior portion of the dentate line. Now remove the Parks retractor. Remove the large blades from the retractor and replace them with small blades. Then carefully insert the blades of the Parks retractor into the lumen of the ileum and open the retractor slowly.

With the Parks retractor blades in place, continue to approximate the ileum to the dentate line with 12–15 interrupted sutures of 4-0 Vicryl. This requires that the retractor be loosened and rotated from time to time to provide exposure of the entire circumference of the anastomosis. Be certain to include the underlying internal sphincter muscle together with the epithelial layer of the anal canal when inserting these sutures.

An alternative, more effective method of exposing the anastomosis is to use a Gelpi retractor with one arm inserted into the tissues immediately distal to the dentate line at about 2 o'clock while the second arm of this retractor is placed at 8 o'clock. A second Gelpi retractor is inserted into the anus with one arm at 5 o'clock and the second at 11 o'clock. If the patient is properly relaxed, these two retractors ensure visibility of the whole circumference of the cut end of the anorectal mucosa at the dentate line. Then draw the ileum down into the anal canal and complete the anastomosis.

## Constructing the Ileal Reservoir

We prefer a J-loop ileal reservoir that is constructed by making a side-to-side anastomosis in the distal segment of the ileum. We do not include the elbow of the J-loop in the staple line, thereby ensuring that there is no possibility of impairing the blood supply to the ileoanal anastomosis. The terminal end of the ileum is occluded with staples. Although it is possible to establish an ileoanal anastomosis using a circular stapler, we prefer to suture this anastomosis because we like to be sure that no rectal mucosa has been left behind.

## OPERATIVE TECHNIQUE

### Mucosal Proctectomy Combined with Total Colectomy

When the mucosa of the distal rectum is devoid of visible ulcerations and significant inflammation, mucosal proctectomy may be performed at the same time as total colectomy. In these cases perform the colectomy as described in Chapter 9. Be certain to divide the mesentery of the rectosigmoid close to the bowel wall to avoid damaging the hypogastric and parasympathetic nerves. Also, divide the branches of the ileocolic vessels close to the cecum to preserve the blood supply of the terminal ileum. It is important to transect the ileum within 1–2 cm of the ileocecal valve. Preserving as much ileum as possible salvages some of the important absorptive functions of this organ.

Use a cutting linear stapler to divide the terminal ileum. Lightly cauterize the everted mucosa. Mobilize the entire colon down to the peritoneal reflection, following the procedures illustrated in Figures 4–5, 4–8, and 9–1 to 9–5. Divide the specimen with a cutting linear stapler at the sigmoid level.

Divide the rectosigmoid mesentery close to the bowel wall to avoid interrupting the hypogastric nerves (see Fig. 11–1). Divide the lateral ligaments close to the rectum and divide Denonvilliers' fascia proximal to the upper border of the prostate. Keep the dissection *close to the anterior and lateral rectal walls* in men to minimize the incidence of sexual impotence. After dividing Waldeyer's fascia (see Fig. 6–10) expose the puborectalis portion of the levator diaphragm (see Fig. 6–25).

At this time, transect the anterior surface of the rectal layer of muscularis in a transverse direction down to the mucosa. Make this incision in the rectal wall about 2–4 cm above the puborectalis muscle. Now dissect the muscular layer away from the mucosa. Injecting a solution of 1:200,000 epinephrine between the mucosa and muscularis expedites this dissection. After the muscle has been separated from 1–2 cm of mucosa anteriorly, extend the incision in the muscularis layer circumferentially around the rectum. Use Metzenbaum scissors and a peanut sponge dissector for this step. Achieve complete hemostasis by accurate electrocoagulation. Continue the mucosal dissection until the middle of the anal canal has been reached. Divided the mucosal cylinder at this point, remove the specimen, and leave an empty cuff of muscle about 2–4 cm in length above the puborectalis, which marks the proximal extent of the anal canal. If any mucosa has been left in the anal canal proximal to the dentate line, it can be removed transanally later in the operation.

Alternatively, one may perform the rectal mucosectomy prior to opening the abdomen. This method is described in the next section of this chapter.

#### *Perineal Approach*

We agree with the suggestion of Sullivan and Garnjobst (1982) that the rectal mucosal dissection is best performed as the initial step in the operation, regardless of whether the procedure is combined with a simultaneous total colectomy. If it is not possible to dissect the mucosa away from the internal sphincter, perform an ileostomy and abdominoperineal total proctectomy instead of a restorative proctocolectomy.

Performing the mucosal proctectomy with the patient in the prone position affords better exposure than is available in the lithotomy position. After inducing endotracheal anesthesia, turn the patient face down and elevate the hips by flexing the operating table or by placing a pillow under the hips. Also place a small pillow under the feet and spread the buttocks apart by applying adhesive tape to the skin and attaching the tape to the sides of the operating table. Gently dilate the anus until it admits three fingers. Obtain exposure by using a large Hill-Ferguson, a narrow Deaver, or a bivalve Pratt (or Parks) retractor. Inject a solution of 1:200,000 epinephrine in saline in the plane just deep to the mucosa, immediately proximal to the dentate line around the circumference of the anal canal **(Fig. 10–1)**. Now make a circumferential incision in the transitional epithelium immediately cephalad to the dentate line. Using Metzenbaum scissors, elevate the mucosa and submucosa for a distance of 1–2 cm circumferentially from the underlying circular fibers of the internal sphincter muscle **(Fig. 10–2)**. Apply several Allis clamps to the cut end of the mucosa. Maintain hemostasis by accurate electrocoagulation using the needle tip attachment on the electrocautery. It is helpful to roll up two 10 × 20 cm moist gauze sponges soaked in a 1:200,000 epinephrine solution and insert this roll into the rectum. This step facilitates the dissection between mucosa and muscle.

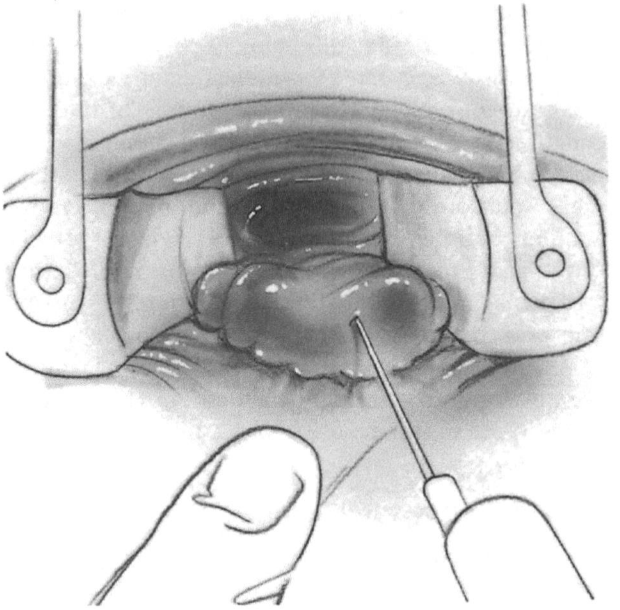

Fig. 10-1

Continue the dissection to a point 4-6 cm above the dentate line **(Fig. 10-3)**. As the dissection continues cephalad, exposure is obtained by inserting two narrow Deaver retractors the assistant holds in varying positions appropriate to the area being dissected.

After an adequate tube of mucosa 4-6 cm in length has been dissected, insert a purse-string suture near the apex of the dissected mucosal tube and amputate the mucosa distal to the suture. Submit this specimen to the pathologist for frozen-section histologic examination. Insert into the denuded rectum a loose gauze pack that has been moistened with an epinephrine solution. Reposition the patient on his or her back with the lower extremities elevated on Lloyd-Davies stirrups (see Figs. 6-3a, 6-3b).

## *Abdominal Incision and Exposure*

In patients who have undergone a previous subtotal colectomy with a mucous fistula and an ileostomy, reopen the previous long vertical incision, free all of the adhesions between the small bowel and the peritoneum, and liberate the mucous fistula from the abdominal wall. Divide the mesentery between Kelly hemostats along a line close to the posterior wall of the sigmoid and rectosigmoid until the peritoneal reflection is reached. Incise the peritoneal reflection to the right and to the left of the rectum. Continue the dissection downward and free the vascular and areolar tissue from the wall of the rectum. Then elevate the rectum out of the presacral space and incise the peritoneum of the rectovesical or rectouterine pouch (see Fig. 6-9). Keep the dissection close to the rectal wall, especially in male patients, to avoid the nervi erigentes and the hypogastric nerves. Pay special attention to dividing the lateral ligaments close to the rectum and avoid the parasympathetic plexus between the prostate and the rectum.

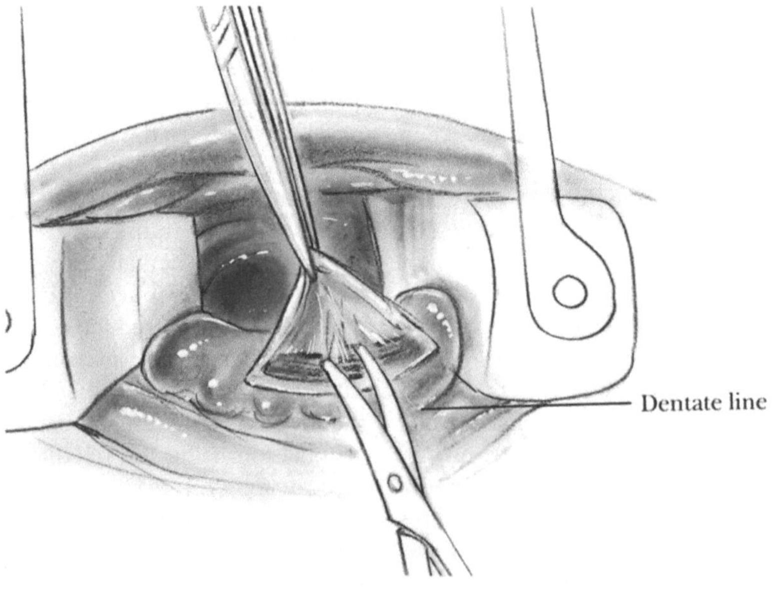


Fig. 10-2

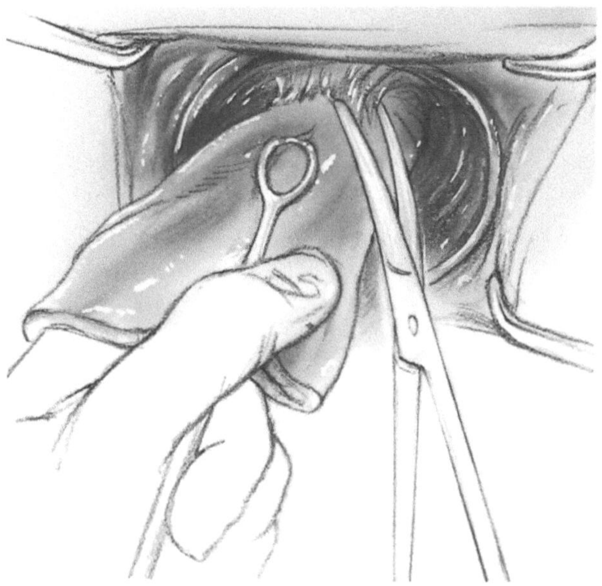

Fig. 10-3

With a long-handled scalpel incise Waldeyer's fascia (see Fig. 6-10) between the tip of the coccyx and the posterior wall of the rectum. Enlarge this incision with long Metzenbaum scissors. In male patients incise Denonvilliers' fascia (see Fig. 6-11) on the anterior wall of the rectum proximal to the prostate and the seminal vesicles. Separate the prostate from the rectum. These last two maneuvers permit exposure of the levator diaphragm. Palpating the rectum at this time should enable the surgeon to detect the level at which the purse-string suture was placed in the mucosa during the first phase of this operation. If this purse-string suture is not palpable, ask the assistant to place a finger in the rectum from the perineal approach to help identify the apex of the previous mucosal dissection. Now transect the rectum with electrocautery and remove the specimen. Remove the gauze packing that was previously placed in the rectal stump and inspect the muscular cylinder, which is all that remains of the rectum. This consists of the circular muscle of the internal sphincter surrounded by the longitudinal muscle of the rectum. All of the mucosa has been removed down to the dentate line. Check for complete hemostasis.

## Constructing the Ileal Reservoir

In patients who have had a previous ileostomy, carefully dissect the ileum away from the abdominal wall, preserving as much ileum as possible. Apply a 55/3.5 mm linear stapler across a healthy portion of the terminal ileum. Fire the stapler and amputate the scarred portion of the ileostomy. Lightly cauterize the everted mucosa and remove the stapling device. Now liberate the mesentery of the ileum from its attachment to the abdominal parietes. For patients who have not undergone a previous ileostomy, divide the terminal ileum with a cutting linear stapling device and divide the mesentery along the path indicated in **Figure 10–4**. Freeing the small bowel mesentery from its posterior attachments and all other adhesions may elongate the mesentery sufficiently that the ileal reservoir reaches the anal canal *without tension*.

Now select a point on the ileum about 20 cm from its distal margin that will serve as the future site of the ileoanal anastomosis. If this point on the ileum can be brought 6 cm beyond the symphysis pubis, one can be assured that there will be no tension on the anastomosis. Otherwise, further lengthen the mesentery by incising the peritoneum on the anterior and posterior surfaces of the ileal mesentery. Burnstein and associates reported that these relaxing incisions each contributed 1 cm to the length of the ileal mesentery. Obtain additional length, if necessary, by applying traction to the anticipated elbow of the J-pouch **(Fig. 10–5)**, transilluminating the mesentery, and selectively dividing branches of the loop formed by the superior mesenteric and ileocolic arteries as shown in **Figure 10–6**.

Be certain that the blood supply to the terminal ileum remains vigorous and that there is no tension on the ileoanal anastomosis. Take great care to isolate and ligate each vessel in the ileal mesentery individually, especially if the mesentery is thickened from scar tissue or obesity, to avoid postoperative bleeding. If an inadequately ligated vessel retracts into the mesentery, the resulting tense hematoma may produce ileal ischemia.

Now align the distal ileum in the shape of a U, each limb of which measures about 18 cm. Create a side-to-side stapled anastomosis between the antimesenteric aspects of the ascending and descending limbs of this U. Make a transverse stab wound 9 cm proximal to the staple line of the terminal ileum. Make a second transverse stab wound in the descending limb of ileum just opposite the first stab wound **(Fig. 10–7)**. Insert an 80 mm linear cutting stapler in a cephalad direction, one fork in the descending limb and one fork in the ascending limb of jejunum. Remember that this anastomosis is created on the *antimesenteric* borders of both limbs of the jejunum. Fire the stapler, creating an 8 cm side-to-side anastomosis. Withdraw the stapling device and inspect the staple line for bleeding. Electrocauterize bleeding points cautiously. Then reinsert the device into the

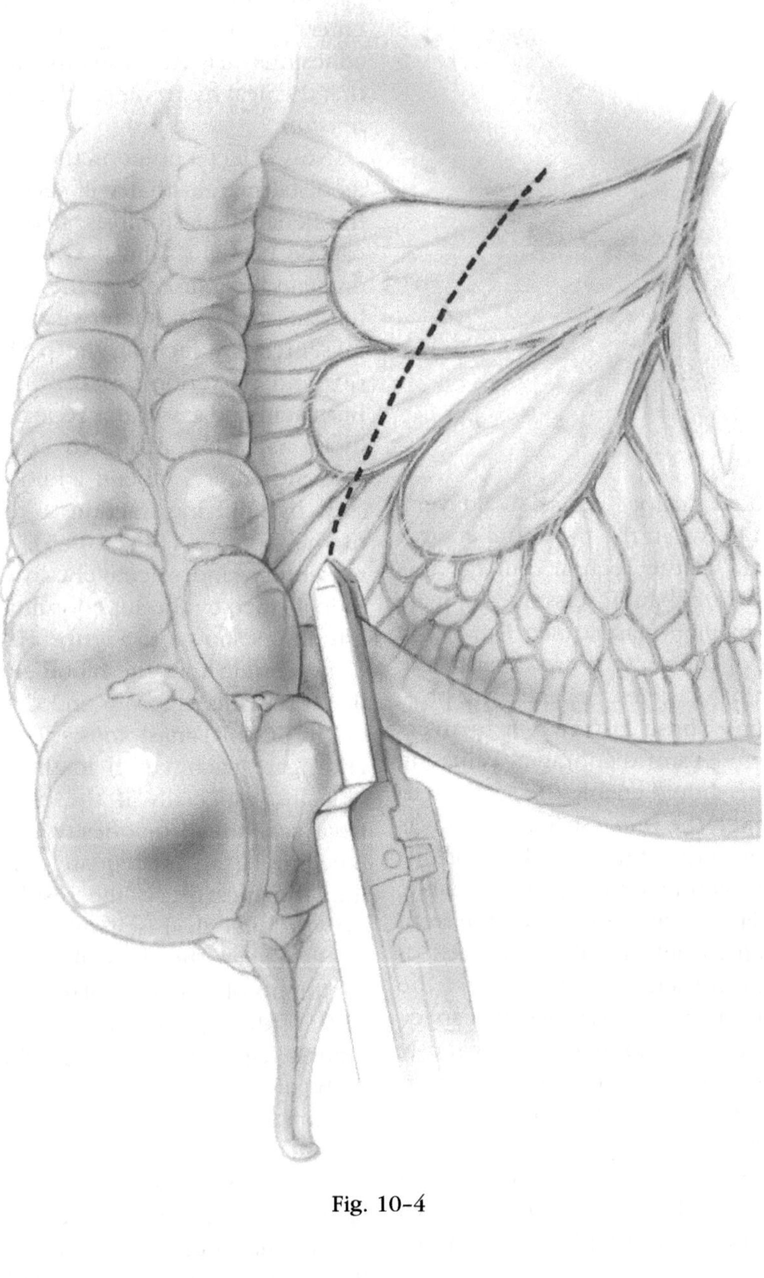

Fig. 10-4

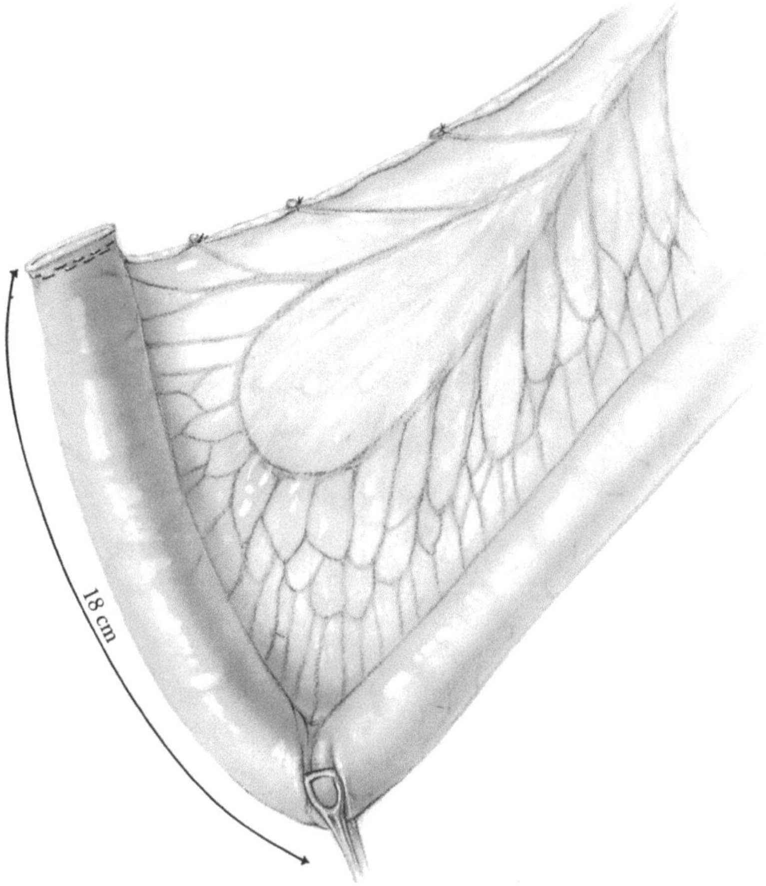


Fig. 10-5

same two stab wounds but direct the stapler in a caudal direction **(Fig. 10–8)**. Lock the device and fire the staples. Remove the stapler and inspect for bleeding. Inspect the staple line via the stab wounds and electrocauterize the bleeding points. The patient should now have a completed side-to-side stapled anastomosis about 16 cm in length. We prefer to leave an intact circular loop of ileum distal to the side-to-side anastomosis to ensure that the bowel to be anastomosed has not been traumatized.

The ileal reservoir is now complete except for the remaining stab wound through which the stapling device was previously inserted. Apply Allis clamps to approximate, in a transverse direction, the walls of the ileum in preparation for transverse application of a 55/3.5 mm linear stapling device, which will accomplish everted closure of the defect. Be certain that the superior and inferior terminations of the previous staple lines are included in the stapler before firing it. Also, avoid the error of trying to fire the linear stapler when the two terminations of the previous staple lines are in exact apposition (see Figs. 2–21 to 2–23). After firing the stapler, lightly electrocauterize the everted mucosa and carefully inspect the staple line to be sure of proper B formation **(Fig. 10–9)**.

Alternatively, *sutures* may be used to construct the side-to-side anastomosis. Make longitudinal incisions along the antimesentric borders of both the ascending and descending limbs of the ileum. Achieve hemostasis with electrocautery. Insert interrupted sutures to approximate the bowel walls at the proximal and distal margins of the anastomosis with 3-0 Vicryl sutures. Insert another suture at the midpoint between these two. Then use a straight atraumatic intestinal needle with 3-0 Vicryl starting at the apex of the posterior portion of the anastomosis and use a continuous locked suture, encompassing all the layers of the bowel. Accomplish closure of the anterior layer of the anastomosis by means of a continuous seromucosal or Lembert suture. Carefully inspect all aspects of the side-to-side anastomosis, both front and back, to be certain there are no defects or technical errors.

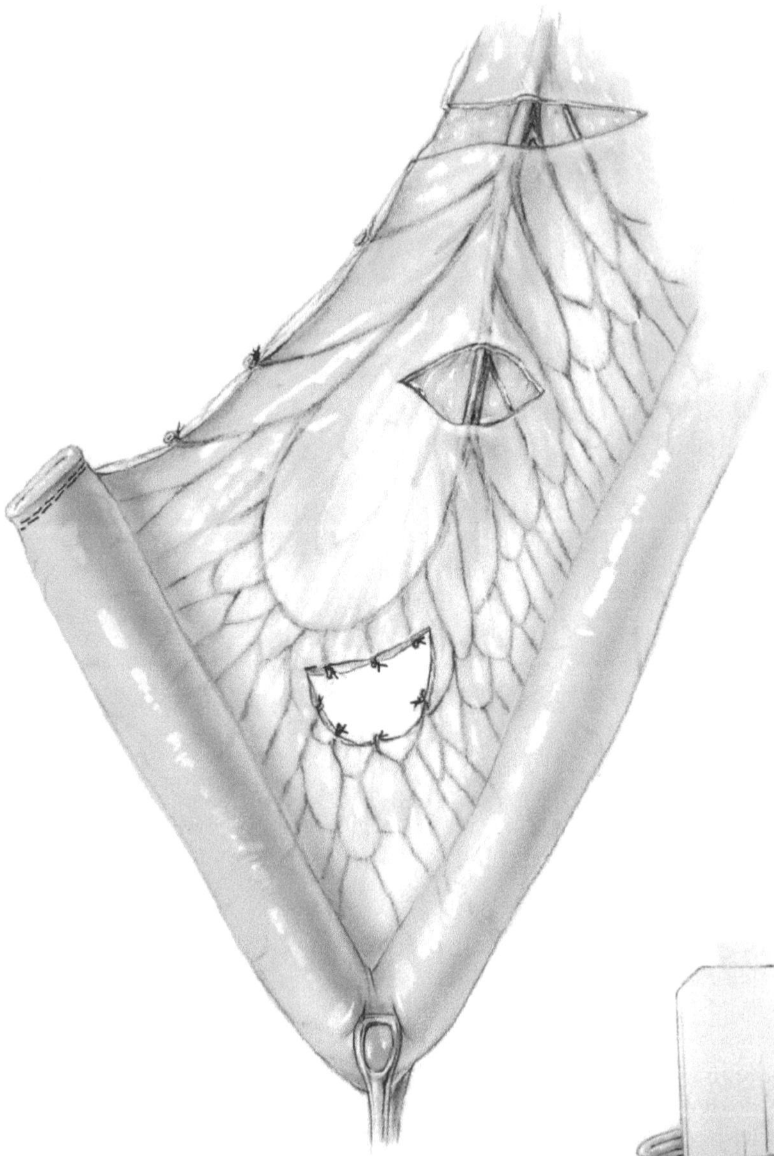

Fig. 10-6

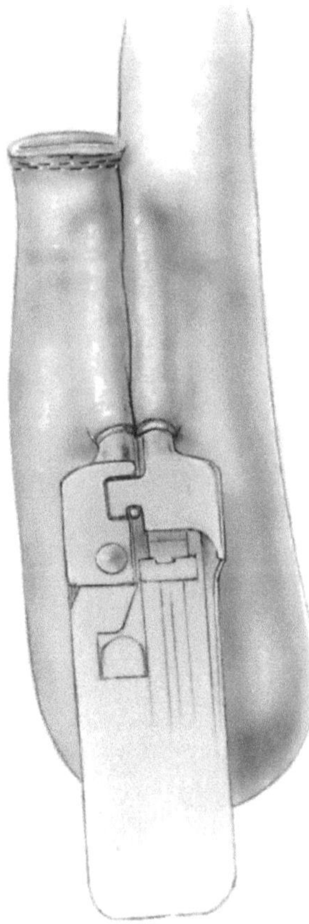

Fig. 10-7

## Ileoanal Anastomosis

Before passing the elbow of the ileal reservoir down through the anus, recheck the position of the pelvis and buttocks on the operating table. The perineum should project beyond the edge of the table. The simplest method for exposing the dentate line for the anastomosis is to insert two Gelpi retractors, one at right angles to the other. The prongs of the retractors should be inserted fairly close to the dentate line so the transected anorectal junction can be seen. Insert the first Gelpi retractor in the axis between 2 and 8 o'clock and the second between 5 and 11 o'clock. If exposure is not adequate, it may be helpful to readjust the stirrups so the thighs are flexed on the

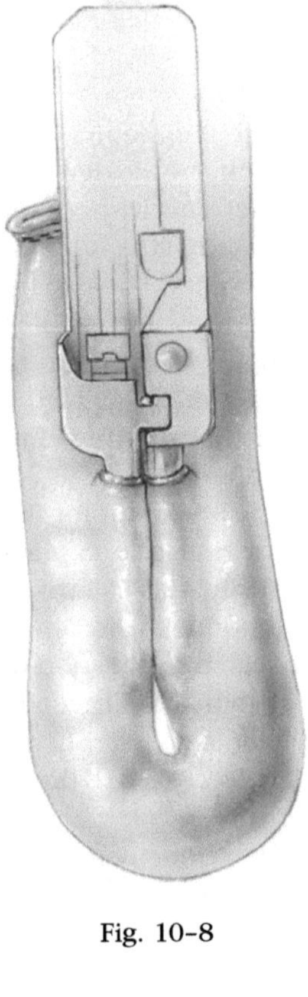

Fig. 10-8

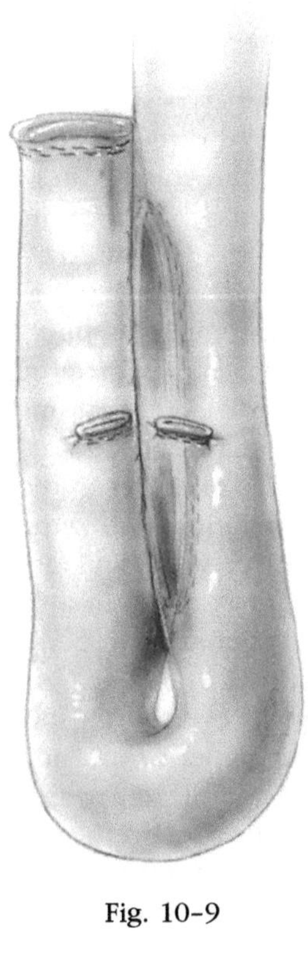

Fig. 10-9

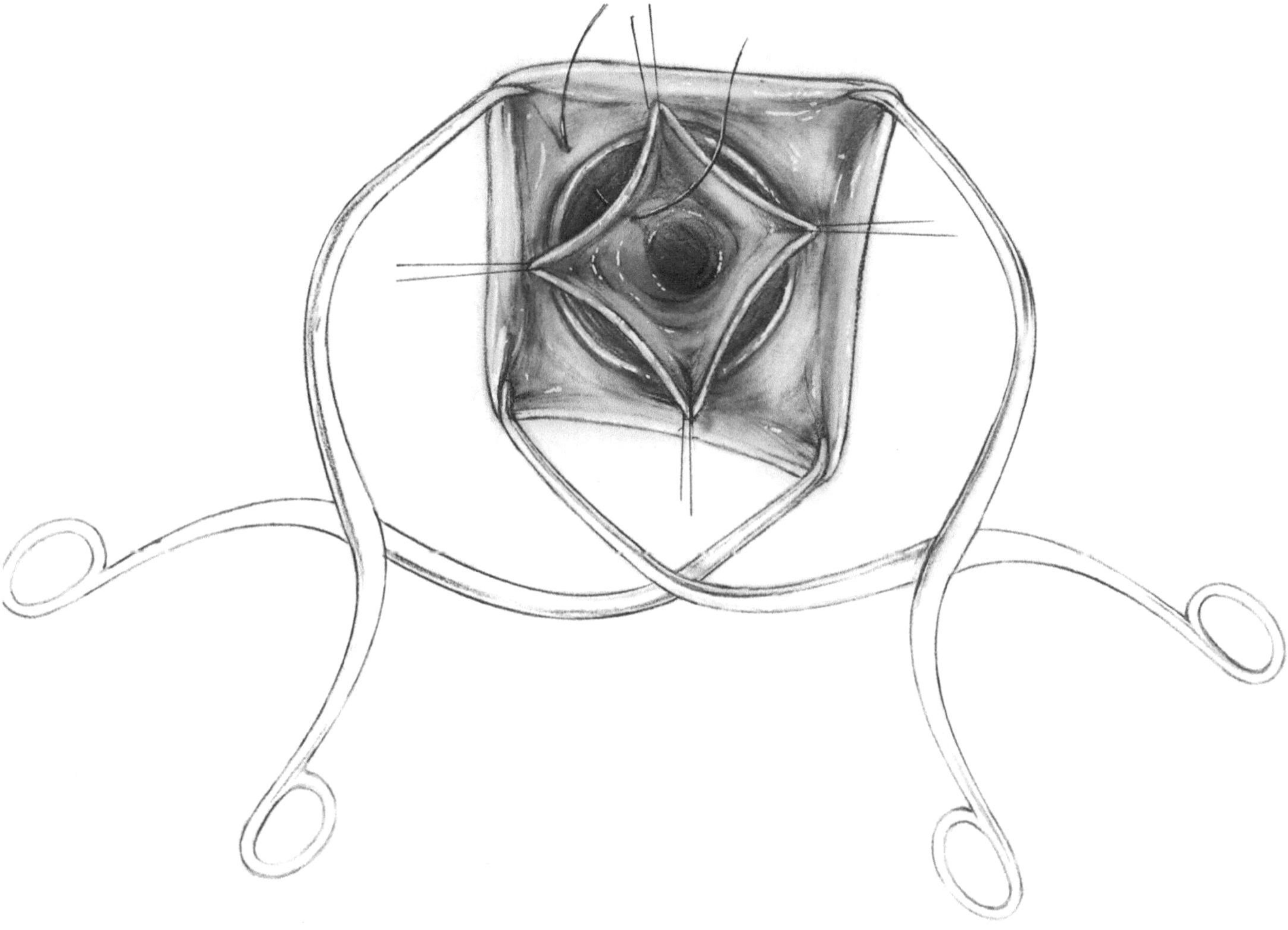

Fig. 10–10

abdomen. This position makes it more convenient to apply retractors to the anus.

After making certain that hemostasis in the pelvis is complete, insert two long Babcock clamps through the anus and grasp the dependent portion of the ileal reservoir. Bring this segment of ileum into the anal canal. Be certain that the bowel has not been twisted during this maneuver and that the mesentery lies flat *without significant tension* on the planned anastomosis. Make a longitudinal incision along the dependent border of the ileal reservoir. Cauterize the bleeding points. Apply traction sutures to the incised ileum, one to each quadrant **(Fig. 10–10)**. Construct a one-layer anastomosis between the ileum and the dentate line of the anus. Be sure to include in each stitch a 4mm bite of underlying internal sphincter muscle as well as anal epithelium. Use atraumatic 4-0 PG or PDS sutures **(Fig. 10–11)**. If the anal canal is deep, a doublecurved Stratte needle-holder (see Figs. G–17, G–18) is helpful. Insert the first four sutures at 12, 6, 3, and 9 o'clock. Then continue to insert sutures by the method of successive bisection. The resulting ileoanal anastomosis should be widely patent (Fig. 10–11). If desired, the ileal reservoir may now be inflated with a methylene blue solution to check for possible defects in the reservoir staple or suture lines. **Figure 10–12** illustrates the completed anastomosis.

## Loop Ileostomy

Until more evidence has accumulated to demonstrate that this step is not necessary, we believe that these patients should have a temporary diverting loop ileostomy (see Chapter 13). If the patient has a defect in the abdominal wall that remains after dismantling

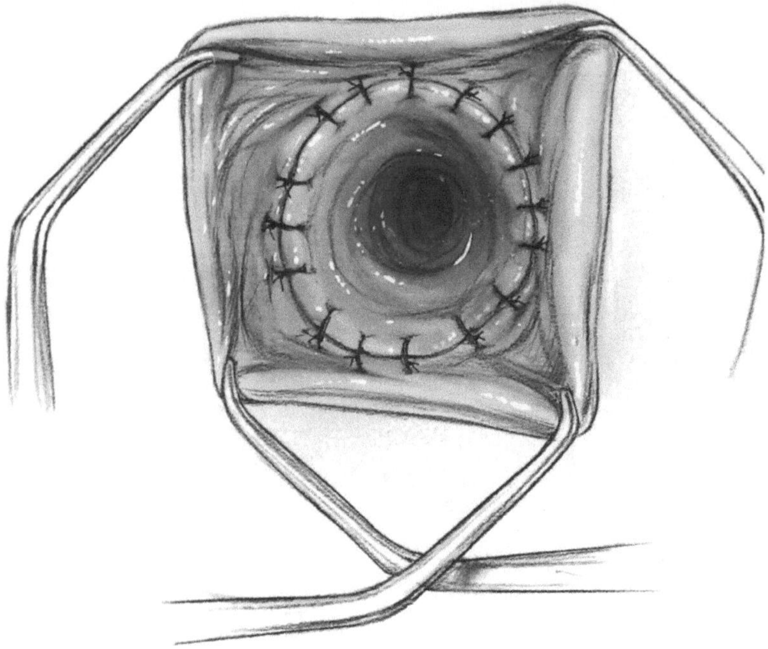

Fig. 10-11

a previous ileostomy, it is generally possible to use the same site for the loop ileostomy. Insert a large Babcock clamp through the opening in the abdominal wall and grasp the antimesenteric aspect of a segment of ileum proximal to the ileal reservoir. Select a segment of ileum that does not exert any tension whatever on the ileal reservoir. Construct the loop ileostomy as described later (see Figs. 13-1 through 13-4).

## Drainage and Closure

Hematoma or infection in the space between the rectal cuff and the ileal reservoir may produce fibrosis and impair fecal continence. Consequently, at this point in the operation make every effort to achieve complete hemostasis in the rectal cuff and in the pelvis. Insert one or two Jackson Pratt silicone closed-suction drains through puncture wounds in the abdominal wall down to the rectal cuff. Some believe it is important to place a layer of sutures between the proximal cut end of the rectal cuff and the ileal reservoir. Although we do not believe that these sutures can compensate for an inadequate ileoanal anastomosis, they may help prevent tension on the pouch.

Close the abdominal wall with interrupted No. 1 PDS by the modified Smead-Jones technique. Close the skin with interrupted fine nylon or skin staples.

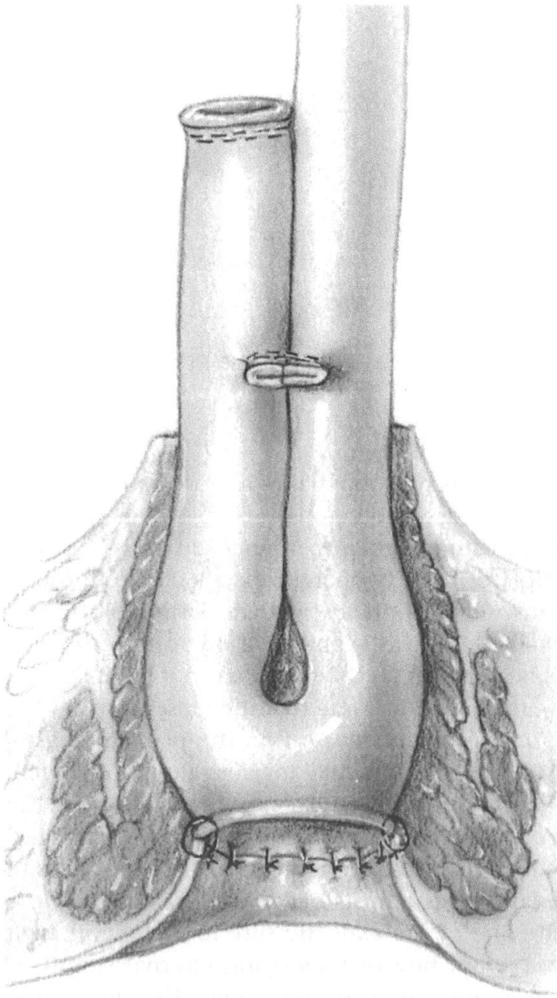

Fig. 10-12

Then mature the loop ileostomy as described above if this step has not already been done.

## POSTOPERATIVE CARE

Continue perioperative antibiotics for 24 hours. Continue nasogastric suction until the ileostomy begins to function. Remove the closed-suction drains from the pelvis between postoperative days 4 and 6, depending on the volume of drainage. (Inject 25 mg kanamycin in 25 ml saline into the drainage catheters every 8 hours.)

Until the loop ileostomy is closed, perform weekly or biweekly digital examinations of the ileoanal anastomosis to prevent the development of a stricture. About 8 weeks following operation, rule out anastomotic defects by direct inspection and palpation. If there has been uneventful healing with no evidence of hematoma or sepsis in the pelvis, perform a barium enema to visualize the ileal reservoir. If both these procedures are negative, close the loop ileostomy. Following closure of the loop ileostomy, regulation of the bowel movements takes time and sometimes requires dietary adjustment and medication to achieve optimum continence.

## COMPLICATIONS

An abscess may occur in the rectal cuff or pelvis. This complication has been reported during the early postoperative period and, remarkably, 2 and 6 months after operation in other cases. If the loop ileostomy is still in place, most cuff abscesses can be treated by drainage directly through the anastomosis. Pelvic abscesses may require laparotomy or computed tomography-guided percutaneous catheter insertion for drainage. With proper precautions postoperative sepsis is rare.

Hematoma in pelvis or in reservoir.

Anastomotic dehiscence or stricture.

Wound infection.

Urinary tract infection.

Excessive number of stools.

Fecal incontinence.

Pouchitis (more likely to occur in patients with inflammatory bowel disease). Treatment with metronidazole may be sufficient.

Pouch surveillance is performed in patients with familial polyposis syndromes. Polyps have been known to form in the ileal reservoir.

Acute intestinal obstruction due to adhesions.

## REFERENCES

Burnstein MJ, Schoetz DJ Jr, Collier JA, et al. Technique of mesenteric lengthening in ileal reservoir-anal anastomosis. Dis Colon Rectum 1987;30:863.

Cohen Z, McLeod RS, Stephen W, et al. Continuing evolution of the pelvic pouch procedure. Ann Surg 1992;216:506.

Dehni N, Schlegel RD, Cunningham C, et al. Influence of a defunctioning stoma on leakage rates after low colorectal anastomosis and colonic J pouch-anal anastomosis. Br J Surg 1998;85:1114.

Fazio VW, O'Riordain MG, Lavery IC, et al. Long-term functional outcome and quality of life after stapled restorative proctocolectomy. Ann Surg 1999;230:575.

McCourtney JS, Finlay IG. Totally stapled restorative proctocolectomy. Br J Surg 1997;84:808.

Meagher AP, Farouk R, Dozois RR, Kelly KA, Pemberton H. J-Ileal pouch-anal anastomosis for chronic ulcerative colitis: complications and long-term outcome in 1310 patients. Br J Surg 1998;85:800.

Michelassi F, Hurst R. Restorative proctocolectomy with J-pouch ileoanal anastomosis. Arch Surg 2000;135:347.

Mowschenson PM, Critchlow JF, Peppercorn MA. Ileoanal pouch operation: long-term outcome with or without diverting ileostomy. Arch Surg 2000;135:463.

Reilly WT, Pemberton JH, Wolff BG, et al. Randomized prospective trial comparing ileal pouch-anal anastomosis performed by excising the anal mucosa to ileal pouch-anal anastomosis performed by preserving the anal mucosa. Ann Surg 1997;225:666.

Sullivan ES, Garnjobst WM. Advantage of initial transanal musocal stripping in ileo-anal pull-through procedures. Dis Colon Rectum 1982;25:170.

Thompson-Fawcett MW, Warren BF, Mortensen NJ. A new look at the anal transitional zone with reference to restorative proctocolectomy and the columnar cuff. Br J Surg 1998;85:1517.

# 11 Abdominoperineal Proctectomy for Benign Disease

## INDICATIONS

Inflammatory bowel disease, including ulcerative colitis and Crohn's colitis with intractable rectal involvement that precludes restorative proctocolectomy.

## PREOPERATIVE PREPARATION

See Chapter 10.

## PITFALLS AND DANGER POINTS

Operative damage to or interruption of pelvic autonomic nerves in male patients, leading to sexual impotence or failure of ejaculation

Pelvis sepsis, especially in patients who have perineal fistulas

Inadequate management of perineal wound, resulting in a chronic perineal draining sinus

## OPERATIVE STRATEGY

Abdominoperineal proctectomy is not a cancer operation. Resection should be conservative, and every attempt should be made to avoid damage to adjacent structures.

Transection of the hypogastric sympathetic nerve trunks that cross over the anterior aorta causes ejaculatory failure in men. Beyond the aortic bifurcation these nerves diverge into two bundles going toward the region of the right and left hypogastric arteries, where they join the inferior hypogastric plexus on each side. According to Lee et al. (1973) the *parasympathetic* sacral autonomic outflow is interrupted if the lateral ligaments are divided too far lateral to the rectum or if the nerve plexus between the rectum and prostate is damaged. Parasympathetic nerve damage results in failure of erection. Proper strategy requires that the mesentery in the region of the rectosigmoid be divided along a line just adjacent to the colon, leaving considerable fat and mesentery in the presacral space to protect the hypogastric nerves. The remainder of the pelvic dissection should be carried out as close to the rectum as possible, *especially in the region of the lateral ligaments and prostate.*

So long as there are no multiple perineal fistulas, it is generally possible to achieve primary healing of the perineum *if deadspace between the closed levators and the peritoneal pelvic floor is eliminated.* Because there is no need for radical excision of the pelvic peritoneum, preserve as much of it as possible and mobilize additional pelvic peritoneum from the lateral walls of the pelvis and the bladder. If there is sufficient peritoneum to permit the pelvic peritoneal suture line to come down easily into contact with the reconstructed levator diaphragm, close this layer. Otherwise it is much better to leave the pelvic peritoneum entirely unsutured to permit the small bowel to fill this space. To aid in preventing perineal sinus formation due to chronic low-grade sepsis, insert closed-suction catheters into the presacral space and instill an antibiotic solution postoperatively.

Lyttle and Parks (1977) advocate *preservation of the external sphincter muscles.* They begin the perineal dissection with an incision near the dentate line of the anal canal and continue the dissection in the intersphincteric space between the internal and external sphincters of the anal canal. Thus the rectum is cored out of the anal canal, leaving the entire levator diaphragm and external sphincters intact. We have used this technique and found that it causes less operative trauma, minimizes deadspace, and may further reduce the incidence of damage to the prerectal nerve plexus.

## OPERATIVE TECHNIQUE

### Abdominal Incision and Position

With the patient positioned on Lloyd-Davies leg rests, thighs abducted and slightly flexed, make a midline incision from the mid-epigastrium to the pubis (see

Fig. 6–3a). If the patient has previously undergone subtotal colectomy with ileostomy and mucous fistula, free the mucous fistula from its attachments to the abdominal wall. Ligate the lumen with umbilical tape and cover it with a sterile rubber glove.

### *Mesenteric Dissection*

Divide the mesentery between sequentially applied Kelly clamps along a line *close to the posterior wall* of the rectosigmoid. Continue the line of dissection well into the presacral space. This leaves a considerable amount of fat and mesentery behind to cover the bifurcation of the aorta and sacrum **(Fig. 11–1)**. The fat and mesentery prevent injury to the hypogastric nerve bundles, which travel from the preaortic area down the promontory of the sacrum toward the hypogastric vessels on each side to join the hypogastric plexuses on each side (see Figs. 6–4, 6–6).

## Rectal Dissection

Incise the pelvic peritoneum along the line where the peritoneum joins the rectum, preserving as much peritoneum as possible. Accomplish this first on the right and then on the left side (see Fig. 6–5). Note the location of each ureter (see Fig. 6–6). Divide the posterior mesentery to the mid-sacral level. The posterior wall of rectum can now be seen, as at this point

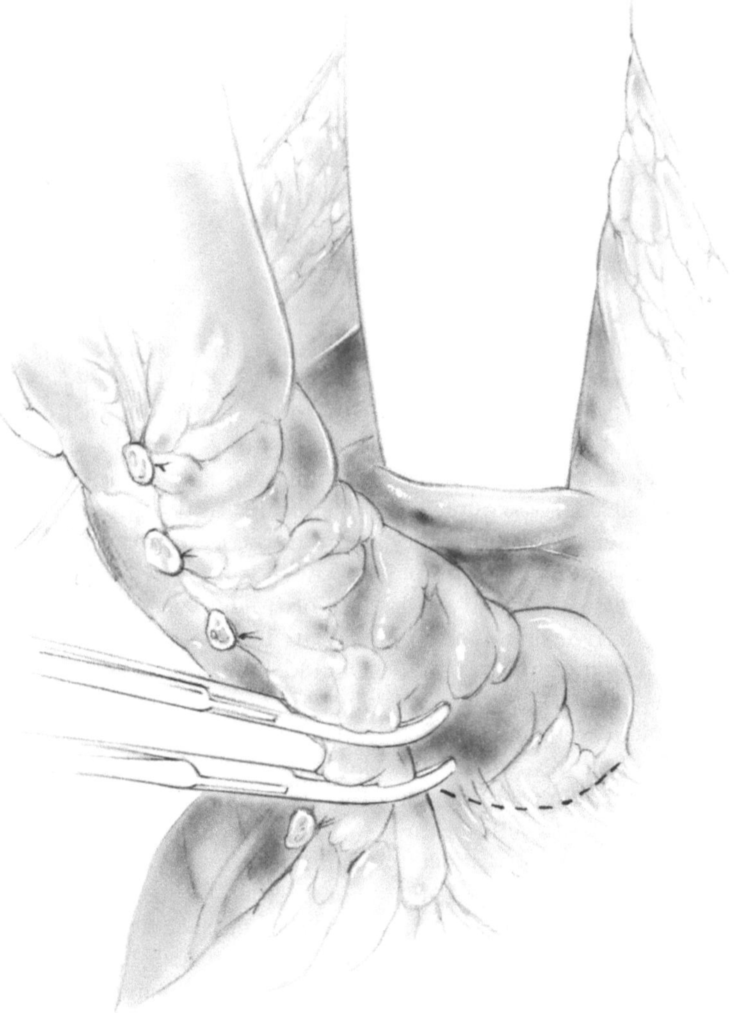

Fig. 11–1

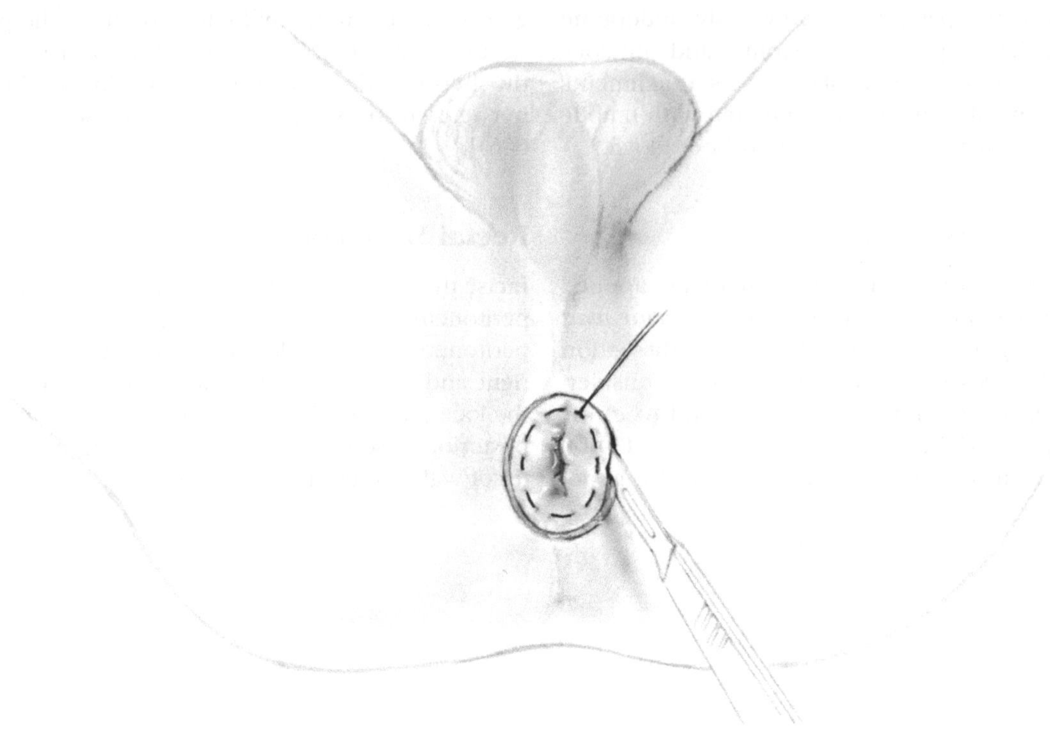

Fig. 11-2

the blood supply of the rectum comes from the lateral wall of the pelvis. Elevate the rectum from the distal sacrum by blunt dissection and with Metzenbaum scissors incise Waldeyer's fascia close to the rectum. Draw the rectum in a cephalad direction and place the peritoneum of the rectovesical or rectouterine pouch on stretch. This peritoneum can now be divided easily with Metzenbaum scissors. Division of the lateral ligament can also be accomplished with good hemostasis by inserting a right-angle clamp underneath the ligament and dividing the overlying tissue with electrocautery (see Fig. 6-9).

With cephalad traction on the rectum and a Lloyd-Davies retractor holding the bladder forward, divide Denonvilliers' fascia at the level of the proximal portion of the prostate (see Fig. 6-11b). Keep the dissection *close to the anterior rectal wall*, which should be bluntly separated from the body of the prostate. In female patients, the dissection separates the rectum from the vagina. When the dissection has continued beyond the tip of the coccyx posteriorly and the prostate anteriorly, initiate the perineal dissection.

## Perineal Incision

Close the skin of the anal canal with a heavy pursestring suture **(Fig. 11–2)**. Then make an incision circumferentially in the skin just outside the sphincter muscles of the anus. Carry the dissection down *close* to the outer margins of the external sphincter to the levator muscles **(Fig. 11–3)**. The inferior hemorrhoidal vessels are encountered running toward the rectum overlying the levator muscles. Occlude these vessels by electrocautery. After the incision has been deepened to the levators on both sides, expose the tip of the coccyx. Transect the anococcygeal ligament by electrocautery and enter the presacral space posteriorly. The fascia of Waldeyer, which attaches to the anterior surfaces of the lower sacrum and coccyx and to the posterior rectum, forms a barrier that blocks entrance into the presacral space from below even after the anococcygeal ligament has been divided. If this fascia is elevated from the sacral periosteum by forceful blunt dissection in the perineum, venous bleeding and damage to the sacral neural

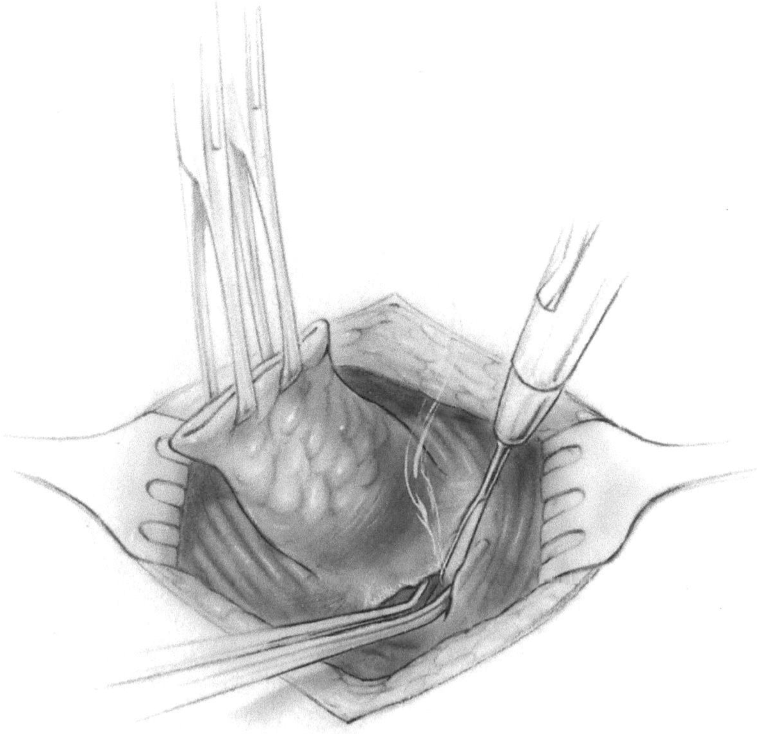

Fig. 11-3

components of the nervi erigentes may occur. Consequently, divide this *sharply* from above (Fig. 6-10) or below before an attempt is made to enter the presacral space from below.

### *Division of Levator Diaphragm*

From the perineal approach, insert the left index finger into the opening to the presacral space and place it in the groove between the rectum and the levator muscles. Use electrocautery to divide the levators close to the rectum on either side. Then deliver the specimen from the presacral space down through the posterior perineum, so the anal canal is attached only anteriorly. Visualize the prostate gland. Using electrocautery, transect the puborectalis and rectourethralis muscles close to the anterior rectal wall. Carry this dissection down to the level of the prostate and remove the specimen.

### *Closure of Pelvic Floor*

Insert one or two large (6mm) plastic catheters through the skin of the perineum and the levator muscles into the presacral space for closed-suction drainage. Alternatively, these drains may be brought up from the presacral space into the pelvis and out through puncture wounds of the abdominal wall.

Close the defect in the levator diaphragm using interrupted sutures of 2-0 PG after thoroughly irrigating the pelvis with an antibiotic solution and achieving perfect hemostasis **(Fig. 11–4)**. Close the skin with subcuticular sutures of 4-0 PG. Attach the catheters to suction for the remainder of the procedure while an assistant closes the peritoneum of the pelvic floor with continuous 2-0 PG sutures using the abdominal approach.

## Ileostomy

Choose a suitable site and construct a terminal ileostomy as described in Chapter 50 (if not already performed during a previous operation).

## Abdominal Closure

After checking the integrity of the peritoneal pelvic suture line and making certain it is contiguous with the pelvic floor, irrigate the abdominal cavity and pelvis. Approximate the abdominal wall with inter-

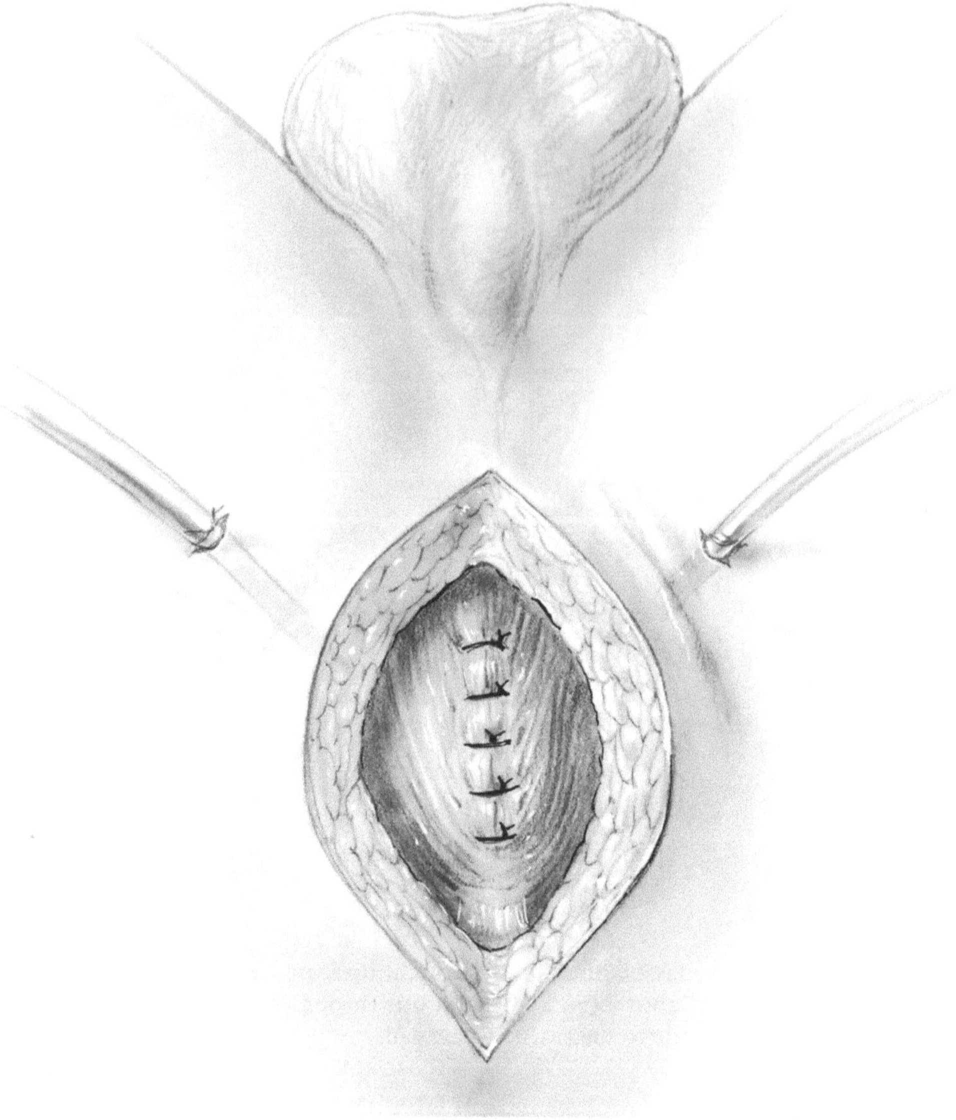

Fig. 11-4

rupted sutures using the modified Smead-Jones technique.

## POSTOPERATIVE CARE

See Chapter 7.

## COMPLICATIONS

See Chapter 7.

## REFERENCES

Lee JF, Maurer VM, Block GE. Anatomic relations of pelvic autonomic nerves to pelvic operations. Arch Surg 1973; 107:324.

Lyttle JA, Parks AG. Intersphincteric excision of the rectum. Br J Surg 1977;64:413.

O'Bichere A, Wilkinson K, Rumbles S, et al. Functional outcome after restorative panproctocolectomy for ulcerative colitis decreases an otherwise enhanced quality of life. Br J Surg 2000;87:802.

# 12 End-Ileostomy

## INDICATIONS

An end-ileostomy is generally done in conjunction with a subtotal or total colectomy for inflammatory bowel disease. Continent alternatives have been developed (see References).

Occasionally a temporary end-ileostomy and mucous fistula of the distal end of the bowel is constructed after resection of a gangrenous segment of intestine or a perforated cecal lesion, when primary anastomosis is contraindicated.

## PITFALLS AND DANGER POINTS

Devascularization of an excessive amount of terminal ileum, with resultant necrosis and stricture formation

Ileocutaneous fistula resulting from a too-deep stitch in the seromuscular layer of the ileum when fashioning the ileostomy

## OPERATIVE STRATEGY

Prevention of peristomal skin excoriation (due to escape of small bowel contents underneath the faceplate of the ileostomy appliance) requires formation of a permanently protruding ileostomy. Properly performed, the ileostomy resembles the cervix of the uterus. A permanent protrusion of 2.0 cm is desirable, which allows for the likelihood that an underweight patient accumulates a subcutaneous layer of fat following successful surgery for colitis. To prevent herniation of the small bowel, close the gap between the cut edge of the ileum and the lateral abdominal wall when fashioning a permanent ileostomy.

## OPERATIVE TECHNIQUE

### Preoperative Selection of Ileostomy Site

Apply the face-plate of an ileostomy appliance tentatively to various positions in the right lower quadrant of the patient to make sure it does not come into contact with the costal margin or the anterosuperior spine when the patient is in a sitting position. The face-plate should not extend beyond the mid-rectus line or the umbilicus. During emergency operations, when an ileostomy has not been contemplated, the site for the ileostomy should be placed approximately 5 cm to the right of the midline and about 4 cm below the umbilicus.

### Incision

Because ileostomy generally is not the main part of the contemplated operation, a midline incision has already been made. Now make a circular incision in the previously selected site in the right lower quadrant and excise a circle of skin the diameter of a nickel (2 cm) **(Fig. 12–1)**. The incision then spontaneously stretches to the proper diameter. Make a linear incision down to the anterior rectus fascia and insert retractors to expose the fascia. Do not excise a core of subcutaneous fat unless the patient is significantly obese.

Make a longitudinal 2 cm incision in the fascia, exposing the rectus muscle **(Fig. 12–2)**. Separate the muscle fibers with a Kelly hemostat **(Fig. 12–3)** and make a longitudinal incision in the peritoneum. Then dilate the opening in the abdominal wall by inserting two fingers **(Fig. 12–4)**.

### Fashioning the Ileal Mesentery

At least 6–7 cm of ileum is required beyond the point at which the ileum meets the peritoneum if a proper

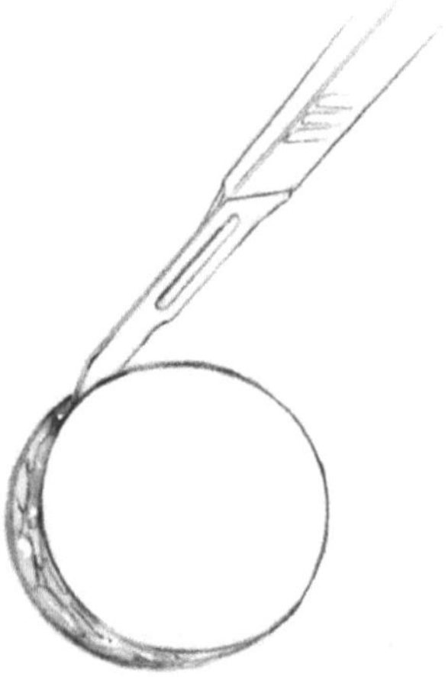

Fig. 12-1

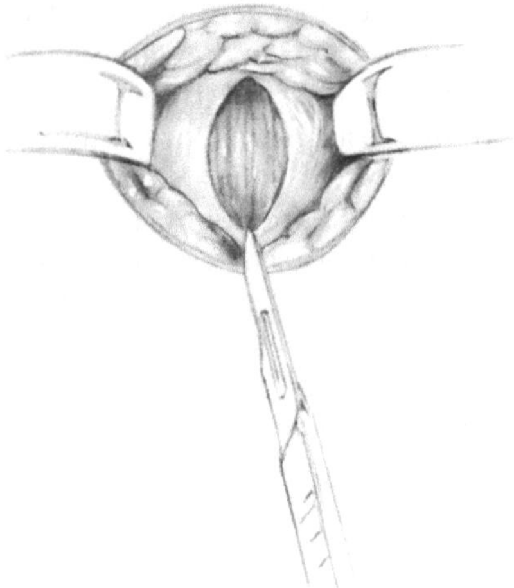

Fig. 12-2

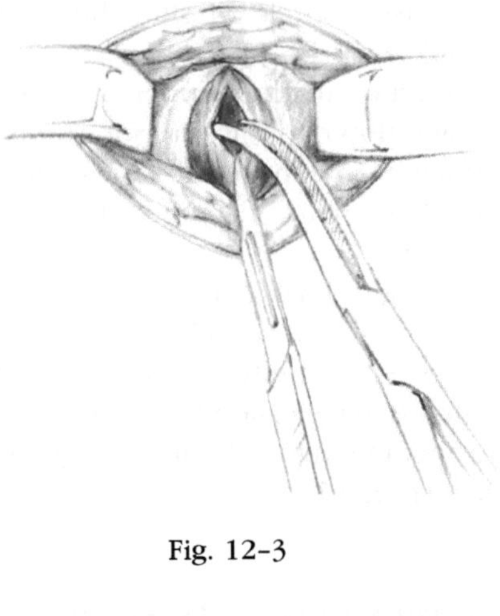

Fig. 12-3

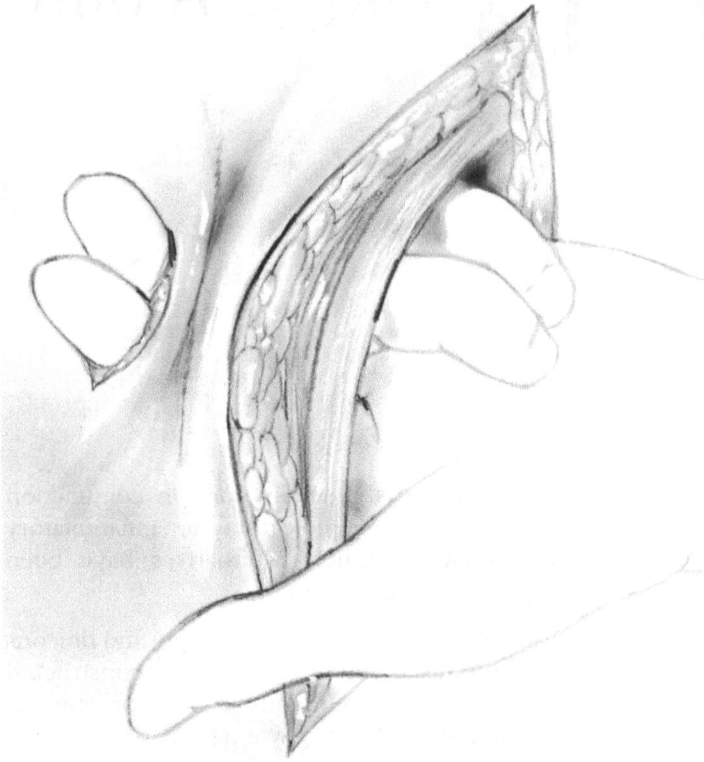

Fig. 12-4

ileostomy of the protruding type is to be made. More length may be required in the obese patient. If the entire mesentery is removed from this length of ileum, necrosis of the distal ileal mucosa takes place in many patients. Consequently, the portion of the ileum that passes through the abdominal wall must retain a sufficient width of mesentery to ensure vascularity. The "marginal" artery can be visualized in the mesentery within 2 cm of the ileal wall. Preserve this segment of vasculature while carefully dividing the mesentery. Complete removal of the mesentery is well tolerated at the distal 2–3 cm of the ileum.

## Closure of Mesenteric Gap

Insert a Babcock clamp into the abdominal cavity through the opening made for the ileostomy. Grasp the terminal ileum with the clamp and gently bring it through this opening, with the mesentery placed in a cephalad direction **(Fig. 12–5)**. Place no sutures between the ileum and the peritoneum or the rectus fascia **(Fig. 12–6)**.

Using a continuous 2-0 PG suture, suture the cut edge of the ileal mesentery to the cut edge of the paracolic peritoneum. This maneuver completely obliterates the mesenteric defect **(Fig. 12–7)**.

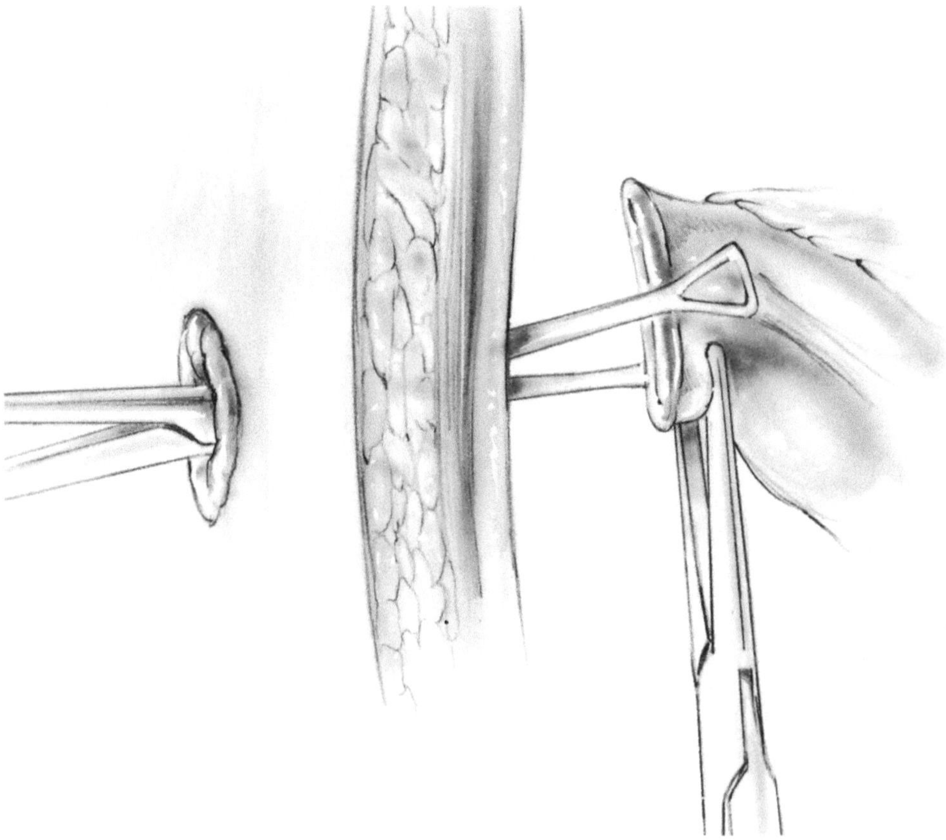

Fig. 12-5

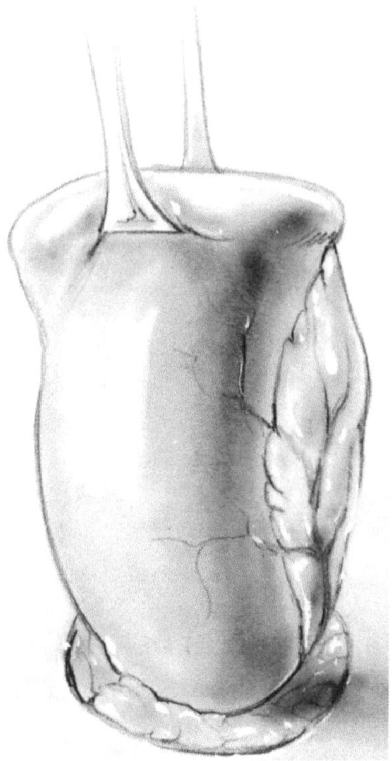

Fig. 12-6

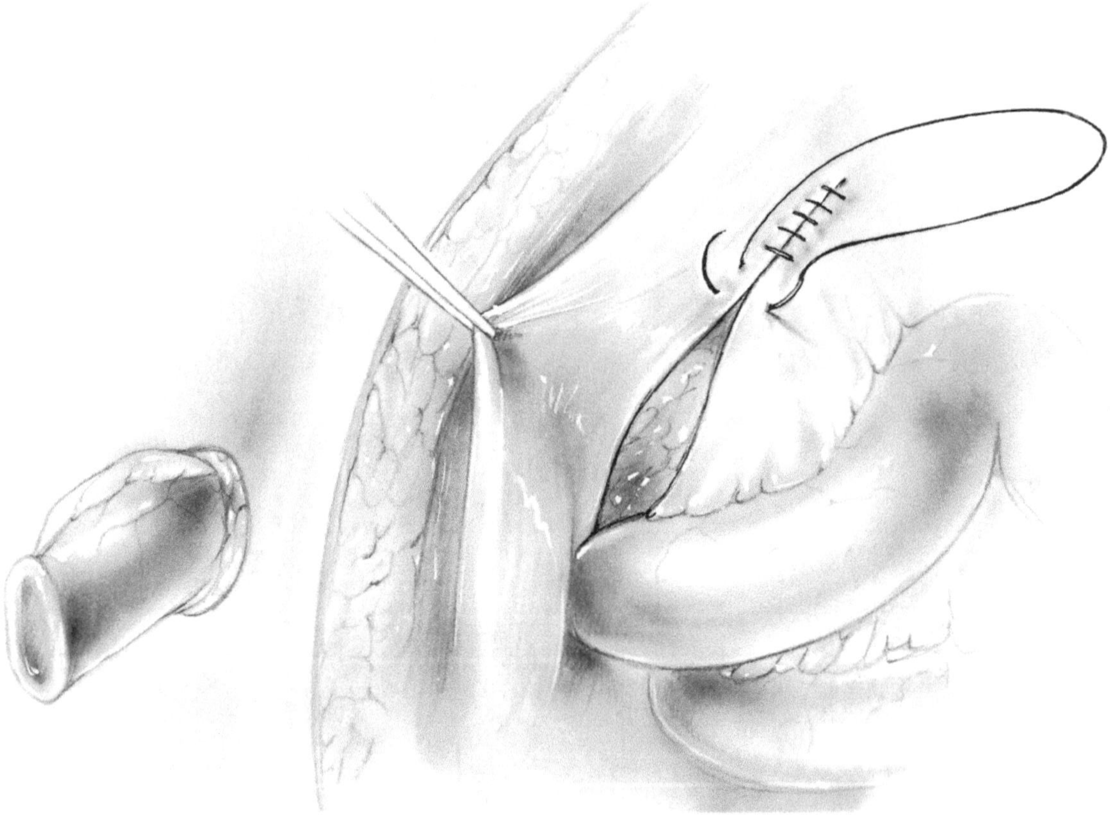

Fig. 12–7

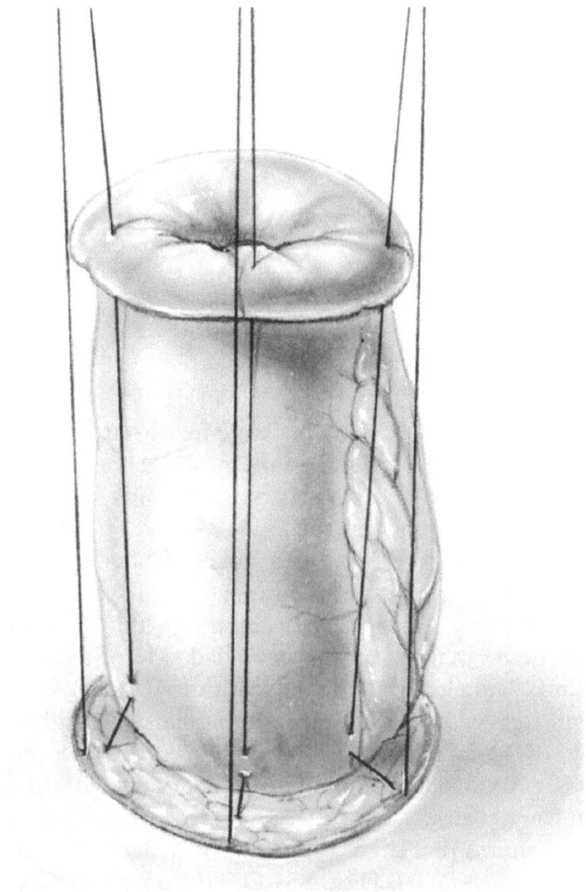

Fig. 12-8

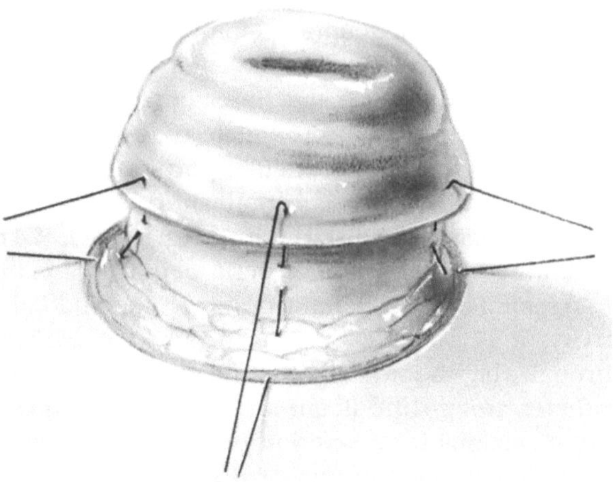

Fig. 12-9

## Mucocutaneous Fixation of Ileostomy

Construct a "cervix" by inserting interrupted 4-0 PG sutures through the full thickness of the terminal ileum; then, using the same needle, take a shallow seromuscular bite of the lateral wall of the ileum, which is situated opposite the level of the skin. Complete the suture by taking a bite of the subcuticular layer of skin **(Fig. 12–8)**. Temporarily hold the stitch in a hemostat and place identical stitches in each of the other quadrants of the ileostomy. After all the sutures have been inserted tighten them gently to evert the ileum **(Fig. 12–9)**. Then tie the sutures. Place one additional suture of the same type between each of the four quadrant sutures, completing the mucocutaneous fixation.

# POSTOPERATIVE CARE

Nasogastric suction may be required, depending on the nature of the primary procedure.

Prescribe perioperative antibiotics.

Apply a Stomahesive disk to the ileostomy in the operating room; place an ileostomy bag over the disk.

Instruct the patient in ileostomy care.

# COMPLICATIONS

Early problems

Occasional necrosis of the distal ileum (although rare when good technique is used)

Peristomal infection or fistula

Late problems

Prolapse of ileostomy

Stricture of ileostomy

Obstruction of ileostomy due to food fiber

Peristomal skin ulceration

# REFERENCE

Dozois RR. Alternative to Conventional Ileostomy. Chicago, Year Book, 1985.

# 13 Loop Ileostomy

## INDICATIONS

Loop ileostomy is performed when temporary diversion of the fecal stream is required. It may be used to protect a tenuous colon anastomosis or as part of the initial treatment of severe inflammatory bowel disease.

In some patients loop ileostomy is easier to construct than end-ileostomy. It allows better preservation of the blood supply to the stoma.

## PITFALLS AND DANGER POINTS

If the ileum is not transected at the proper point, to make the proximal stoma the dominant one, total fecal diversion is not accomplished.

See Chapter 12.

## OPERATIVE STRATEGY

Properly performed, this technique is a good method for achieving temporary but complete diversion of the intestinal contents. Because the entire mesentery is preserved, the blood supply to the stoma is optimized. Closure can be accomplished by a local plastic procedure or by local resection and anastomosis.

## OPERATIVE TECHNIQUE

If a loop ileostomy is being performed as a primary procedure, a midline incision beginning at the umbilicus and proceeding caudally for 8–10 cm is adequate. Identify the distal ileum and the segment selected for ileostomy by applying a single marking suture to that segment of the ileum that will form the *proximal* limb of the loop ileostomy.

Select the proper site in the right lower quadrant (see Chapter 12) and excise a nickel-size circle of skin. Expose the anterior rectus fascia and make a 2 cm longitudinal incision in it (see Fig. 12–1). Separate the rectus fibers with a large hemostat and make a similar vertical incision in the peritoneum (see Figs. 12–2, 12–3). Then stretch the ileostomy orifice by inserting two fingers (see Fig. 12–4).

After this step has been accomplished, insert a Babcock clamp through the aperture into the abdominal cavity. Arrange the ileum so the proximal segment emerges on the cephalad side of the ileostomy. Then grasp the ileum with the Babcock clamp and deliver it through the abdominal wall with the aid of digital manipulation from inside the abdomen. The proximal limb should be on the cephalad surface of the ileostomy.

Confirm that there is no tension whatever on any distal anastomosis **(Fig. 13–1)**. Position the ileum so the afferent or proximal limb of ileum enters the stoma from its cephalad aspect and the distal ileum leaves the stoma at its inferior aspect. To ensure that the proximal stoma dominates the distal stoma and completely diverts the fecal stream, transect the anterior half of the ileum at a point 2 cm distal to the apex of the loop **(Fig. 13–2)**. Then evert the ileostomy **(Fig. 13–3)**. Insert interrupted atraumatic sutures of 4-0 PG to approximate the full thickness of the ileum to the subcuticular portion of the skin. The end result should be a dominant proximal stoma that compresses the distal stoma **(Fig. 13–4)**. We do not suture the ileum to the peritoneum or fascia.

To minimize contamination of the abdominal cavity, it is possible to deliver the loop of ileum through the abdominal wall and then pass a small catheter around the ileum and through the mesentery to maintain the position of the ileum. Division of the ileum and suturing of the ileostomy may be postponed until the abdominal incision has been completely closed. After suturing the ileum to the subcutis, remove the catheter.

Close the abdominal wall with interrupted No. 1 PDS sutures by the modified Smead-Jones technique. Close the skin with interrupted fine nylon or skin staples. Then mature the loop ileostomy as described above if this step has not already been done.

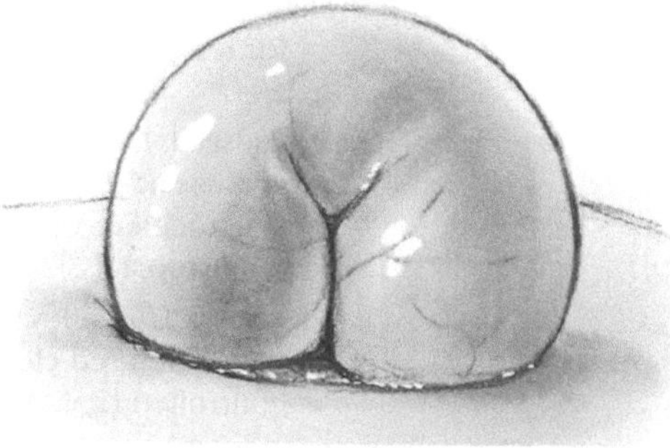

Fig. 13-1

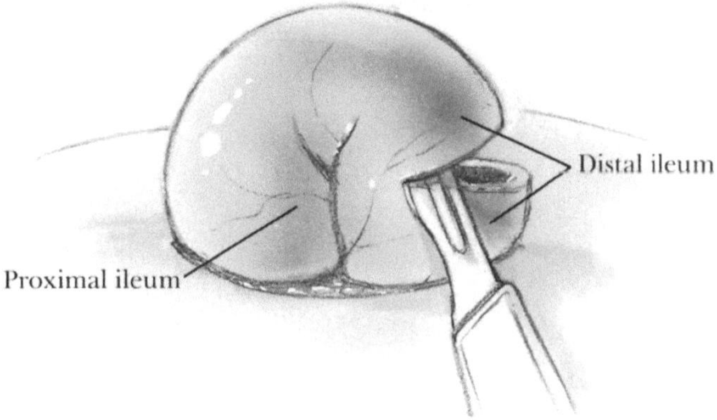


Fig. 13-2

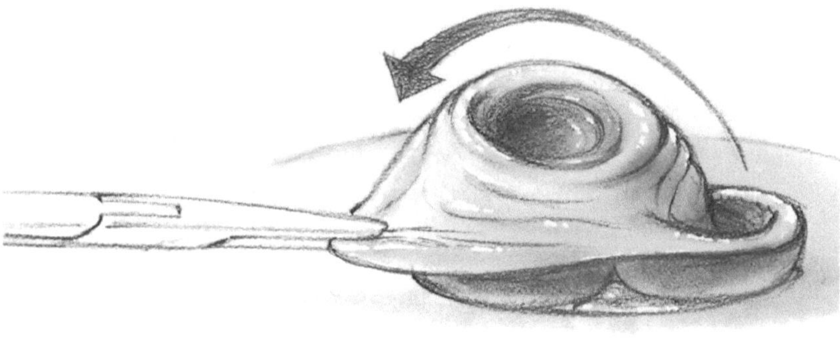

Fig. 13-3

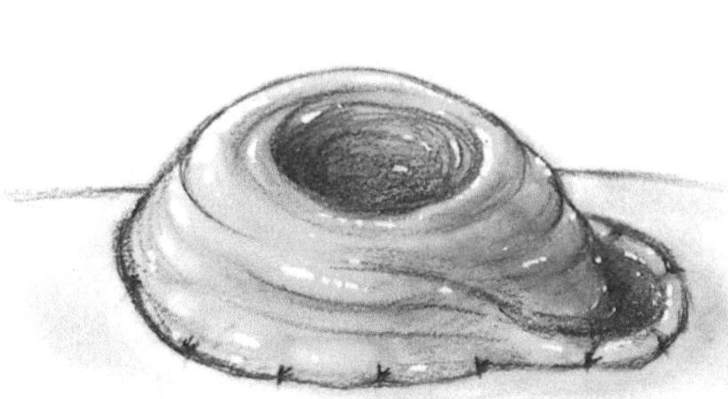

Fig. 13-4

## POSTOPERATIVE CARE

See Chapter 12.

## COMPLICATIONS

See Chapter 12.

## REFERENCES

Beagley MJ, Poole G, Peat BG, Rees MJ. The use of temporary laparoscopic loop ileostomy in lumbosacral burns. Burns 2000;26:298.

Flati G, Talarico C, Carboni M. An improved technique for temporary diverting ileostomy. Surg Today 2000;30:104.

Fonkalsrud EW, Thakur A, Roof L. Comparison of loop versus end ileostomy for fecal diversion after restorative proctocolectomy for ulcerative colitis. J Am Coll Surg 2000;190:418.

Hasegawa H, Radley S, Morton DG, Keighley MR. Stapled versus sutured closure of loop ileostomy: a randomized controlled trial. Ann Surg 2000;231:202.

Lane JS, Kwan D, Chandler CF, et al. Diverting loop versus end ileostomy during ileoanal pullthrough procedure for ulcerative colitis. Am Surg 1998;64:979.

Turnbull R, Weakley FL. Surgical treatment of toxic megacolon: ileostomy and colostomy to prepare patients for colectomy. Am J Surg 1971;122:325.

# 14 Cecostomy

## Surgical Legacy Technique

## INDICATIONS

Cecostomy is an alternative to resection when there is impending perforation of the cecum secondary to a colonic obstruction or ileus. Colonoscopic decompression is a better alternative for cases of pseudo-obstruction. Cecostomy is used only when other methods have failed.

## PREOPERATIVE PREPARATION

Perioperative antibiotics

Nasogastric suction

Fluid resuscitation

## PITFALLS AND DANGER POINTS

Cecostomy may fail to produce adequate decompression.

Limited exploration through a small incision may miss an area of perforation elsewhere.

Fecal matter may spill into the peritoneal cavity.

## OPERATIVE STRATEGY

There are two kinds of cecostomy. A simple tube cecostomy is constructed in a manner analogous to a Stamm gastrostomy. Even a large tube is easily plugged by fecal debris, and this kind of cecostomy primarily allows decompression of gas and liquid. The main advantage of tube cecostomy is that when the cecostomy is no longer needed removing the tube frequently results in spontaneous closure. The skin-sutured cecostomy described here provides more certain decompression but requires formal closure. In the attempt to avoid fecal contamination of the abdominal cavity during this operation, the cecum is sutured to the external oblique aponeurosis before being incised.

## OPERATIVE TECHNIQUE

### Skin-Sutured Cecostomy

#### *Incision*

Make a transverse incision about 4–5 cm long over McBurney's point and carry it in the same line through the skin, external oblique aponeurosis, the internal oblique and transversus muscles, and the peritoneum. Do not attempt to split the muscles along the line of their fibers.

#### *Exploration of Cecum*

Rule out patches of necrosis in areas beyond the line of incision by carefully exploring the cecum. To accomplish this without the danger of rupturing the cecum, insert a 16-gauge needle attached to an empty 50 cc syringe, which releases some of the pressure. After this has been accomplished, close the puncture wound with a fine suture. Elevate the abdominal wall with a retractor to expose the anterior and lateral walls of the cecum. If the exposure is inadequate, make a larger incision. If a necrotic patch of cecum can be identified, use this region as the site for the cecostomy and excise it during the procedure.

#### *Cecal Fixation*

Suture the wall of the cecum to the external oblique aponeurosis with a continuous 4-0 PG suture on a fine needle to prevent any fecal spillage from reaching the peritoneal cavity **(Fig. 14–1)**. If the incision in the external oblique aponeurosis is longer than 4–5 cm, narrow it with several PG sutures. Narrow the skin incision also to the same length with several fine PG subcuticular sutures.

#### *Mucocutaneous Suture*

Make a transverse incision in the anterior wall of the cecum 4 cm long **(Fig. 14–2)** and aspirate liquid stool and gas. Then suture the full thickness of the

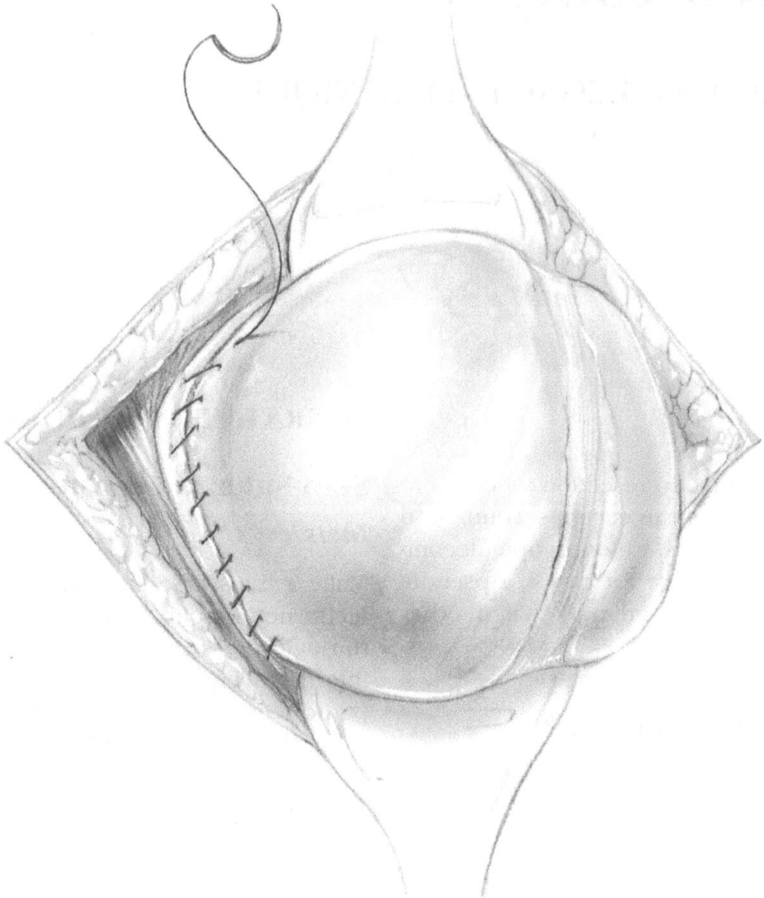

Fig. 14–1

cecal wall to the subcuticular layer of the skin with a continuous or interrupted suture of 4-0 PG on an atraumatic needle **(Fig. 14–3)**. Place a properly fitted ileostomy bag over the cecostomy at the conclusion of the operation.

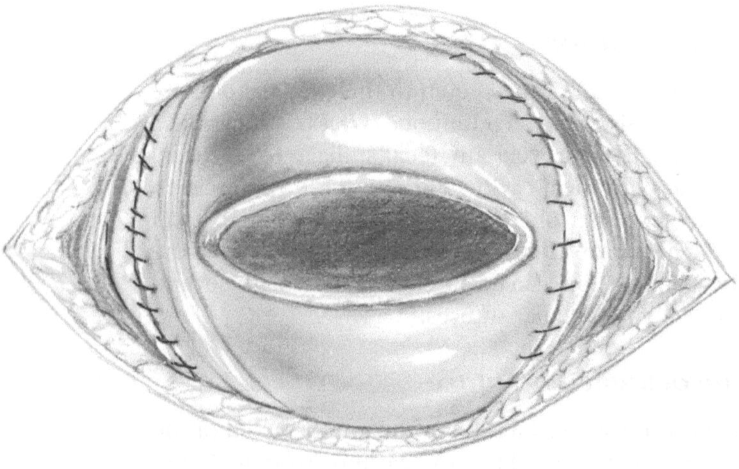

Fig. 14–2

## Tube Cecostomy

The abdominal incision and exploration of the cecum for a tube cecostomy are identical to those done for a skin-sutured cecostomy. Insert a purse-string suture in a circular fashion on the anterior wall of the cecum using 3-0 atraumatic PG. The diameter of the circle should be 1.5 cm. Insert a second purse-string suture outside the first, using the same suture material. Then make a stab wound in the middle of the purse-string suture; insert a 36F soft-rubber tube into the suture and for about 5–6 cm into the ascending

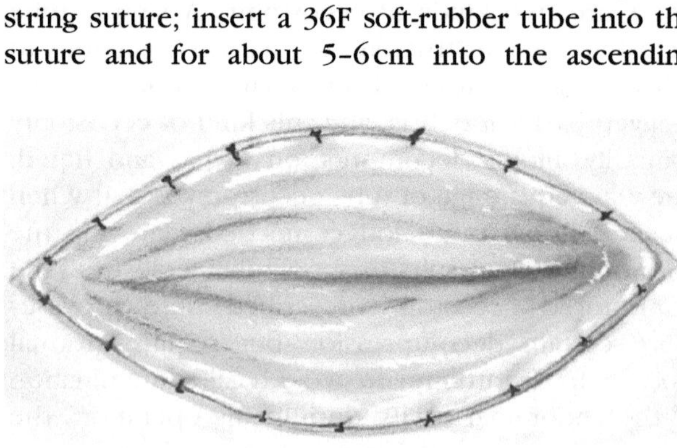

Fig. 14–3

colon. Tie the first purse-string suture around the rubber tube; then tie the second purse-string suture so as to invert the first. It is helpful if several large side-holes have been cut first in the distal 3–4 cm of the rubber tube.

Select a site about 3 cm above the incision for a stab wound. Bring out the rubber tube through this stab wound and suture the cecum to the peritoneum around the stab wound. Use four interrupted 3-0 PG atraumatic sutures to keep the peritoneal cavity free of any fecal matter that may leak around the tube.

Close the abdominal incision in a single layer by the modified Smead-Jones technique using interrupted 1-0 PDS sutures. Do not close the skin wound; insert several 4-0 nylon interrupted skin sutures, which will be tied 3–5 days after operation.

## POSTOPERATIVE CARE

Manage the skin-sutured cecostomy in the operating room by applying an adhesive-backed ileostomy-type disposable plastic appliance to it. The tube cecostomy requires repeated irrigation with saline to prevent it from being plugged by fecal particles. It may be removed after the tenth postoperative day if it is no longer needed.

## COMPLICATIONS

The major postoperative complication of this procedure is peristomal sepsis, as the possibility of bacterial contamination of the abdominal incision cannot be completely eliminated. Nevertheless, peristomal sepsis is much less common than one would anticipate with an operation of this type.

## REFERENCE

Duh QY, Way LW. Diagnostic laparoscopy and laparoscopic cecostomy for colonic pseudoobstruction. Dis Colon Rectum 1993;36:65.

# 15 Transverse Colostomy

## INDICATIONS

Relief of obstruction due to lesions of the left colon

Diversion of fecal stream

Complementary to left colon anastomosis (see also Chapter 13)

## PREOPERATIVE PREPARATION

Before performing a colostomy for colonic obstruction, confirm the diagnosis by barium enema, colonoscopy, or computed tomography (CT) of the abdomen.

Use a preoperative flat radiograph of the abdomen to identify the position of the transverse colon relative to a fixed point, such as a coin placed over the umbilicus.

Apply fluid resuscitation.

Place a nasogastric tube.

Prescribe perioperative antibiotics.

## PITFALLS AND DANGER POINTS

Performing colostomy in error for diagnoses such as fecal impaction or pseudo-obstruction

Be certain the "ostomy" is, in fact, being constructed in the transverse colon, not in the redundant sigmoid colon, jejunum, or even the gastric antrum.

With advanced colonic obstruction, be aware of the possibility of impending cecal rupture for which transverse colostomy is an inadequate operation unless the cecum is seen to be viable.

## OPERATIVE STRATEGY

### Impending Rupture of Cecum

For routine cases of left colon obstruction, with the diagnosis confirmed by barium enema radiography, the colon may be approached through a small transverse incision in the right rectus muscle. This incision should be made for the colostomy alone; the rest of the abdominal cavity does not have to be explored. Exceptions to this policy should be made for patients with a sigmoid volvulus, those suspected to have ischemic colitis or perforation, and those in whom an advanced obstruction threatens cecal rupture.

When impending rupture is suspected, direct visual inspection of the cecum is mandatory. This may be accomplished with a midline laparotomy incision or a transverse right lower quadrant incision made over the cecum. Cecal necrosis or perforation mandates resection, usually with ileostomy and mucous fistula.

### Diversion of Fecal Stream

Contrary to widespread medical opinion, it is not necessary to construct a double-barreled colostomy with complete transection of the colon to divert the stool from entering the left colon. We agree with Turnbull and Weakley (1967) that if a 5 cm longitudinal incision is made on the antimesenteric wall of the transverse colon and is followed by immediate maturation, fecal diversion is accomplished even in the absence of a supporting glass rod. The long incision in the colon permits the posterior wall to prolapse, resulting in functionally separate distal and proximal stomas.

## OPERATIVE TECHNIQUE

### Incision

Make a transverse incision over the middle and lateral thirds of the upper right rectus muscle **(Fig. 15–1)**. Ideally the length of the skin incision equals the length of the longitudinal incision to be made in the colon (5-6 cm). To accomplish this it is necessary to identify the level at which the transverse colon

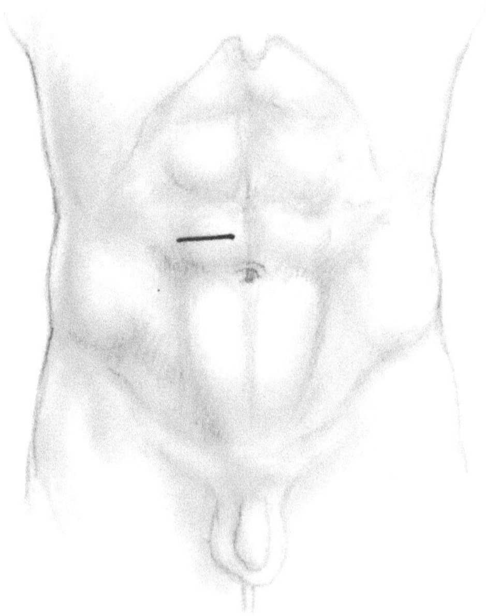

Fig. 15-1

crosses the path of the right rectus muscle. It may be done on a preoperative flat radiograph of the abdomen, followed by confirmation using percussion of the upper abdomen in the operating room. Make the transverse incision sufficiently long to accomplish accurate identification of the transverse colon. The incision will be partially closed, leaving a 5 cm gap to accommodate the colostomy.

When the transverse colostomy is to precede a subsequent laparotomy for removal of colon pathology, begin the transverse incision 2 cm to the right of the midline and extend it laterally. If this is done, the colostomy does not prevent the surgeon from using a long midline incision for the second stage of the operation.

After the skin incision is made, incise the anterior rectus fascia with a scalpel. Insert a Kelly hemostat between the muscle belly and the posterior rectus sheath. Incise the rectus muscle transversely over the hemostat with coagulating electrocautery for a distance of 6 cm. Then enter the abdomen in the usual manner by incising the posterior rectus sheath and peritoneum.

## Identification of Transverse Colon

Even though the transverse colon is covered by omentum, in the average patient the omentum is thin enough that the colon can be seen through it. Positive identification can be made by observing the taenia. Divide the omentum for 6–7 cm over the colon. If colon is not clearly visible, extend the length of the incision.

Exteriorize the omentum and draw it in a cephalad direction; its undersurface leads to its junction with the transverse colon. At this point make a window in the overlying omentum so the transverse colon may protrude through the incision. Then replace the omentum into the abdomen.

## Immediate Maturation of Colostomy

In patients who undergo operations for colon obstruction, the transverse colon is often so tensely distended it is difficult to deliver the anterior wall of the colon from the abdominal cavity without causing damage. To solve this problem, apply two Babcock clamps 2 cm apart to the anterior wall of the transverse colon. Insert a 16 gauge needle attached to a low-pressure suction line into the colon between the Babcock clamps **(Fig. 15–2)**. After gas has been allowed to escape through the needle, the colon can be exteriorized easily.

The incision in the abdominal wall should be about 6 cm long. If it is longer than 6 cm, close the lateral portion with interrupted No. 1 PDS sutures of the Smead-Jones type. Shorten the skin incision with interrupted 4-0 nylon skin sutures as needed.

Make a 5- to 6-cm longitudinal incision along the anterior wall of the colon, preferably in the taenia **(Fig. 15–3)**. Aspirate the bowel gas. Irrigate the operative field with 0.1% kanamycin solution. Then suture the full thickness of the colon wall to the

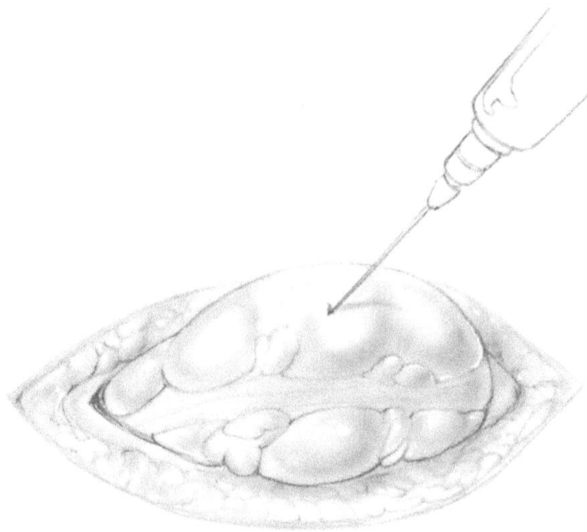

Fig. 15-2

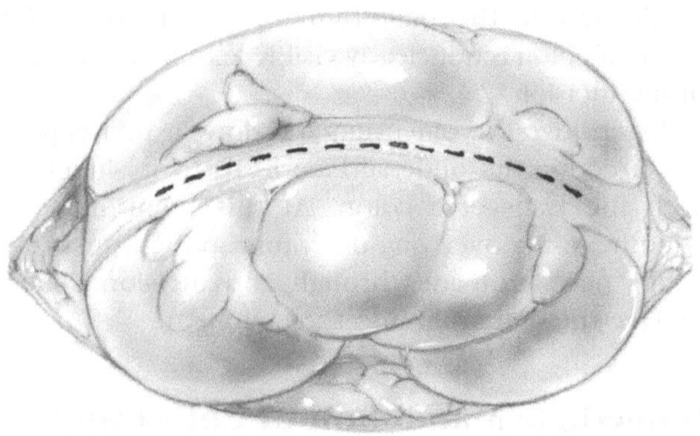

Fig. 15-3

*subcuticular* layer of the skin with 4-0 PG sutures, either interrupted or continuous **(Fig. 15–4)**. Attach a disposable ileostomy or colostomy bag to the colostomy.

## Modification of Technique Using a Glass Rod

We prefer not to interrupt the suture line between the colon and skin by use of a glass rod. In markedly obese patients who have a short mesentery, a modified glass rod technique may be used to prevent retraction while keeping the colocutaneous suture line intact. Make a stab wound through the skin at a point about 4 cm caudal to the midpoint of the proposed colostomy. By blunt dissection pass a glass or plastic rod between the subcutaneous fat and the anterior rectus fascia, proceeding in a cephalad direction. Pass the rod deep to the colon and have it emerge from a second stab wound 4 cm cephalad to the colostomy **(Fig. 15–5)**. This technique permits the subcutaneous fat to be protected from postoperative contamination by stool and greatly simplifies application of the colostomy bag.

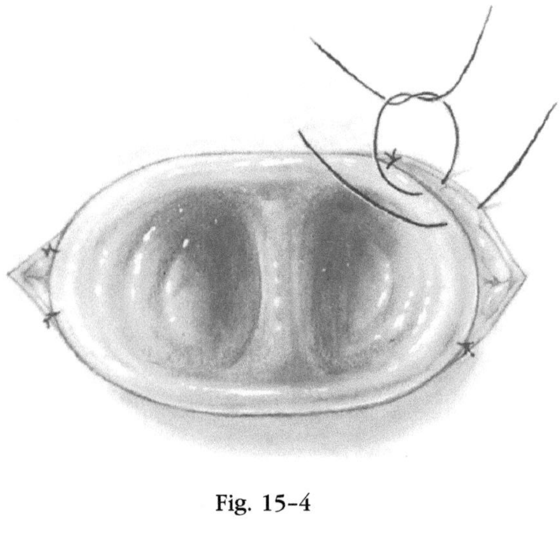

Fig. 15-4

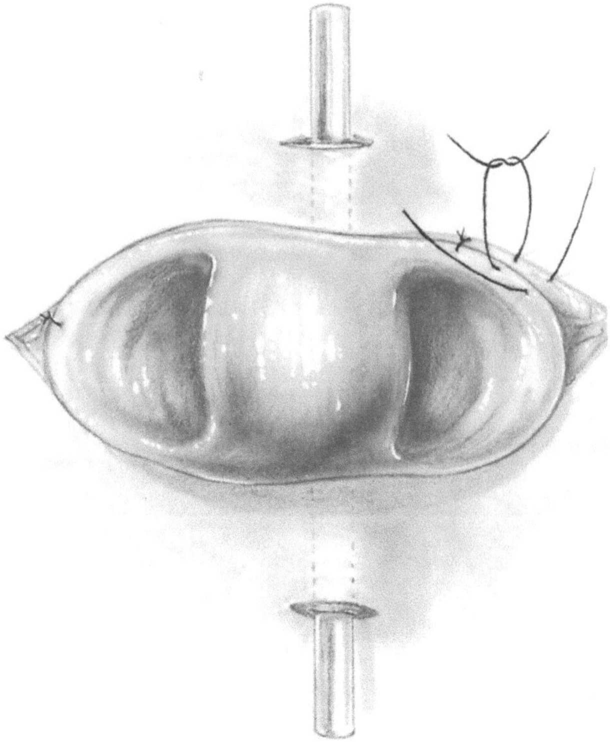

Fig. 15-5

An alternative to the solid rod is a thick Silastic tube, 6 mm in diameter, such as a nonperforated segment of a closed-suction drain tube. We prefer this method because it produces minimal inflammatory tissue response. However, because this tube is soft, it must be fixed to the skin of the two stab wounds with nylon sutures.

## POSTOPERATIVE CARE

In the operating room apply a plastic disposable adhesive-type colostomy bag.

Apply nasogastric suction until the colostomy functions.

## COMPLICATIONS

*Peristomal sepsis* is surprisingly uncommon. Treatment requires local incision and drainage. Massive sepsis would require moving the colostomy to another site.

*Prolapse of the defunctionalized limb* is fairly common when a loop colostomy is allowed to remain for months or years. It is managed by resection of the colostomy with restoration of gastrointestinal continuity or conversion to an end-colostomy. Careful tacking of both limbs at the peritoneal level helps prevent this complication but renders mobilization and subsequent closure more difficult.

## REFERENCES

Abcarian H, Pearl RK. Stomas. Surg Clin North Am 1988; 68:1295.

Bergren CT, Laws HL. Modified technique of colostomy bridging. Surg Gynecol Obstet 1990;170:453.

Doberneck RC. Revision and closure of the colostomy. Surg Clin North Am 1991;71:193.

Fitzgibbons RJ Jr, Schmitz GD, Bailey RT Jr. A simple technique for constructing a loop enterostomy which allows immediate placement of an ostomy appliance. Surg Gynecol Obstet 1987;164:78.

Gooszen AW, Geelkerken RH, Hermans J, Lagaay MB, Gooszen HG. Temporary decompression after colorectal surgery: randomized comparison of loop ileostomy and loop colostomy. Br J Surg 1998;85:76.

Kyzer S, Gordon PH. Hidden colostomy. Surg Gynecol Obstet 1993;177:181.

Majno PE, Lees VC, Goodwin K, Everett WG. Siting a transverse colostomy. Br J Surg 1992;79:576.

Morris DM, Rayburn D. Loop colostomies are totally diverting in adults. Am J Surg 1991;161:668.

Ng WT, Book KS, Wong MK, Cheng PW, Cheung CH. Prevention of colostomy prolapse by peritoneal tethering. J Am Coll Surg 1997;184:313.

Turnball RB Jr, Weakly FL. Atlas of Intestinal Stomas. St. Louis, Mosby, 1967.

# 16 Closure of Temporary Colostomy

## INDICATIONS

A temporary colostomy should be closed when it is no longer needed. Anastomotic healing and absence of a distal obstruction should be demonstrated by contrast studies. Suitably prepared patients may undergo colostomy closure as early as 2-3 weeks after surgery.

## PREOPERATIVE PREPARATION

Barium colon enema radiography to demonstrate patency of distal colon

Nasogastric tube

Routine mechanical and antibiotic bowel preparation (saline enemas to cleanse the inactivated left colon segment may be required as well)

Perioperative systemic antibiotics

## PITFALLS AND DANGER POINTS

Suture-line leak

Intraabdominal abscess

Wound abscess

## OPERATIVE STRATEGY

To avoid suture-line leakage, use only healthy, well vascularized tissue for colostomy closure. Adequate lysis of the adhesions between the transverse colon and surrounding structures allows a sufficient segment of transverse colon to be mobilized, avoiding tension on the suture line. If necessary, the incision in the abdominal wall should be enlarged to provide exposure. If the tissue in the vicinity of the colostomy has been devascularized by operative trauma, do not hesitate to resect a segment of bowel and perform an end-to-end anastomosis instead of a local reconstruction. Proper suturing or stapling of healthy colon tissue and minimizing fecal contamination combined with perioperative antibiotics helps prevent formation of abscesses.

Infection of the operative incision is rather common following colostomy closure, owing in part to failure to minimize the bacterial inoculum into the wound. Another phenomenon that contributes to wound infection is retraction of subcutaneous fat that occurs around the colostomy. This can produce a gap between the fascia and the epidermis when the skin is sutured closed, creating deadspace. Avoid this problem by leaving the skin open at the conclusion of the operation.

## OPERATIVE TECHNIQUE

### Incision

Occlude the colostomy by inserting small gauze packing moistened with povidone-iodine solution. Make an incision in the skin around the colostomy 3-4 mm from the mucocutaneous junction **(Fig. 16–1)**. Continue this incision parallel to the mucocutaneous junction until the entire colostomy has been encircled. Applying three Allis clamps to the lips of the defect in the colon expedites this dissection and helps prevent contamination. Deepen the incision by scalpel dissection until the seromuscular coat of colon can be identified. Then separate the serosa and surrounding subcutaneous fat by Metzenbaum scissors dissection **(Fig. 16–2)**. Perform this dissection with meticulous care to avoid trauma to the colon wall. Continue down to the point where the colon meets the anterior rectus fascia.

### Fascial Dissection

Identify the fascial ring and use a scalpel to dissect the subcutaneous fat off the anterior wall of the fascia for a width of 1-2 cm until a clean rim of fascia is visible all around the colostomy. Then dissect the

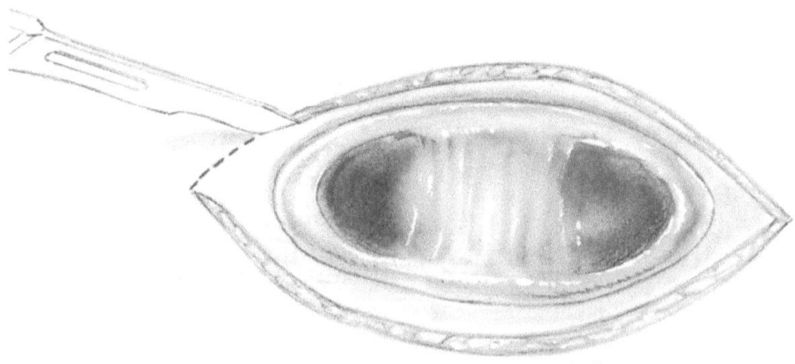

Fig. 16-1

colon away from the fascial ring until the peritoneal cavity is entered.

## Peritoneal Dissection

Once the peritoneal cavity has been identified, it is often possible to insert an index finger and gently dissect the transverse colon away from the adjoining peritoneal attachments. Using the index finger as a guide, separate the remainder of the colon from its attachments to the anterior abdominal wall. This can often be accomplished without appreciably enlarging the defect in the abdominal wall. However, if any difficulty whatever is encountered while freeing the adhesions between the colon and peritoneum, extend the incision laterally by dividing the remainder of the rectus muscle with electrocautery for a distance adequate to accomplish the dissection safely.

## Closure of Colon Defect by Suture

After the colostomy has been freed from all attachments for a distance of 5–6 cm **(Fig. 16–3)**, detach the rim of skin from the colon. Carefully inspect the wall of the colon for injury. A few small superficial patches of serosal damage are of no significance so long as they are not accompanied by devascularization. In most cases, merely freshening the edge of the colostomy by excising a rim of 3–4 mm of scarred colon reveals healthy tissue.

The colon wall should now be of relatively normal thickness. In these cases the colostomy defect, which resulted from a longitudinal incision in the transverse

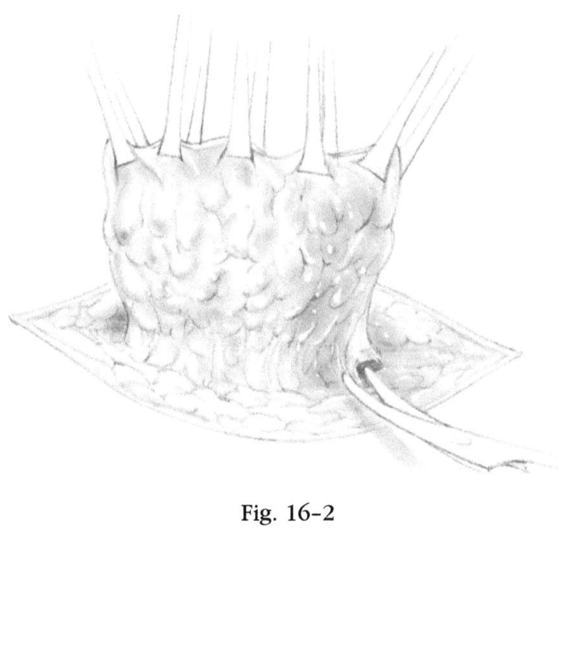

Fig. 16-2

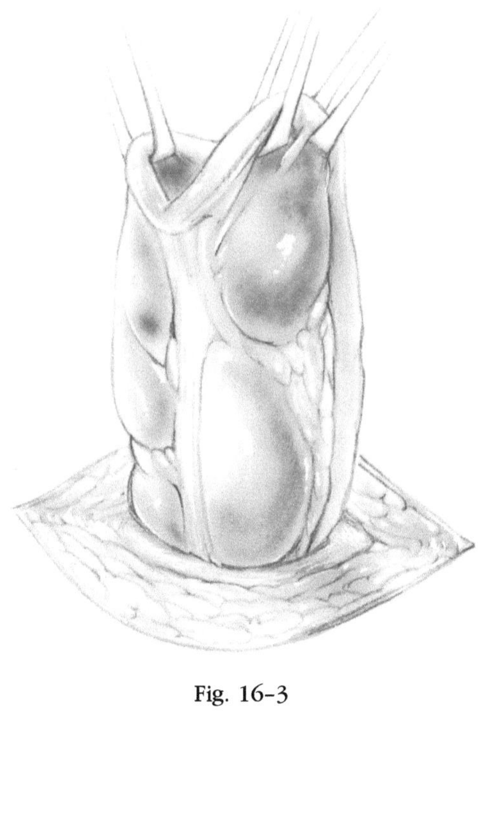

Fig. 16-3

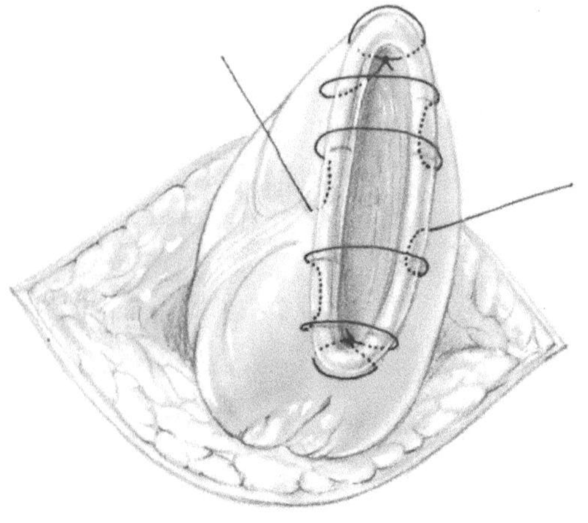

Fig. 16-4

colon at the initial operation, should be closed in a transverse direction. Initiate an inverting stitch of 4-0 PG on an atraumatic curved needle at the caudal margin of the colonic defect and pursue it as a continuous Connell or continuous Cushing suture to the midpoint of the defect **(Fig. 16–4)**. Then initiate a second suture of the same material on the cephalad margin of the defect and continue it also to the midpoint; terminate the suture line here (Fig. 16–4). Invert this layer with another layer of interrupted 4-0 silk atraumatic seromuscular Lembert sutures **(Fig. 16–5)**. Because of the transverse direction of the suture line, the lumen of the colon is quite commodious at the conclusion of the closure. There should be no tension whatever on this suture line. Finally, irrigate the operative field and reduce the colon into the abdominal cavity.

## Closure of Colonic Defect by Staples

If the colon wall is not so thick that compressing it to 2 mm produces necrosis, stapling is an excellent method for closing the colon defect. Align the defect so the closure can take place in a transverse direction. Place a single guy suture to mark the midpoint of the transverse closure **(Fig. 16–6)** and apply Allis clamps to approximate the colon staple line with the bowel wall in eversion.

Carry out stapling by triangulation with two applications of the 55 mm linear stapling device, rather than attempting a single application of a 90 mm

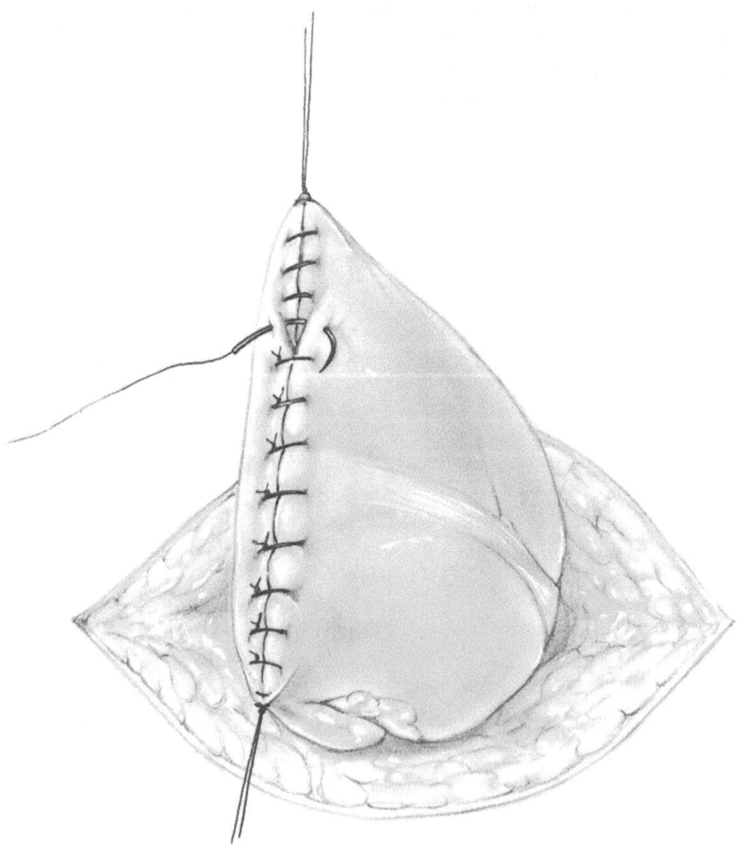

Fig. 16-5

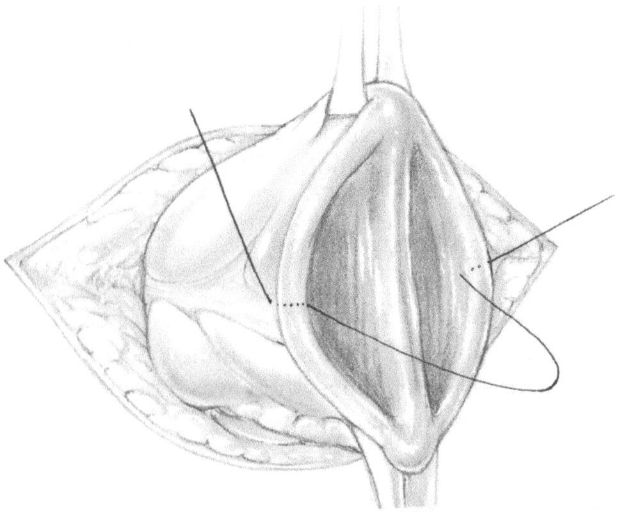

Fig. 16-6

device. This minimizes the chance of catching the back wall of the colon in the staple line. First, apply the stapler across the everted mucosa supported by the Allis clamps on the caudal aspect of the defect and the guy suture. Fire the staples and use Mayo scissors to excise the redundant everted mucosa flush with the stapler. Leave the guy suture at the midpoint of the closure intact.

Make the second application of the 55 mm linear stapler with the device positioned deep to the Allis clamps on the cephalad portion of the defect **(Fig. 16–7)**. It is important to position the guy suture to include the previous staple line in this second line of staples, ensuring that no gap exists between the two staple lines. Then fire the staples. Remove any redundant mucosa by excising it with Mayo scissors flush with the stapler. Lightly electrocoagulate the everted mucosa. Carefully inspect the integrity of the staple line to ensure that proper B formation has taken place. It is important, especially with stapling, to ascertain that no tension is exerted on the closure.

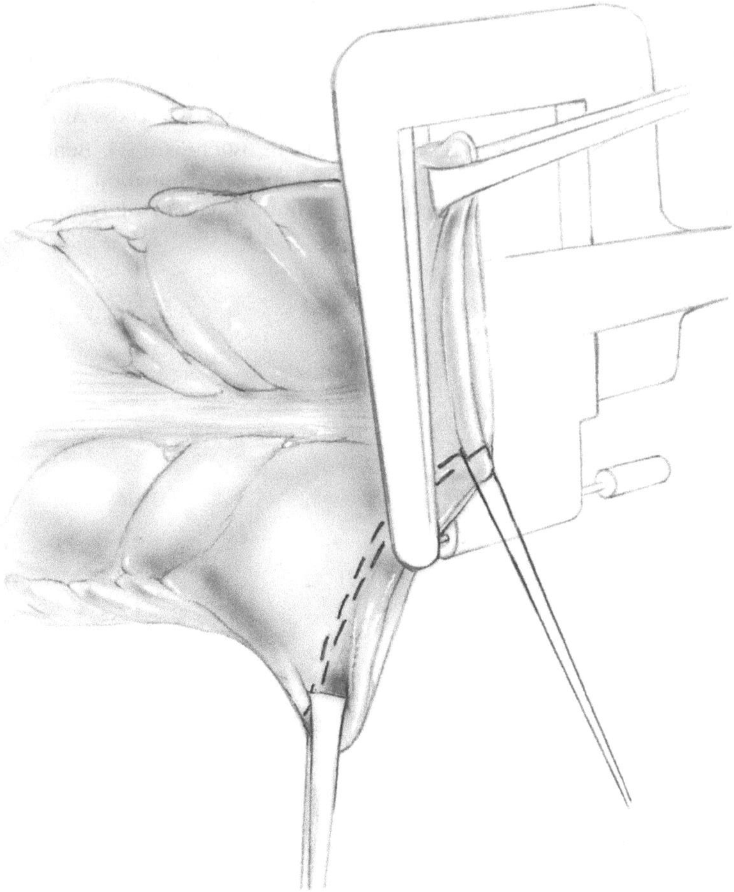

Fig. 16-7

### Resection and Anastomosis of Colostomy

Whenever the tissue is of inadequate quality for simple transverse closure, enlarge the incision in the abdominal wall and resect a segment of colon. Mobilize a sufficient section of the right transverse colon, occasionally including the hepatic flexure. Dissect the omentum off the transverse colon proximal and distal to the defect. After the proximal and distal segments of the colon have been sufficiently mobilized and the traumatized tissue excised, an end-to-end anastomosis can be constructed by the usual twolayer suture technique (see Figs. 4-18 through 4-26) or the staple technique (see Figs. 4-35 through 4-38).

### Closure of Abdominal Wall

Irrigate the area with a dilute antibiotic solution and apply an Allis clamp to the midpoint of the abdominal wall on the caudal and cephalad aspects of the wound. Then close the incision by the modified Smead-Jones technique.

### Management of Skin Wound

Frequently the colostomy can be closed without enlarging the skin incision, which was no longer than 5-6 cm. There is a high incidence of wound infection following primary closure of the skin. In such cases we simply insert loosely packed gauze into the subcutaneous space, which we allow to heal by granulation and contraction. If desired, several interrupted vertical mattress sutures of nylon may be inserted, but do not tie them until the eighth or tenth postoperative day. Keep the subcutaneous tissue separated with moist gauze packing and approximate the skin by previously placed sutures or tape strips when healthy granulation tissue has formed.

## POSTOPERATIVE CARE

Apply nasogastric suction if necessary.

Systemic antibiotics are not continued beyond the perioperative period unless there was serious wound contamination during surgery.

## COMPLICATIONS

Wound infection

Abdominal abscess

Colocutaneous fistula

## REFERENCES

Doberneck RC. Revision and closure of the colostomy. Surg Clin North Am 1991;71:193.

Renz BM, Feliciano DV, Sherman R. Same admission colostomy closure (SACC): a new approach to rectal wounds: a prospective study. Ann Surg 1993;218:279.

Sola JE, Buchman TG, Bender JS. Limited role of barium enema examination preceding colostomy closure in trauma patients. J Trauma 1994;36:245.

# 17 Laparoscopic Stoma Construction and Closure

Dan Enger Ruiz
Steven D. Wexner

## INDICATIONS

Obstructing tumors

Colonic inflammation (diverticulitis, inflammatory bowel disease, radiation)

Perineal sepsis (Crohn's disease, complex fistula, Fournier's disease)

Trauma (perineal injury, rectal perforation)

Dysfunction (fecal incontinence, dysmotility)

## PREOPERATIVE PREPARATION

Enterostomal therapist consultation for marking

In elective setting, standard bowel preparation. (selected cases)

Oral and/or intravenous antibiotic preparation. (elective cases with bowel preparation)

Sequential compression stockings

Subcutaneous heparin

## PITFALLS AND DANGER POINTS

Appropriate stoma location

Adequate abdominal opening to avoid outlet obstruction ischemia, parastomal hernia, prolapses

Injury to the spleen

Injury to the ureters

Injury to the bowel

Adequate orientation of the bowel (as mesentery must not be torsed)

## OPERATIVE STRATEGY

Deciding the best place for stoma placement is the key issue in stoma formation. The stoma site should be carefully preoperatively determined to avoid post-operative complications.

Another important issue is which stoma to use. Loop stomas are often preferred over end stomas because they vent the intestine and they are relatively easy to close. For protection of an anastomosis or colonic diseases an end ileostomy is preferred. An end ileostomy is the only choice after colectomy for fulminant inflammatory disease.

Loop ileostomies are selected over colostomies for easier management and less major complications after subsequent closure. Moreover, performing a loop colostomy places the marginal artery at risk during stoma closure, potentially devascularizing the distal colon and therefore the proximal anastomosis.

The surgeon must keep in mind that the area of manipulation has to form a semicircle or a triangle with the laparoscope between the two operating ports. For a loop ileostomy the most distal segment that can be used without tension is chosen. For a left colostomy a left paracolic dissection may be necessary and a gentle dissection is done to avoid splenic injuries. Identification of the ureter is required when dissecting the mesentery from the retroperitonium. Placement of ureteric catheters can be useful in cases of major inflammatory processes or tumors encroaching on the ureter(s).

## OPERATIVE TECHNIQUE

### Loop Ileostomy

#### *Room Setup and Trocar Placement*

The patient is placed in the supine position **(Figure 17–1)** and monitors are placed near the patient's right knee and left shoulder. The surgeon is operating from the opposite side of the stoma site. Pneumoperitonium is raised in the standard fashion using a Hasson's technique and a 10 mm laparoscope is introduced at the supraumbilical port. This initial part is deliberately placed midway between the umbilicus and xiphoid to allow adequate working space. Traditional placement near the umbilicus will result insufficient

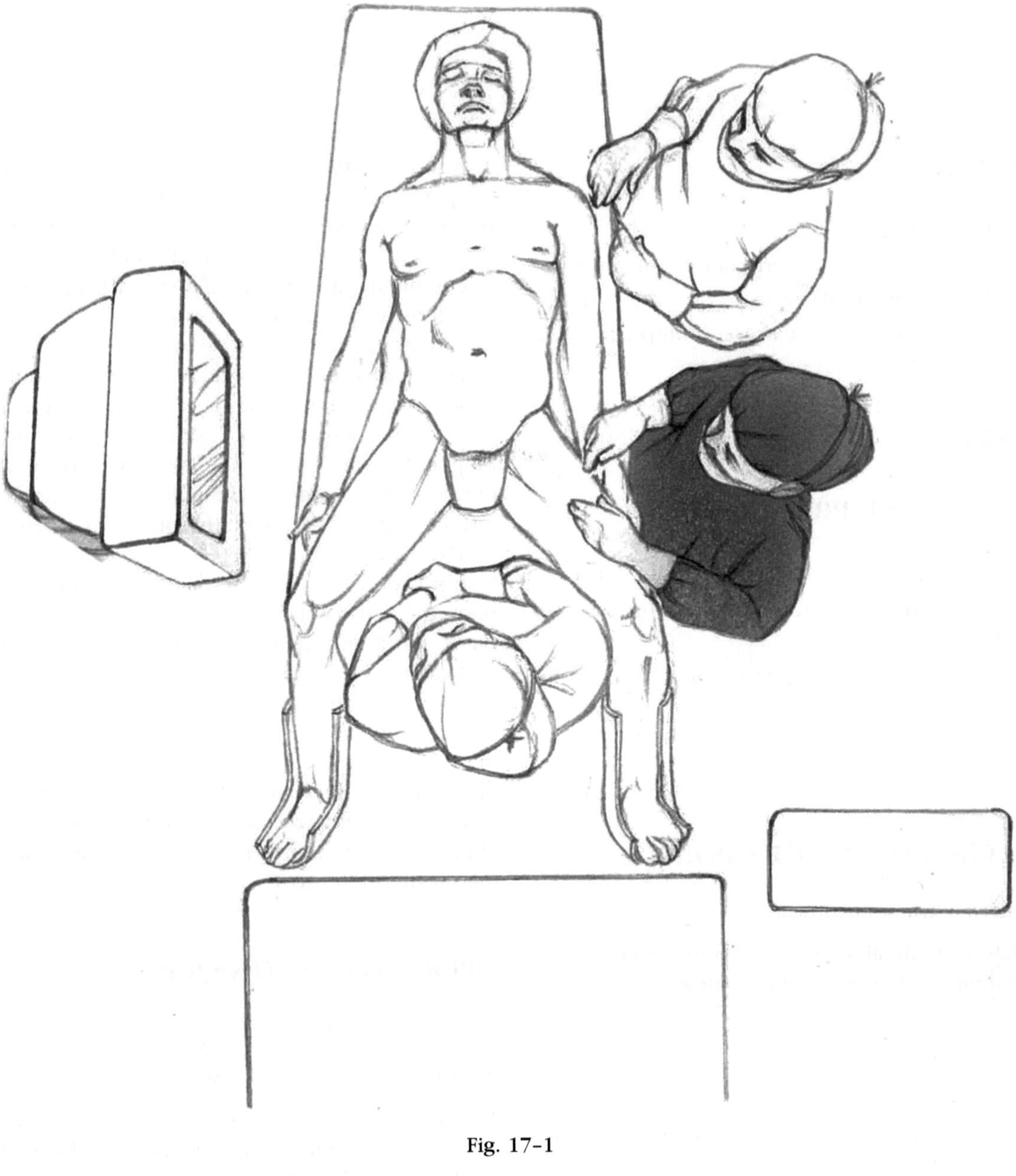

Fig. 17-1

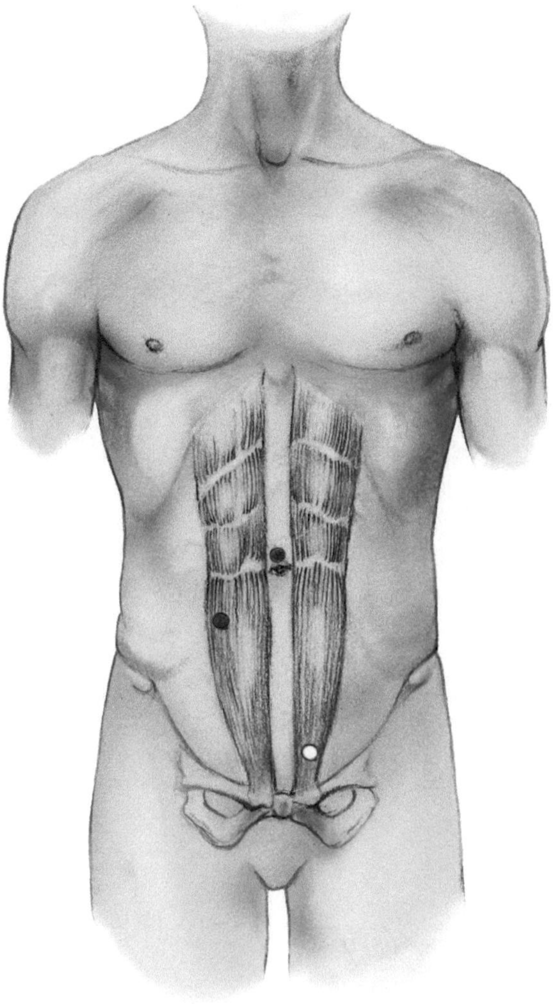

Fig. 17–2

space between the instruments for triangulation. The next 10 mm port is placed right in the ileostomy site assuring avoidance of epigastric vessels that may be damaged by transiluminating the chosen stoma site. Before the trocar is placed, a 2 cm circular skin and subcutaneous tissue disc is resected around the stoma mark **(Figure 17–2)**. An extra 10 mm cannula can be placed contralateral to the stoma in the iliac fossa, if needed, to facilitate the dissection.

### *Choosing a Loop of Terminal Ileum*

The patient is placed in the Trendelenburg position to displace the small bowel out of the pelvis. Using a 10 mm diameter laparoscopic Babcock-type clamp, the surgeon identifies an appropriate loop of bowel (20–30 cm) proximal to the cecum and lifts it to the stoma site, verifying it is tension-free **(Figure 17–3)**. Special care must be taken to avoid torsing of the bowel. Gently grasping the cecum and elevating it anteriorly to expose the ileocecal junction and thus the terminal ileum can facilitate this maneuver.

### *Exposing the Ileum*

After slowly grasping the ileum, desulflating the pneumoperitonium, and without rotating the bowel the ileum is exteriorized through the stoma site

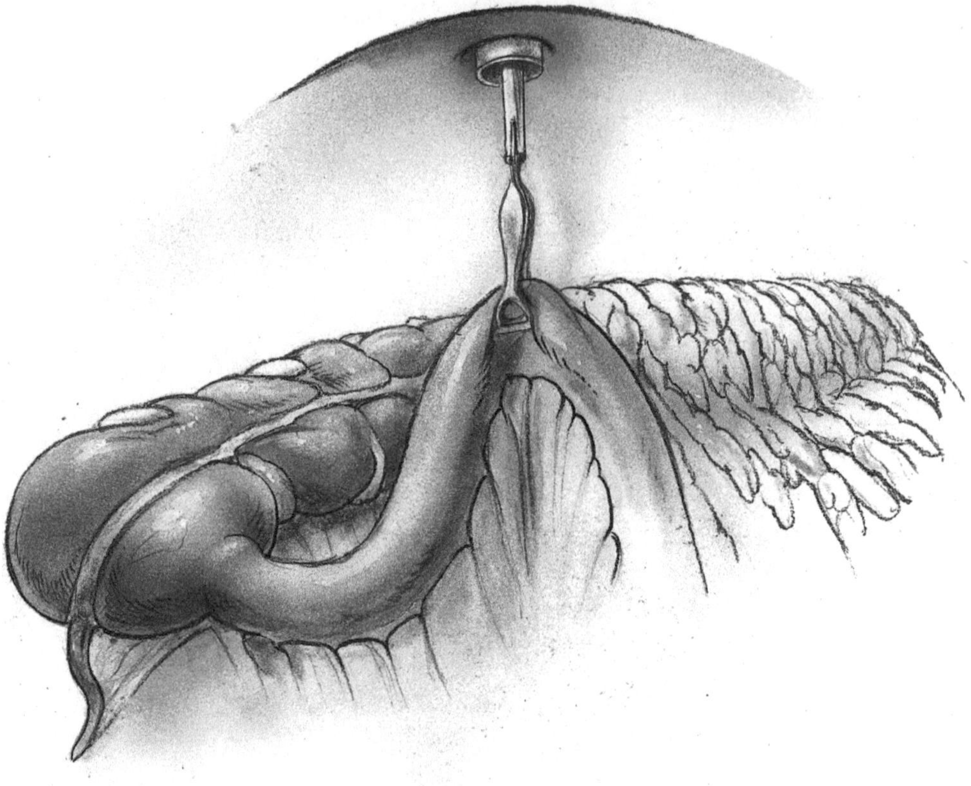

Fig. 17-3

**(Figure 17–4)**. The loop of bowel occluding the stoma site is used to reinsulflate the abdomen and confirm orientation of the bowel and mesentery. The ostomy is then matured using standard techniques.

## Loop Sigmoid Colostomy

### *Room Setup and Trocar Placement*

Position the patient in the supine modified lithotomy position; monitors are placed lateral to each patient's knee. The surgeon and first assistant position is on the right side of the patient and the second assistant between patient's legs **(Figure 17–5)**. Pneumoperitonium is established in the standard fashion through a 10 mm port introduced at the supraumbilical port. This initial port is deliberated placed midway between the umbilicus and xiphoid. A second 10 mm trocar is placed at the stoma site after exploration of the abdomen. If a third 10 mm cannula is needed for dissection it is placed in between umbilicus and right iliac spina on the right side **(Figure 17–6)**.

### *Dissecting the Left Parietocolic Attachment*

In many cases the sigmoid colon must be mobilized from its lateral peritoneal attachments to achieve the stoma site without tension. In this case, a 5 mm port is placed suprapubically from the right side and laparoscopic scissors are used to dissect and mobilize the colon from its lateral attachments **(Figure 17–7)**. If the descending colon requires mobilization, the surgeon should move from the right side to between the patient's legs.

### *Exteriorizing the Sigmoid Loop*

A 10 mm diameter Babcock is used to gently grasp the loop of sigmoid colon that best reaches above the stoma site at the skin level. The sigmoid is withdrawn and trocar removed simultaneously

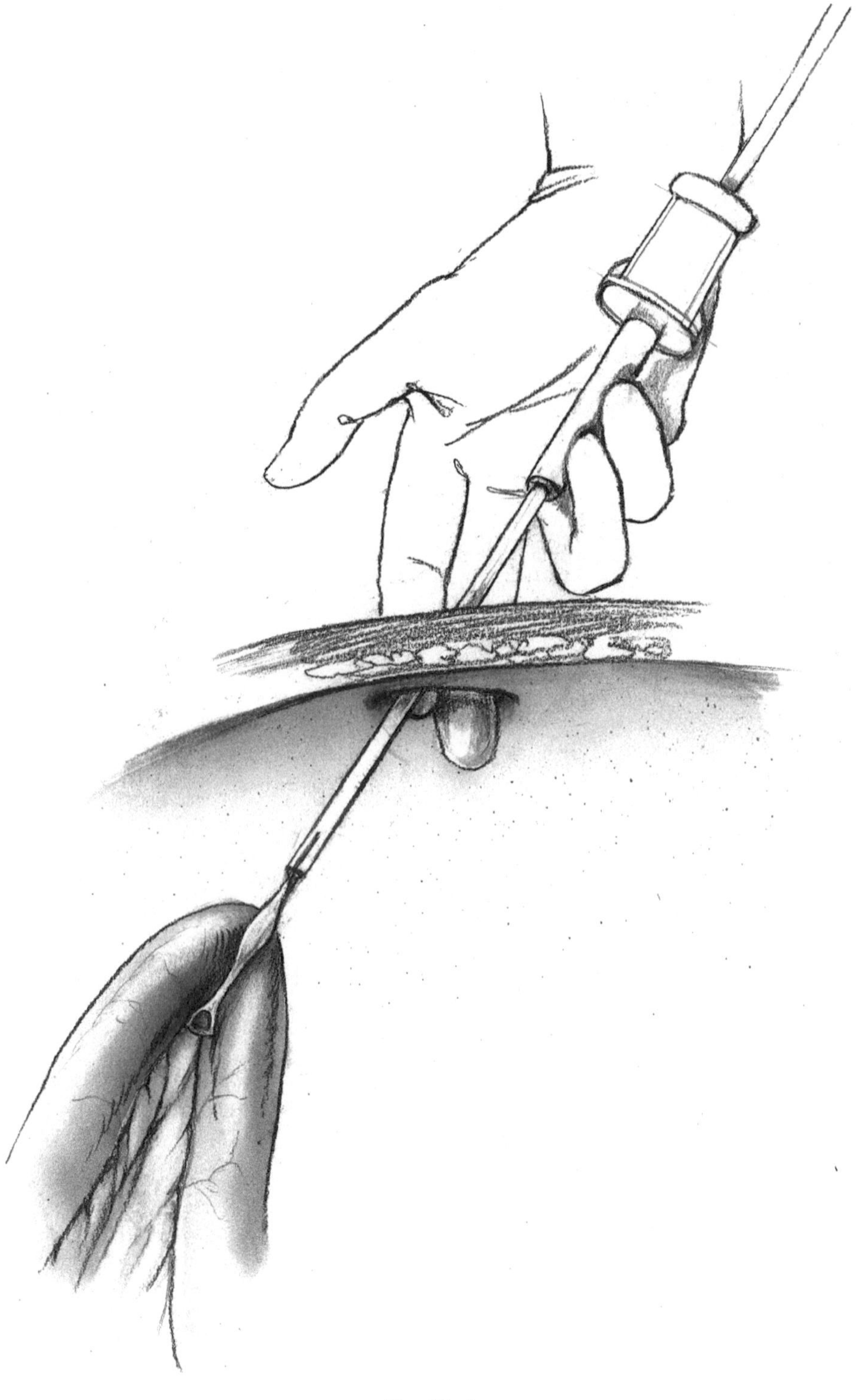

Fig. 17-4

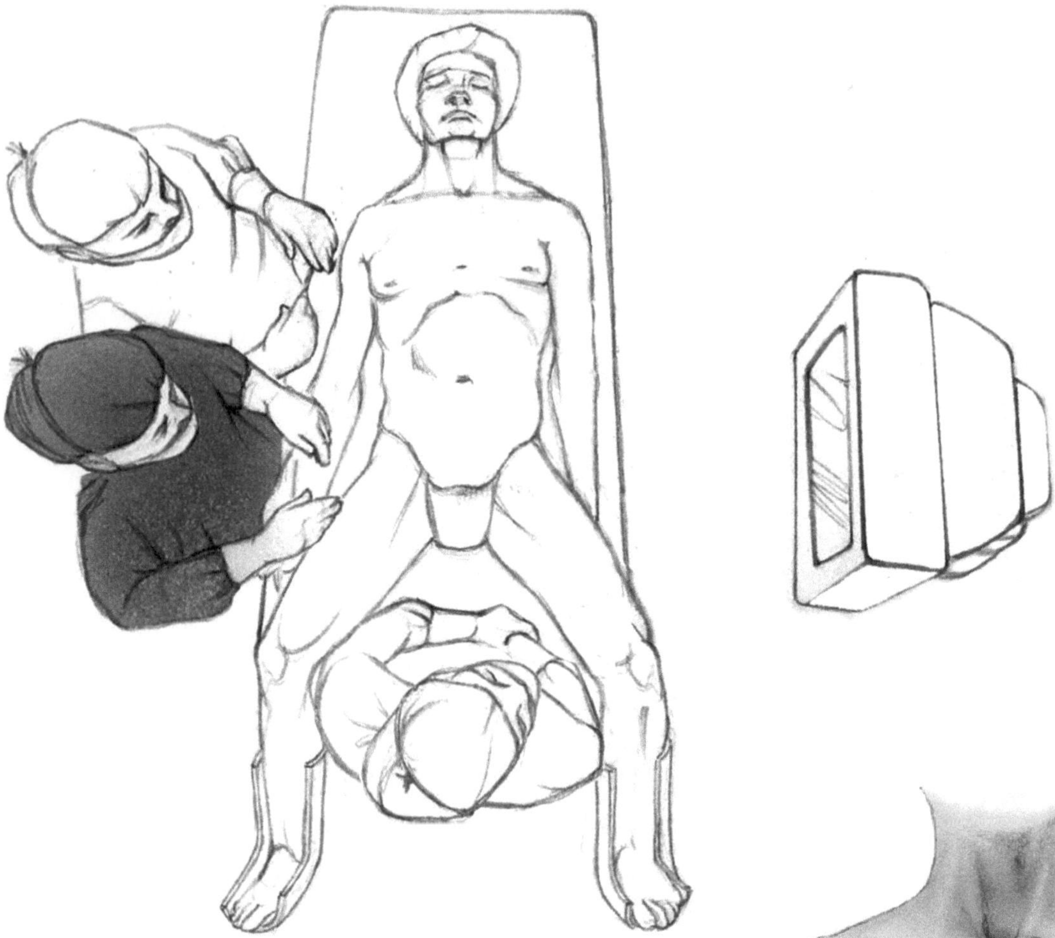

Fig. 17-5

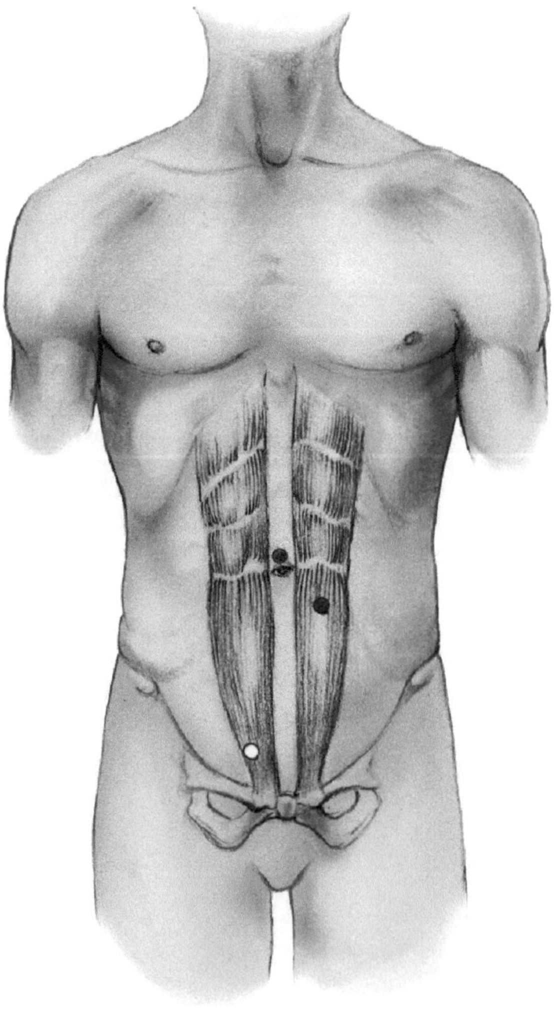

Fig. 17-6

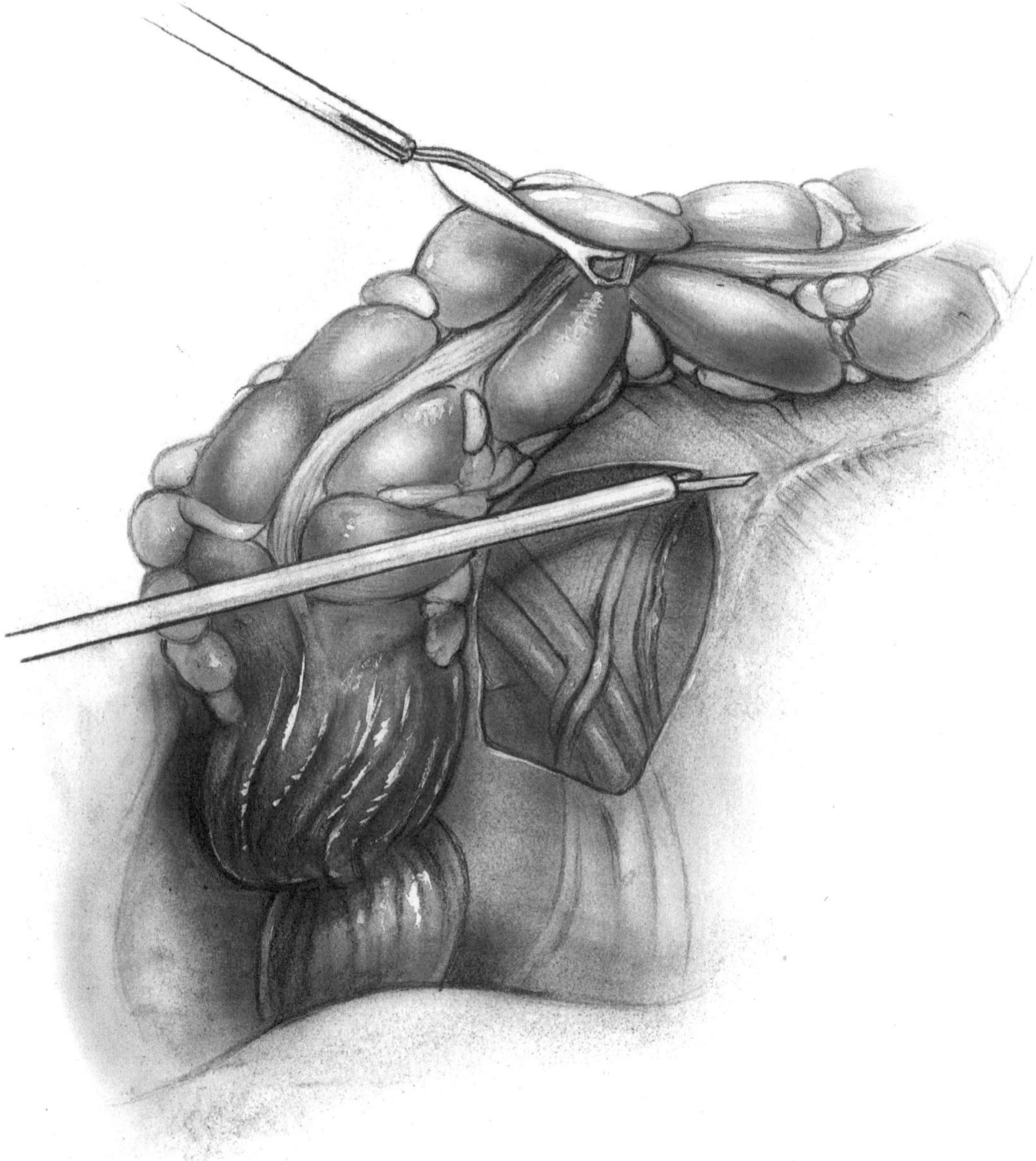

Fig. 17-7

**(Figure 17–8)**. Delivery of the sigmoid loop through the stoma site reveals the peritoneal cavity and pneumoperitonium is then reestablished. Visual inspection of the cavity and mesentery should be performed to ensure that there is no tension or torsion of the sigmoid colon. The stoma is then matured using standard techniques.

## End Sigmoid Colostomy/Mucous Fistula

### *Operating Room Setup and Trocar Placement*

The operating room set up is the same as that depicted for loop sigmoidostomy (Figure 17–7).

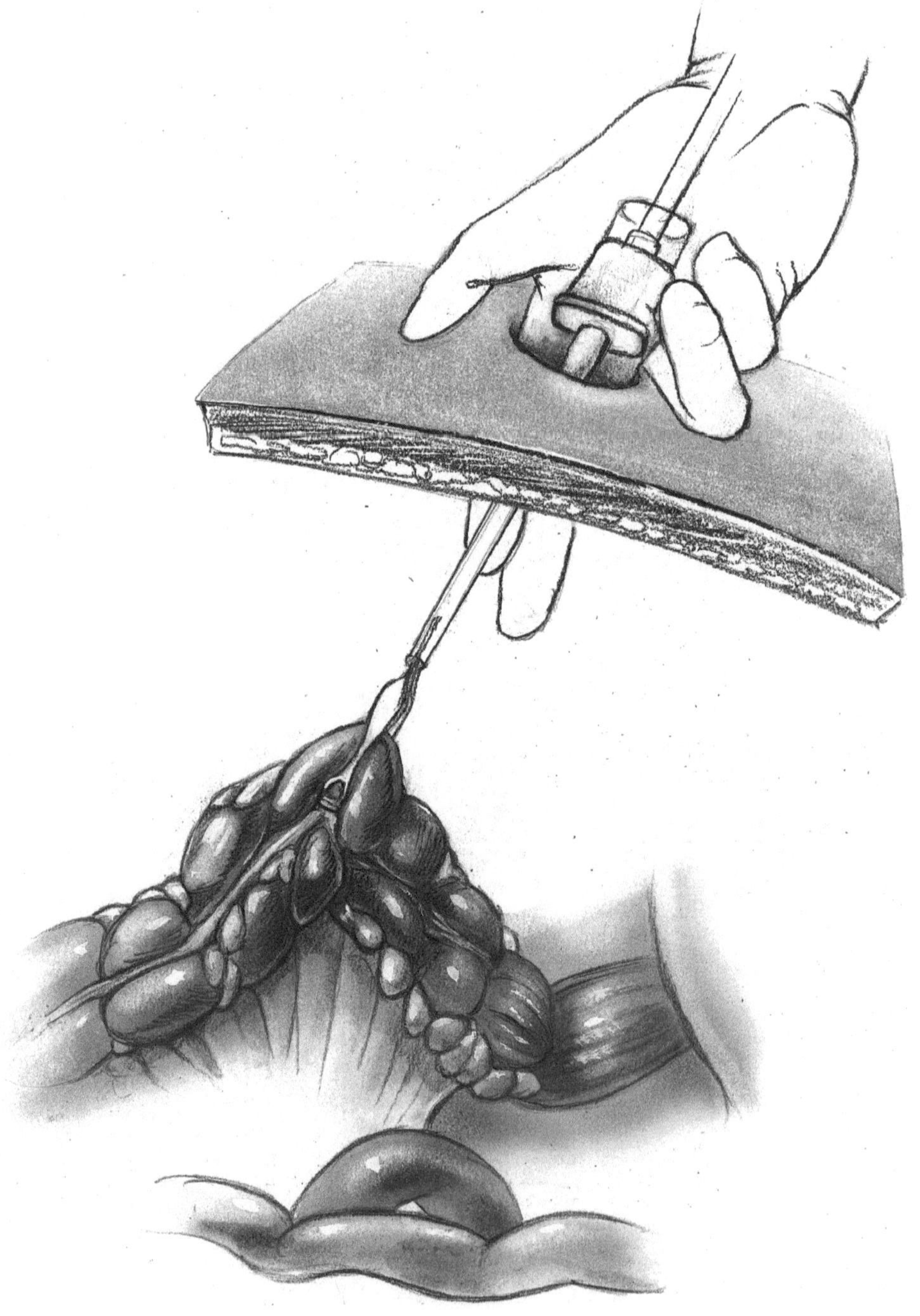

Fig. 17–8

Pneumoperitonium is established through the umbilical site. The second port is placed at the stoma site and the third port can be placed on the ipsilateral side of the stoma. In case of extensive adhesions, the contralateral ports may be needed to facilitate the enterolysis.

### *Identification of the Ureter*

If the ureter cannot be identified, the lateral attachments of the sigmoid are incised. The peritoneum is incised cephalad toward the direction of the origin of the inferior mesenteric artery. The inferior mesenteric artery and vein are swept ventrally away from the preaortic hypogastric neural plexus which is swept dorsally to prevent injury. The sigmoid colon is mobilized lateral to medial and the gonadal vessels and the ureters are then identified and dissected free of the mesentery **(Figure 17–9)**.

### *Incision of the Mesocolon and Division of the Sigmoid Colon*

The ability to mobilize the colon to the anterior abdominal wall is ensured and a window is created in the mesentery **(Figure 17–10)**. A laparoscopic linear 30mm stapler is introduced and used to divide the sigmoid colon **(Figure 17–11)**. After division of the sigmoid colon, a vascular stapler is used to divide the mesentery of the sigmoid colon. This second line stapler allows the two ends of the colon to be separated and used as an end colostomy and mucous

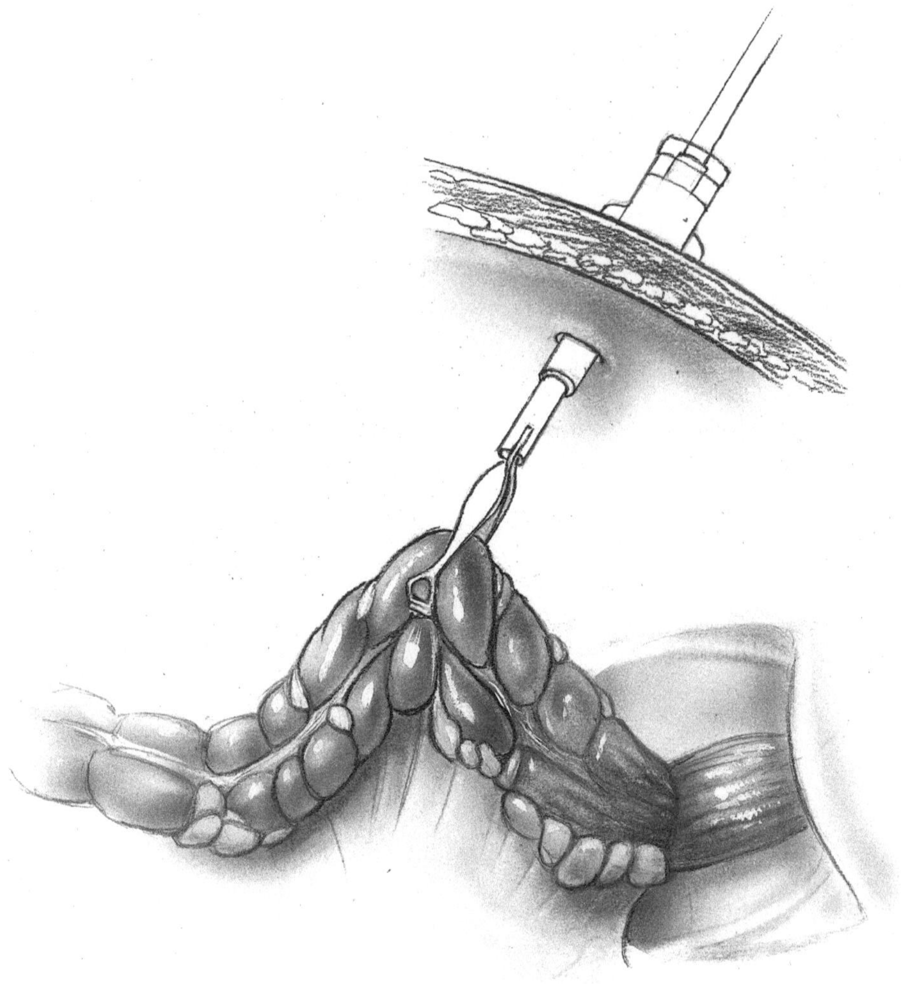

Fig. 17-9

Fig. 17-10

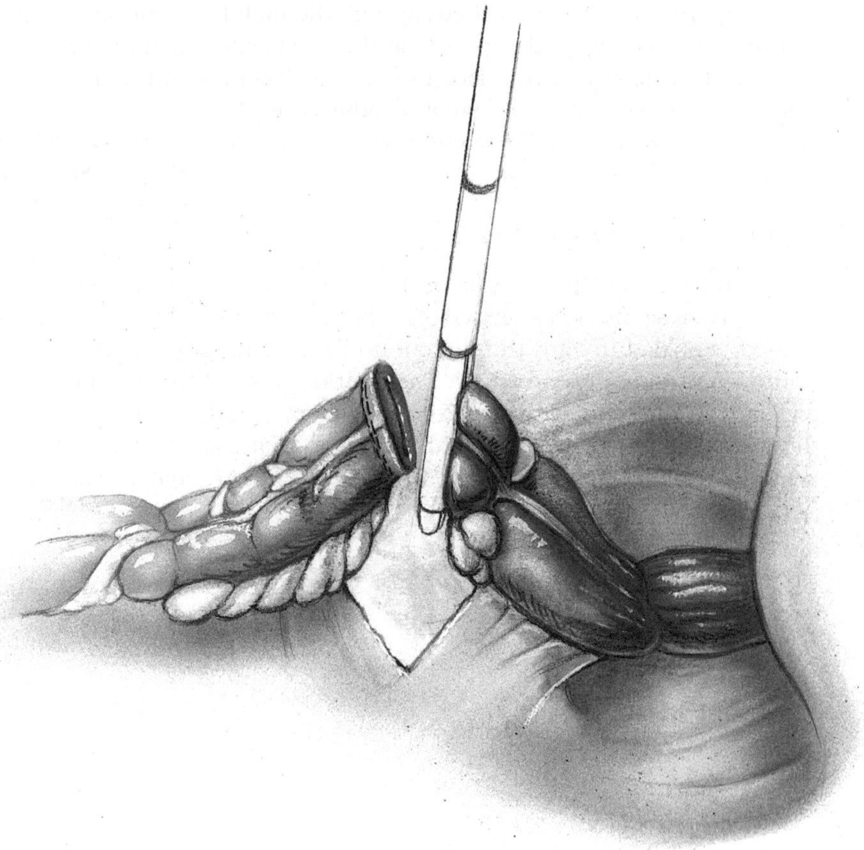

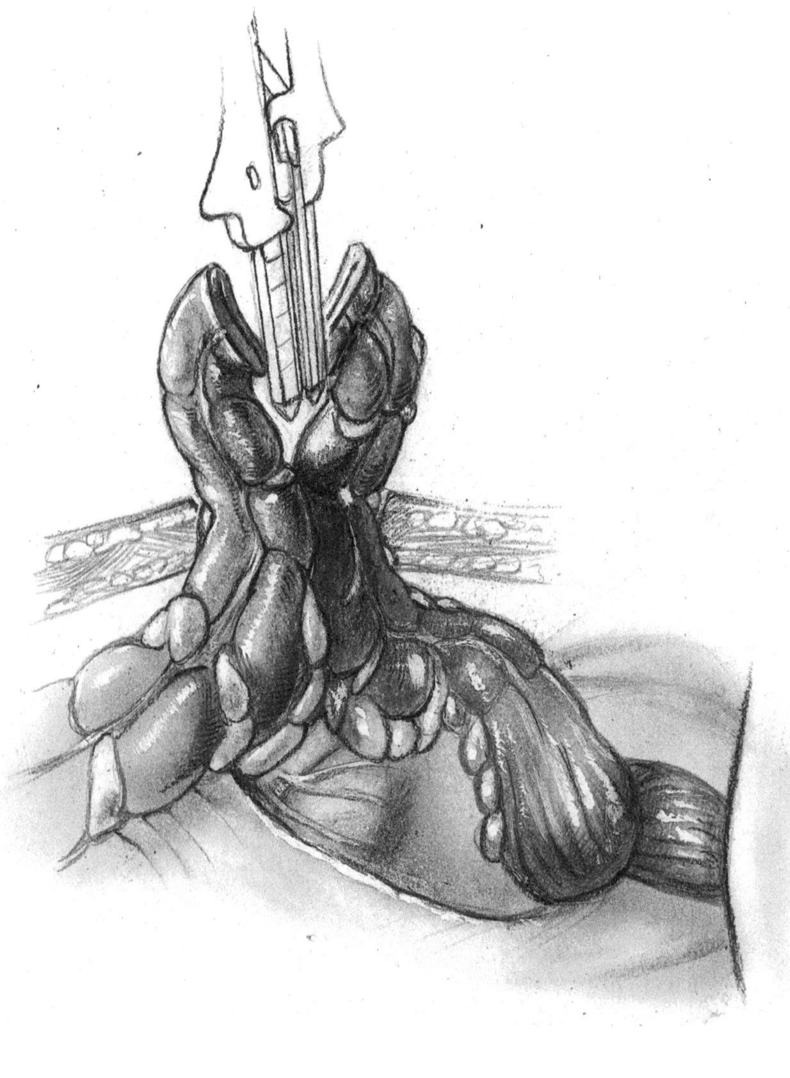

Fig. 17-11

fistula. Alternatively, a loop of sigmoid can be delivered through the stoma site and then extracorporelly divided after insuring appropriate orientation.

### *Exteriorizating the Proximal Sigmoid Colon*

A Babcock clamp is passed though the trocar to deliver the proximal colon. Simultaneous withdrawal of the trocar with a second Babcock is used to withdraw the distal end of the colon after enlarging the peritoneal defect **(Figure 17–12)**. To create the mucous fistula, the mesentery should be divided to allow physical separation of the two loops of colon. Reestablishment of the pneumoperitonium after placement of the stoma as an end colostomy and mucous fistula allows inspection of the abdominal cavity to exclude torsion or tension. Alternatively, the mucus fistula can be matured though the same stoma site, usually at its inferior aspect.

## Transverse Colostmy

### *Operating Room Setup and Trocar Placement*

The patient is placed in the supine or modified lithotomy position. The surgeon stands between patient's legs and the first assistant stands to the right side of the patient **(Figure 17–13)**. Pneumoperitonium is raised through the umbilical port where a 10 mm trocar is placed to introduce the laparoscope; a second 10 mm trocar is placed in the right iliac fossa and a third in the left iliac fossa **(Figure 17–14)**; one of iliac fossa ports should be placed through the selected stoma site.

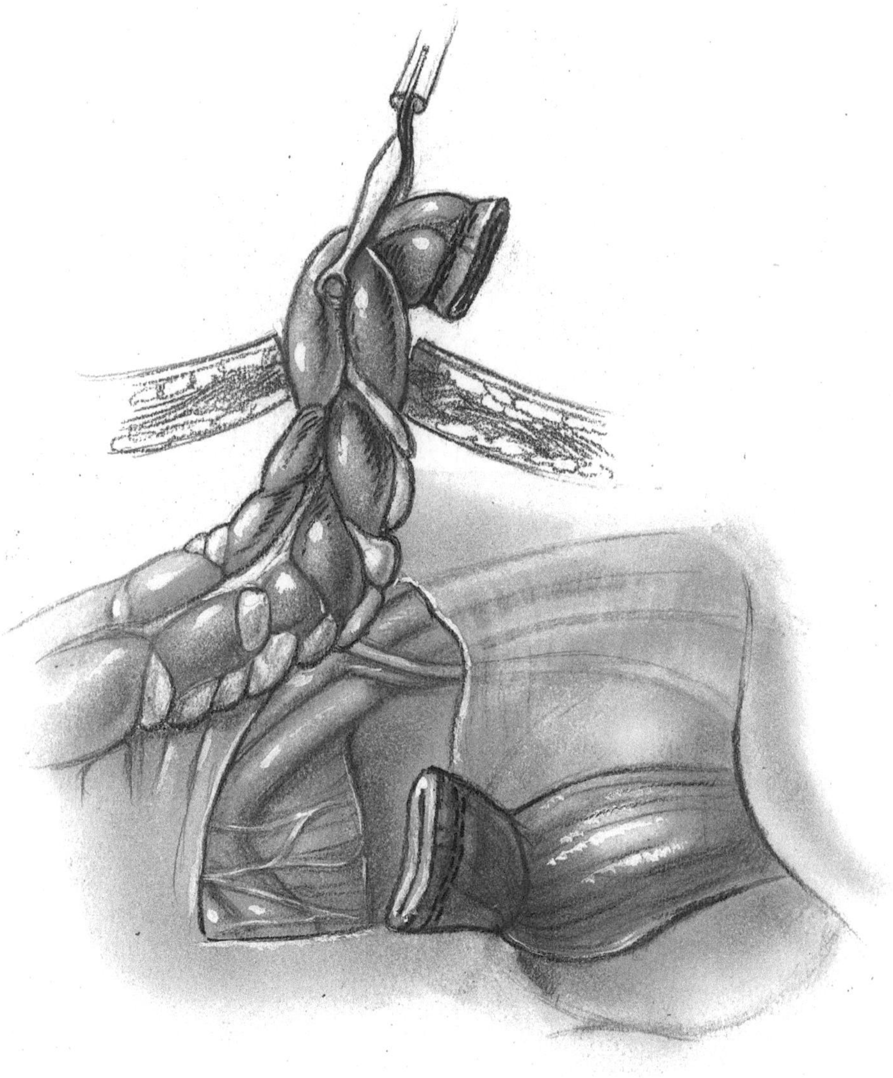

Fig. 17–12

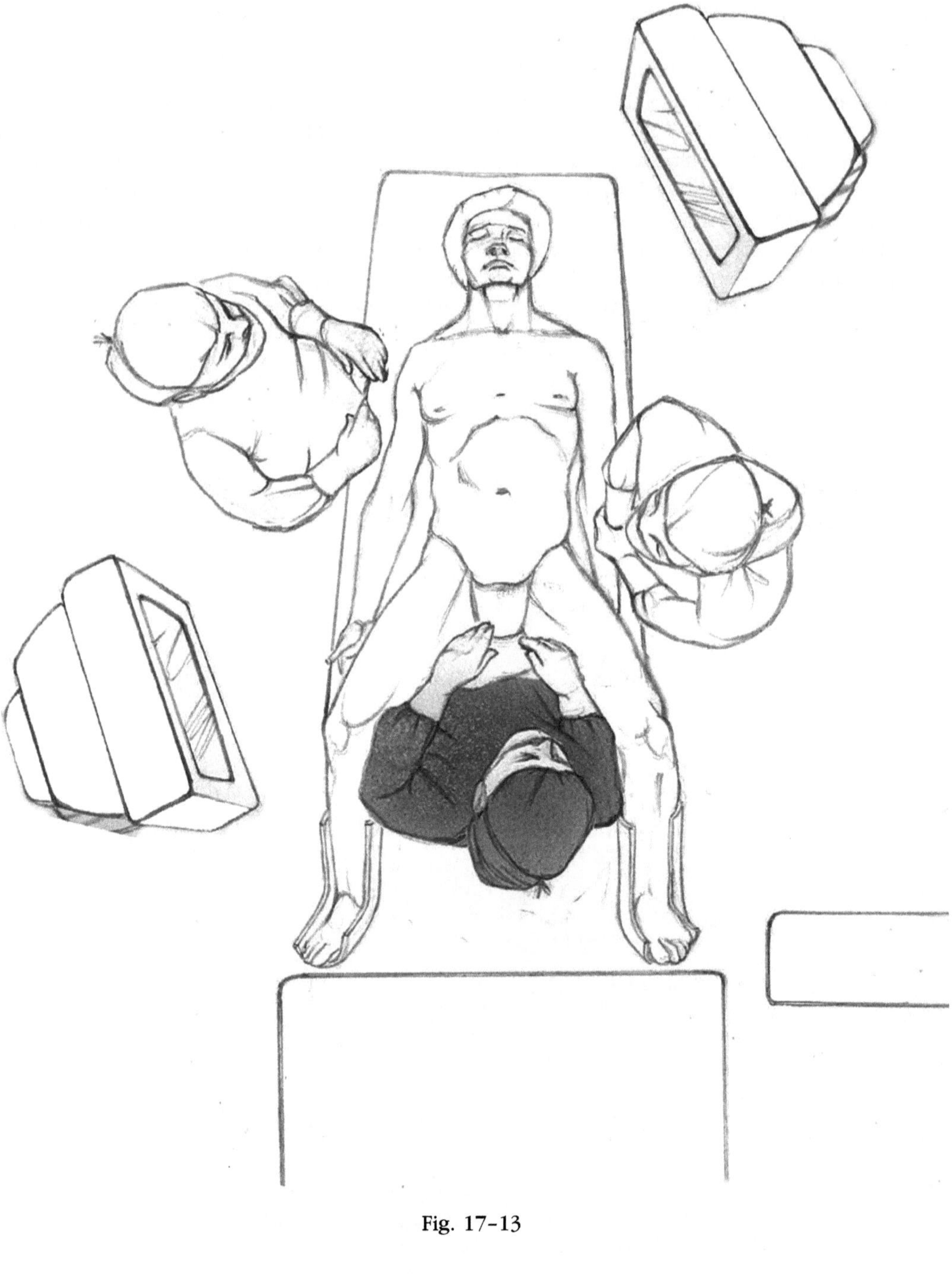

Fig. 17-13

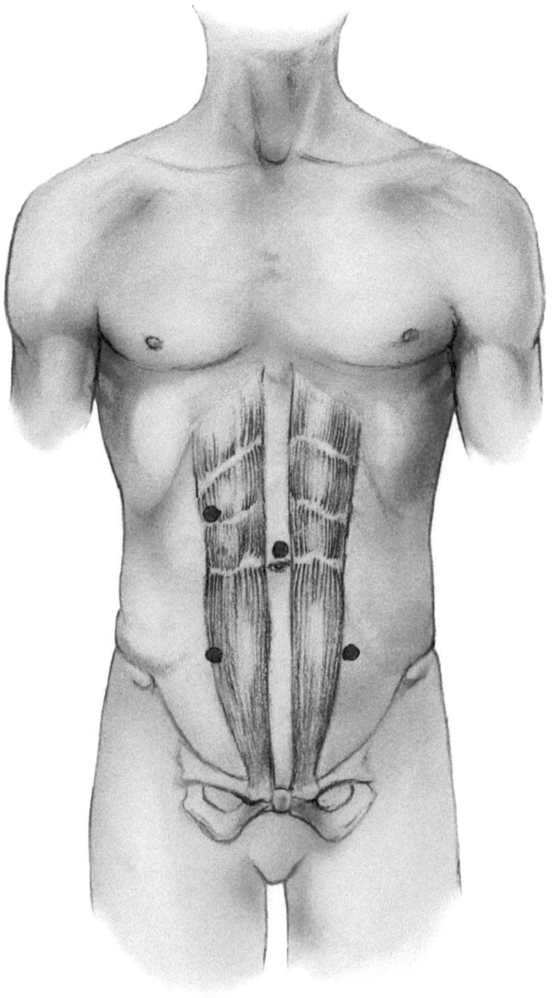

Fig. 17–14

### *Dissecting the Omentum*

The omentum is gently grasped and retracted cephalad. The weight of the transverse colon provides adequate countertraction, thus allowing dissection with the harmonic scalpel. After the bowel has been dissected, the transverse colon is gently grasped and exteriorized through the chosen stoma site; maturation is effected in the standard manner.

## Hartmann's Take Down

## Operating Room Setup, Trocar Placement, and Stoma Mobilization

The patient is placed in the modified dorsal lithotomy position. The rectum is gently irrigated using a soft rubber catheter and warm saline solution. The surgeon stands on the patient's right side and the first assistant and the camera operator next to the surgeon **(Figure 17–15)**. The monitors are placed next to each of the patient's knees.

The stoma is mobilized in the usual fashion, after which the anvil of a 29 cm, or preferably a 33 cm stapler, is secured in place. The proximal colon and anvil are then returned into the peritoneal cavity. Under direct manual and visual guidance, any midline adhesions are sharply divided after which a 10 mm supra or infraumbilical port is placed. The stoma site can be either completely closed or closed around a 10 mm port. Care must be taken to resect any residual proximal diverticular narrowing to ensure that healthy, supple, compliant, well vascularized bowel will be used for the anastomosis. Introduction of pneumoperitonium and placement of distal 10 mm port, as needed are usually in the right iliac fossa and right upper quadrant **(Figure 17–16)**.

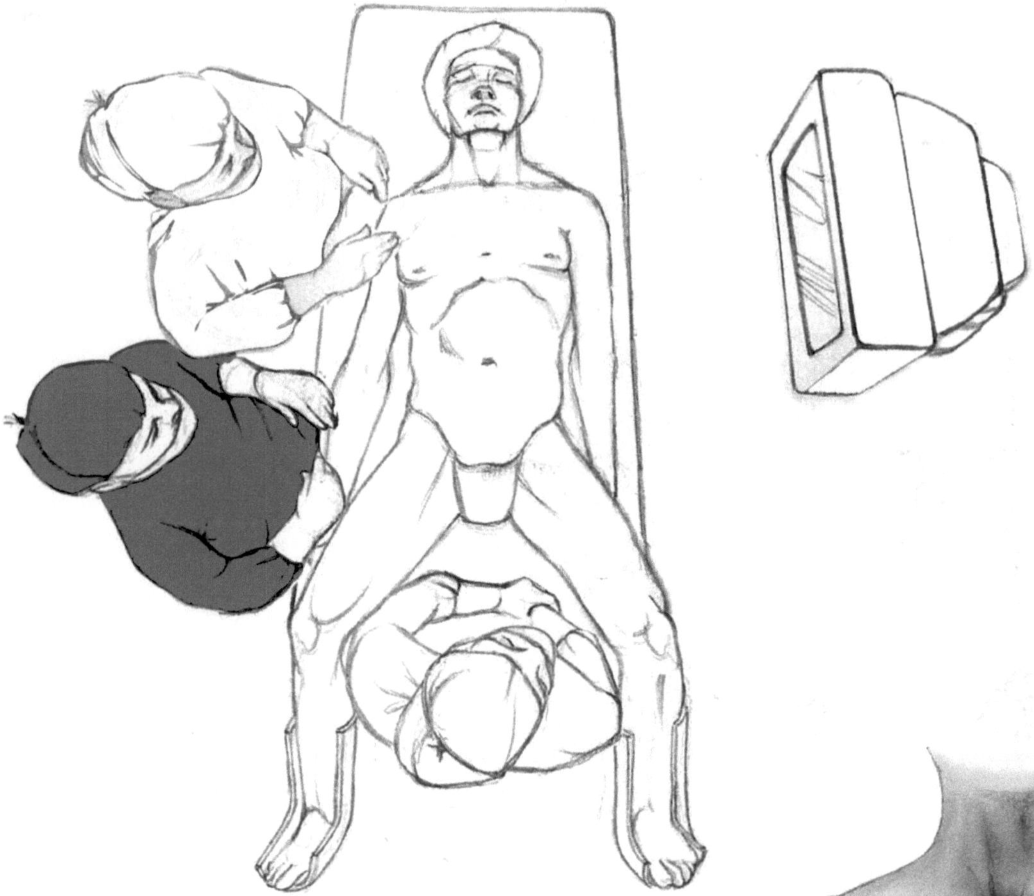

Fig. 17-15

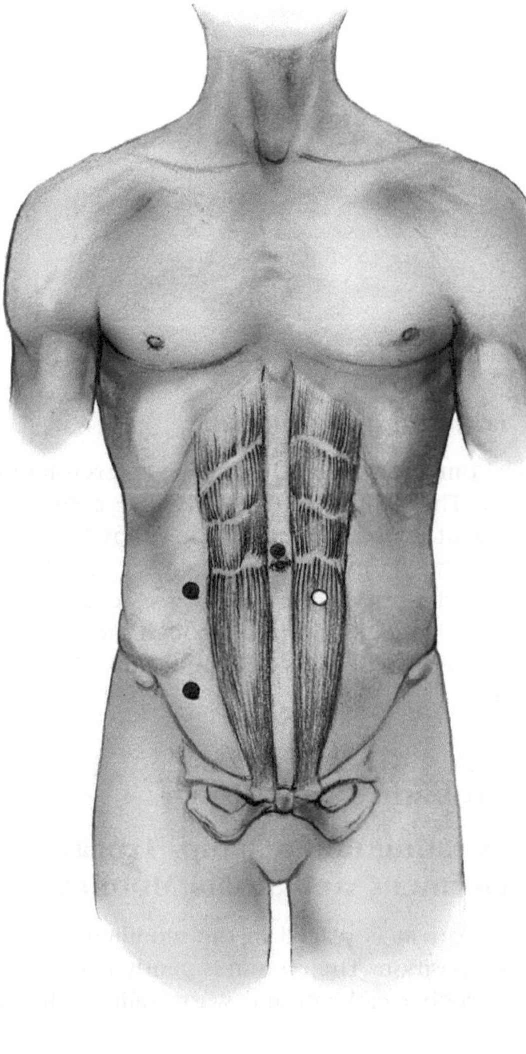

Fig. 17-16

### *Dissecting the Rectal Stump*

With the use of a rigid sigmoidoscope through the anus, the rectal stump can be identified and dissected from the surrounding structures (Figure 17-1). Adhesions must be lysed so that small intestinal loops can be cleared away from the pelvis. The rectal stump is then circumferentially mobilized for 3-5 cm from surrounding pelvic tissues. Any residual sigmoid colon should be resected to insure anastomosis of the descending colon to the top of the rectum and not to residual diseased sigmoid colon. A preoperative contrast enema radiograph is helpful in this regard. Anastomotic landmarks are identified to insure appropriate height, including dissipation of the appendices epiplocae and the confluence of teniae coli as well as proctographic verification of the 15 cm level from the dentate line as being at the sacral promontory and free of any diverticular openings.

### *Mobilization of the Left Colon*

Mobilization of the left colon is often necessary to insure a tension free anastomosis. This mobilization proceeds as described earlier.

### *Performing the Anastomosis*

Before proceeding with the anastomosis, the surgeon must establish that it can be created without tension. A purse string suture is placed at the proximal end and a detached anvil (from an intraluminal stapler) is inserted into the bowel **(Figure 17–18)**. The transanal device is passed through the rectal stump and the anastomosis is accomplished **(Figure 17–19)**. The anastomosis is best viewed from the right iliac fossa port; care must be taken to insure appropriate orientation of the bowel and its mesentery.

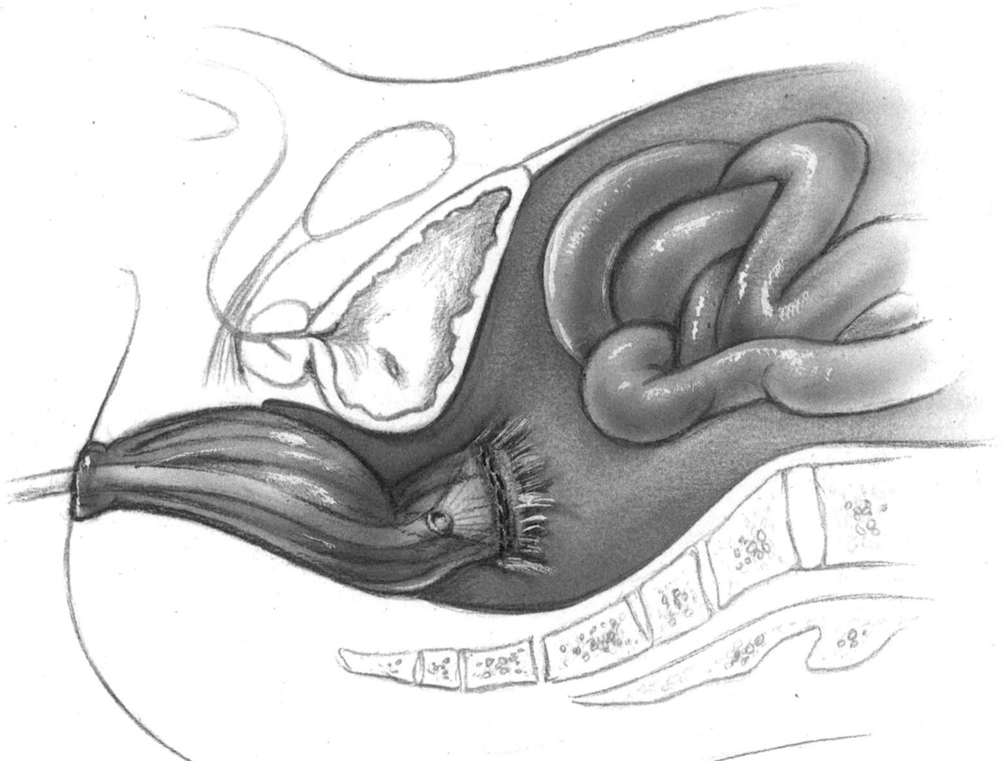

Fig. 17-17

Fig. 17-18

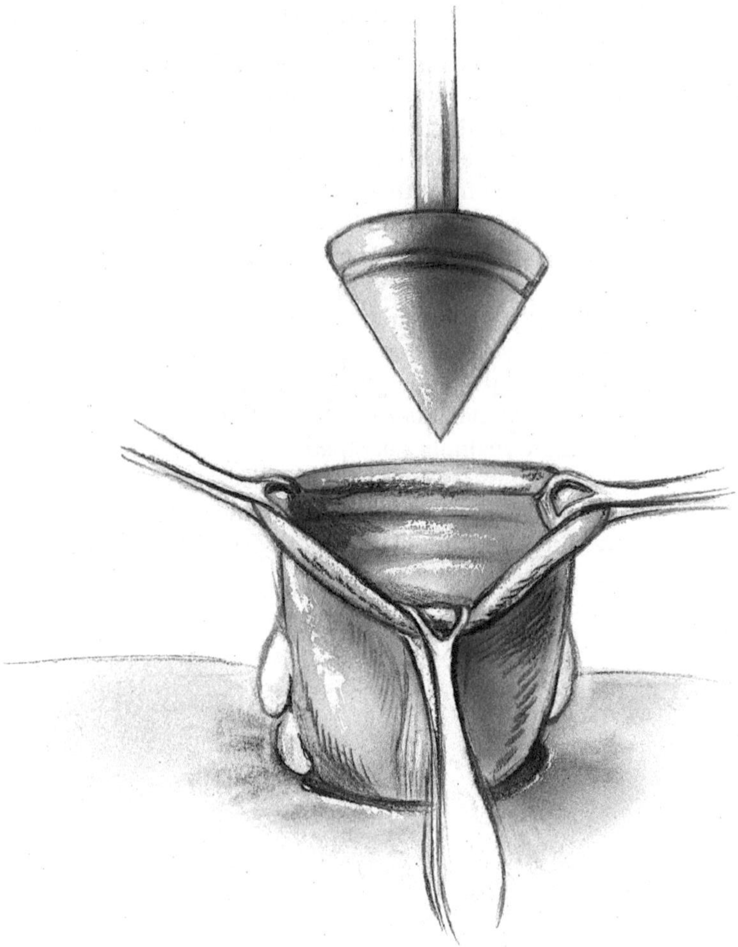

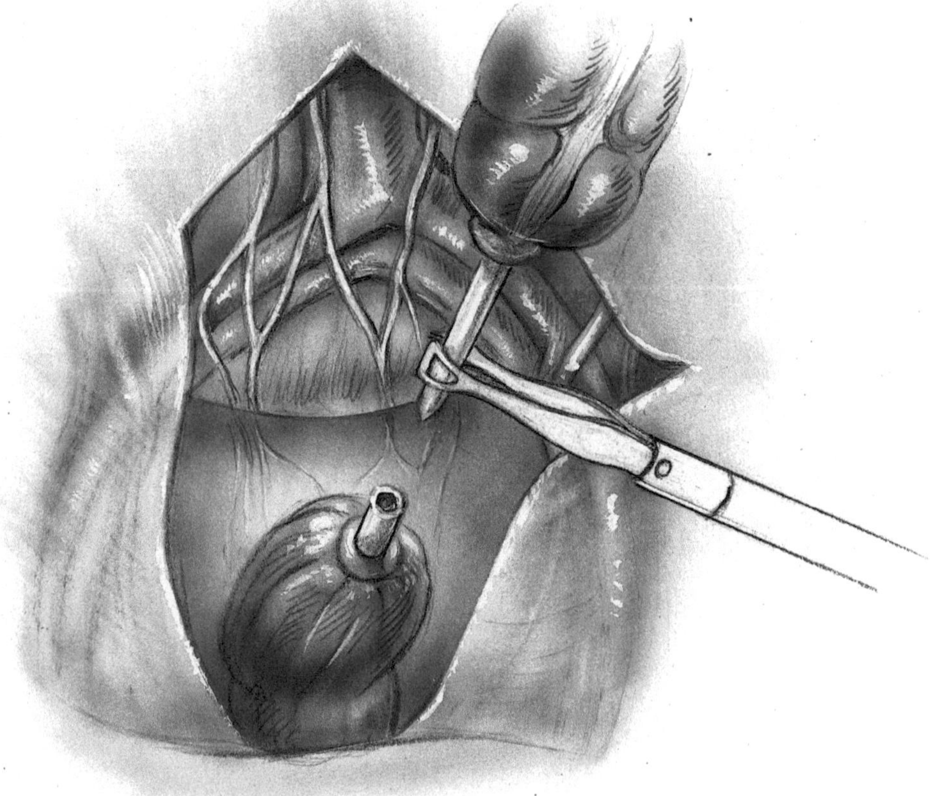

Fig. 17-19

### *Testing the Anastomosis*

The proximal bowel is gently occluded and anastomotic integrity is tested by insufflating air through a sigmoidoscope while filling the pelvis with warm saline solution. Endoscopic verification of a widely patent circumferentially intact anastomosis is undertaken. The anastomosis should be free of any tension and any diverticular distal to the staple line. The same procedure can be employed to anastomose the transverse colon and ileum to the rectum.

## POSTOPERATIVE CARE

A transparent ostomy pouch should be available and applied in the operating room and the stoma can be regularly inspected in the postoperative period. If the margin of the stoma becomes edematous during the first 24 to 72 hours, it is usually not necessary to revise the stoma. However a dark or black stoma needs to be evaluated for extensive necrosis and potentially reconstructed. Oral fluids are usually given during the first 24-hour postoperative period. The patient is discharged following tolerance of a regular diet and stoma education has progressed.

## COMPLICATIONS

### General Complications

Port site bleeding

Wound infection

Obstruction

Ileus

### Complications Related to Stoma Construction

Parastomal hernia

Incisional hernia

Prolapse

Skin problems (stoma formation)

### Complication Related to Stoma Closure

Anastomotic leak (stoma takedown)

## REFERENCES

Ludwig KA, Strong SA.Stoma creation: North American point of view. In Wexner SD (ed). Laparoscopic Colorectal Surgery. New York, Springer-Verlag, 1999, pp 189–202.

Oliveira, L. Stoma creation: South American point of view. In Wexner SD (ed). Laparoscopic Colorectal Surgery. New York, Springer-Verlag, 1999, pp 203–212.

Luchtefeldt MA. Hartmann's take down. In Wexner SD (ed). Laparoscopic Colorectal Surgery. New York, Springer-Verlag, 1999, pp 213–222.

Milson WJ, Bohm B. Stoma construction and closure using laparoscopic techniques. In Wexner SD (ed). Laparoscopic colorectal surgery. New York, Springer-Verlag, 1995, pp 195–214.

MacFadyen B Jr. Laparoscopic stoma creation and reversal In Wexner SD (ed). Laparoscopic Surgery of the Abdomen. New York, Springer-Verlag, 2003, pp 389–396.

# 18 Operations for Colonic Diverticulitis (Including Lower Gastrointestinal Bleeding)

## INDICATIONS

Elective

Recurrent diverticulitis

Colovesical fistula

Urgent

Diverticular abscess or phlegmon unresponsive to medical management

Complete colon obstruction

Suspicion of coexistent carcinoma

Emergent

Spreading or generalized peritonitis

Massive hemorrhage

## PREOPERATIVE PREPARATION

See Chapter 1.

## OPERATIVE STRATEGY

This operation is applicable to elective surgery for diverticular disease and may be used during emergency surgery for lower gastrointestinal bleeding. In the latter case, it is crucial to localize the bleeding source before surgery.

The operative technique for resecting the left colon and for the anastomosis is similar to that described for left colectomy for carcinoma but with a number of important exceptions.

1. Because there is no need to perform a high lymphovascular dissection in the absence of cancer, the mesentery may be divided at a point much closer to the bowel unless the mesentery is so inflamed and edematous it cannot hold ligatures.

2. In most cases it is not necessary to elevate the rectum from the presacral space, as this area is rarely the site of diverticula. The anastomosis can be done at the promontory of the sacrum.

3. Though it is important to remove the greatest concentration of diverticula, in elderly patients it is not necessary to perform an extensive colectomy just because there are some innocent diverticula in the ascending or transverse colon. The site selected for anastomosis should be free of diverticula and gross muscle hypertrophy.

4. Primary anastomosis should be performed only if the proximal and distal bowel segments selected for anastomosis are free of cellulitis and of marked muscle hypertrophy. If an abscess has been encountered in the pelvis, so that the anastomosis would lie on the wall of an evacuated abscess cavity, it is wise to delay the anastomosis for a secondstage operation.

## OPERATIVE TECHNIQUE

### Primary Resection and Anastomosis

#### *Incision*

Make a midline incision from the upper epigastrium to the pubis.

#### *Liberation of Sigmoid and Left Colon*

Initiate the dissection in the region of the upper descending colon by incising the peritoneum in the paracolic gutter. Then insert the left hand behind the colon (**Fig. 18–1**) in an area above the diverticulitis to elevate the mesocolon. Continue the incision in the paracolic peritoneum down to the descending colon and sigmoid to the brim of the pelvis.

At this point, to safeguard the left ureter from damage, it is essential to locate it in the upper portion of the dissection, where the absence of inflammation simplifies its identification. Then trace the ureter down into the pelvis. It may have to be dissected off an area of fibrosis in the sigmoid. When this dissection has been completed, the sigmoid is free down to the promontory of the sacrum.

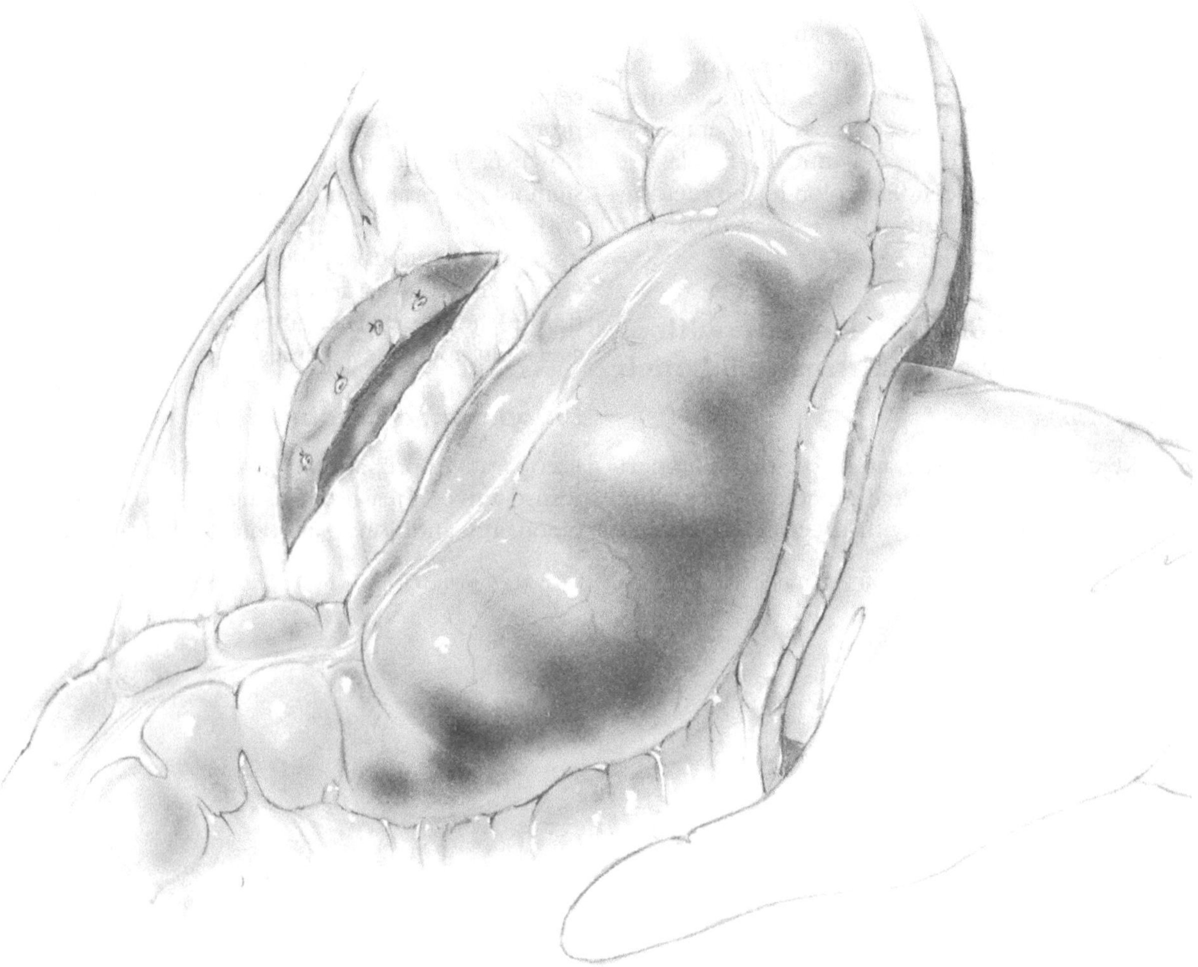

Fig. 18-1

### *Division of Mesocolon*

In elective cases the mesentery generally can be divided serially between Kelly hemostats at a point no more than 4-6 cm from the bowel wall (Fig. 18-1). Initiate the line of division at a point on the left colon that is free of pathology. This sometimes requires liberation of the splenic flexure and distal transverse colon. Continue the dissection to the rectosigmoid. Remove the specimen after applying Allen clamps.

### *Anastomosis*

Perform an open-type anastomosis in one or two layers or by stapling as described in Chapter 4 (see Figs. 4-12 through 4-38). In rare cases it is necessary to make the anastomosis at a lower level, where the ampulla of the rectum is significantly larger in diameter than the proximal colon. In that case a side-to-end Baker anastomosis is preferable, as described in Chapter 6 (see Figs. 6-12 through 6-22).

### *Abdominal Closure*

In the absence of intraabdominal or pelvic abscesses, close the abdomen in the useful fashion. Intraperitoneal drains are not needed.

## Primary Resection with End-Colostomy and Mucous Fistula

If it is decided to delay the anastomosis for a second stage, it is not necessary to excise every bit of inflamed bowel, as this frequently requires a Hartmann pouch at the site of the rectosigmoid transaction and makes the second stage more difficult than if a mucous fistula can be constructed. In almost every case, proper planning of the operation permits exteriorization of the distal sigmoid as a mucous fistula, which can be brought out through the lower margin of the midline incision after a De Martel clamp or stapled closure is secured **(Fig. 18–2)**. Divide the mesocolon to preserve the vascularity of the mucous fistula. Then bring out an uninflamed area of the descending colon as an end-colostomy through a separate incision in the lateral portion of the left rectus muscle and excise the intervening diseased colon. The second stage of this operation—removal of the colostomy and mucous fistula and anastomosis of the descending colon to the rectosigmoid—may be carried out after a delay of several weeks.

## Emergency Sigmoid Colectomy with End-Colostomy and Hartmann's Pouch

### *Indications*

For patients suffering generalized or spreading peritonitis secondary to perforated sigmoid diverticulitis, a conservative approach with diverting transverse colostomy and local drainage is associated with a mortality rate of more than 50%. Immediate excision of the perforated bowel is necessary to remove the septic focus. Following this excision the preferred procedure is a mucous fistula and endcolostomy. However, if excising the perforated portion of the sigmoid leaves an insufficient amount of distal bowel with which to form a mucous fistula, Hartmann's operation is indicated. It is not wise to attempt to create a mucous fistula by extensive presacral dissection in the hope of lengthening the distal segment, as it only opens new planes to potential sepsis.

### *Preoperative Preparation*

Preoperative preparation primarily involves rapid resuscitative measures using intravenous fluids, blood, and antibiotics, as some patients are admitted

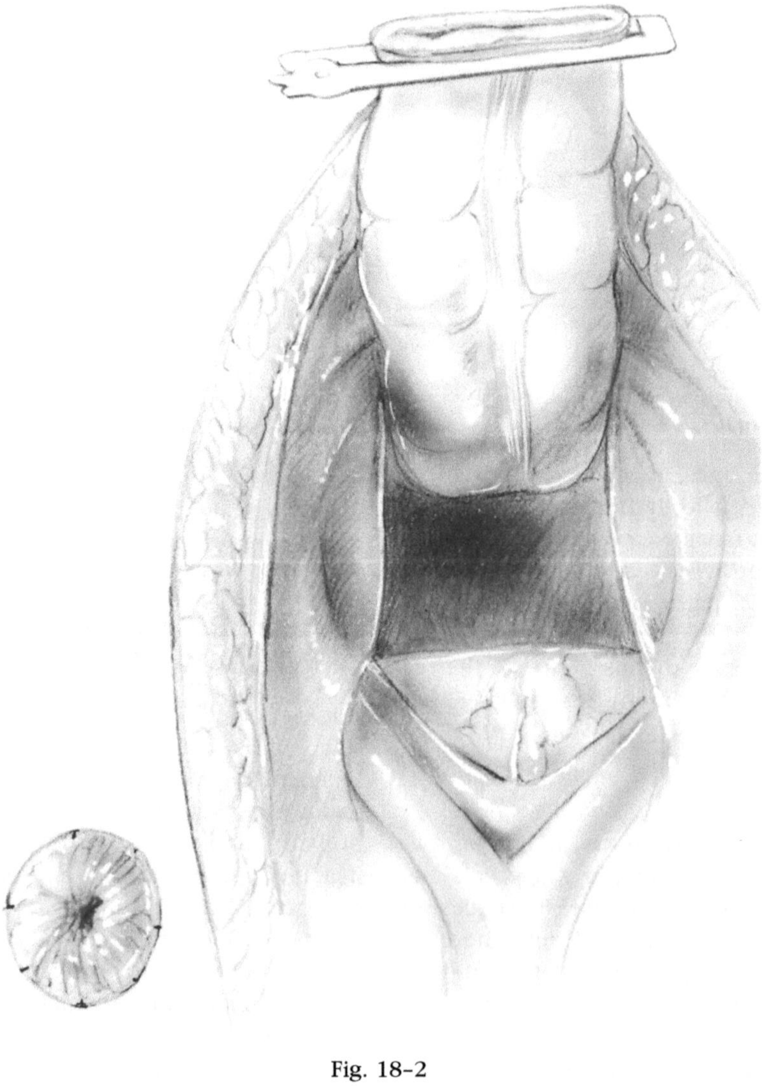

Fig. 18–2

to the hospital in septic shock. Complete colon preparation may not be possible, although many patients are given a modified dose of GoLYTELY for colonic cleansing. Nasogastric suction and bladder drainage with a Foley catheter should be instituted.

## *Operative Technique*

### *Incision and Liberation of Left Colon*

The steps for incision and liberation of the left colon are identical to those described above. It is essential to find the proper retromesenteric plane by initiating the dissection above the area of maximal inflammation. Once this has been achieved, with the left hand elevate the sigmoid colon and the diseased mesocolon (generally the site of a phlegmon) so the left paracolic peritoneum may be incised safely (Fig. 18-1). Again, it is essential to identify the left ureter in the upper abdomen to safeguard it from damage. Sometimes a considerable amount of blood oozes from the retroperitoneal dissection, but it can often be controlled by moist gauze packs while the dissection continues. After the left colon has been liberated, divide the mesentery serially between hemostats, as above.

### *Hartmann's Pouch*

Often with acute diverticulitis the rectosigmoid is not involved to a great extent in the inflammatory process. Mesenteric dissection should be terminated at this point. If the rectosigmoid is not excessively thick, occlude it by applying a 55/4.8mm linear stapler. Place an Allen clamp on the specimen side of the sigmoid and divide the bowel flush with the stapler. After the stapling device is removed there should be slight oozing of blood through the staples, which is evidence that excessively thickened tissue has not been necrotized by using the stapling technique on it **(Fig. 18–3)**.

If the tissue is so thick that compression to 2mm by the stapling device would result in necrosis, the technique is contraindicated. The rectal stump should then be closed by a continuous layer of locked sutures of 3-0 PG. Invert this layer with a second layer of continuous 3-0 PG Lembert sutures. Suture

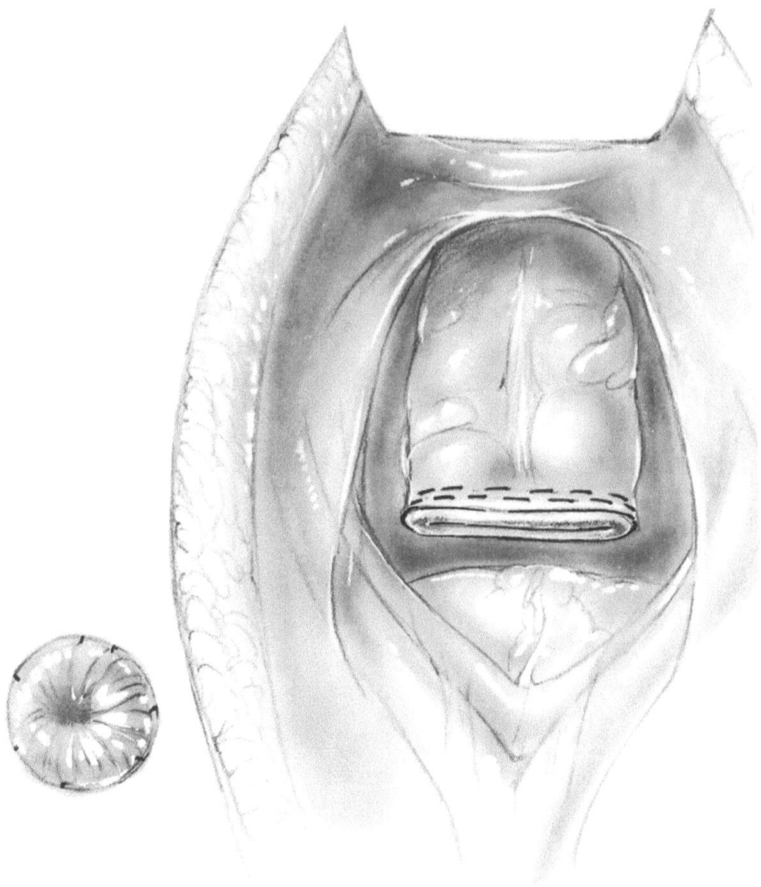

Fig. 18-3

the apex of the Hartmann pouch to the pelvic fascia near, or if possible higher than, the promontory of the sacrum to prevent retraction low into the pelvis, which would make a secondary anastomosis more difficult.

### *End-Colostomy*

Use an uninflamed area of the left colon for an end-colostomy. In a patient who is desperately ill, the colostomy may be brought out through the upper portion of the midline incision if it can save time. Otherwise, bring it out through a transverse incision over the lateral portion of left rectus muscle. The incision should admit two fingers. Bring out the cut end of the colon and immediately suture it with 4-0 PG, either interrupted or continuous, to the subcuticular layer of the skin incision.

### *Wound Closure*

Any rigid abscess cavities that cannot be excised should be managed by insertion of sump drains. If no rigid abscess walls have been left behind, the abdomen should be copiously irrigated and closed in the usual fashion without drainage. The skin can be managed by delayed primary closure.

## REFERENCES

Bergamaschi R, Arnaud JP. Intracorporeal colorectal anastomosis following laparoscopic left colon resection. Surg Endosc 1997;11:800.

Bouillot JL, Aouad K, Badawy A, Alamowitch B, Alexandre JH. Elective laparoscopic-assisted colectomy for diverticular disease: a prospective study in 50 patients. Surg Endosc 1998;12:1393.

Eng K, Ranson JH, Localio SA. Resection of the perforated segment: a significant advance in the treatment of diverticulitis with free perforation of abscess. Am J Surg 1977;133:67.

Smadja C, Sbai Idrissi M, Tahrat M, et al. Elective laparoscopic sigmoid colectomy for diverticulitis: results of a prospective study. Surg Endosc 1999;13:645.

Wexner SD, Moscovitz ID. Laparoscopic colectomy in diverticular and Crohn's disease. Surg Clin North Am 2000;80:1299.

# 19 Ripstein Operation for Rectal Prolapse

## INDICATIONS

Complete prolapse of the rectum

## PREOPERATIVE PREPARATION

Mechanical and antibiotic bowel preparation

Sigmoidoscopy

Barium colon enema

Foley catheter in bladder

Perioperative antibiotics

## PITFALLS AND DANGER POINTS

Excessive constriction of the rectum by mesh, which may result in partial obstruction or, rarely, erosion of mesh into the rectal lumen

Disruption of suture line between mesh and presacral space

Presacral hemorrhage

## OPERATIVE STRATEGY

The Ripstein operation uses permanent polypropylene mesh to fix the rectum to the presacral fascia, thereby restoring the normal posterior curve of the rectum and eliminating intussusception and prolapse. This operation is indicated only in patients who are not also suffering from significant constipation. Constipated patients do better with resection of the redundant sigmoid colon and colorectal anastomosis with sutures attaching the lateral ligaments of the rectum to the sacral fascia. For extremely poor-risk patients with rectal prolapse, a Thiersch operation (see Chapter 26) or perineal resection (see References) may be performed.

To prevent undue constriction of the rectum when the mesh is placed around it, *leave sufficient room to pass two fingers behind the rectum* after the mesh has been fixed in place. The success of the Ripstein operation is *not predicated on any degree of constriction* of the rectum. It suffices if the mesh simply prevents the rectum from advancing in an anterior direction away from the hollow of the sacrum.

The site on the rectum selected for placing the mesh is important. The upper level of the mesh should be 5 cm below the promontory of the sacrum, which requires opening the rectovesical or rectouterine peritoneum. In most cases the lateral ligaments of the rectum need not be divided. Avoid damage to the hypogastric nerves in the presacral area, especially in male patients, in whom nerve transection produces retrograde ejaculation.

## OPERATIVE TECHNIQUE

### Incision

A midline incision between the umbilicus and pubis provides excellent exposure in most patients. In young women the operation is accompanied by improved cosmetic results if it is performed through a Pfannenstiel incision. Place the 12- to 15-cm long Pfannenstiel incision just inside the public hairline, in the crease that goes from one anterior superior iliac spine to the other **(Fig. 19–1)**. With the scalpel, divide the subcutaneous fat down to the anterior rectus sheath and the external oblique aponeurosis. Divide the anterior rectus sheath in the line of the incision about 2 cm above the pubis **(Fig. 19–2)**. Extend the incision in the rectus sheath laterally in both directions into the external oblique aponeurosis. Apply Allis clamps to the cephalad portion of this fascial layer and bluntly dissect it off the underlying rectus muscles almost to the level of the umbilicus **(Fig. 19–3)**. Separate the rectus muscles in the midline, exposing the preperitoneal fat and peritoneum. Grasp the fat and peritoneum in an area sufficiently cephalad to the bladder to not endanger that

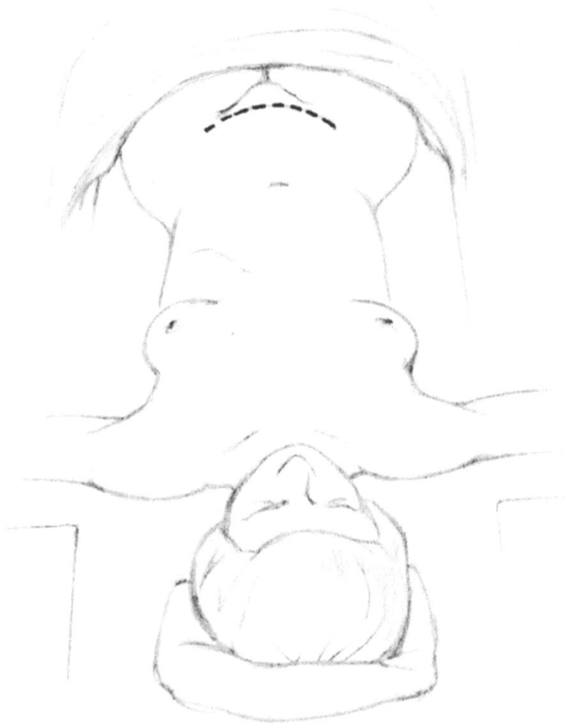

Fig. 19-1

organ. Incise the peritoneum, open the abdominal cavity, and explore it for coincidental pathology. A moderate Trendelenburg position is helpful.

## Incision of Pelvic Peritoneum

Retract the small intestine in a cephalad direction. Make an incision in the pelvic peritoneum beginning at the promontory of the sacrum and proceed along the left side of the mesorectum down as far as the cul-de-sac. Identify the left ureter.

Make a second incision in the peritoneum on the right side of the mesorectum, where the mesorectum meets the pelvic peritoneum. Extend this incision also down to the cul-de-sac and identify and preserve the right ureter. Join these two incisions by dividing the peritoneum at the depth of the rectovesical or rectouterine pouch using Metzenbaum scissors (see Figs. 6-4 through 6-6). Frequently, the cul-de-sac is deep in patients with rectal prolapse. Further dissection between the rectum and the prostate or vagina is generally not necessary.

## Presacral Dissection

For rectal prolapse the rectum can be elevated with ease from the hollow of the sacrum. Enter the presacral space via a Metzenbaum dissection, a method similar to that described for anterior resection (see Chapter 6). Take the usual precautions to avoid

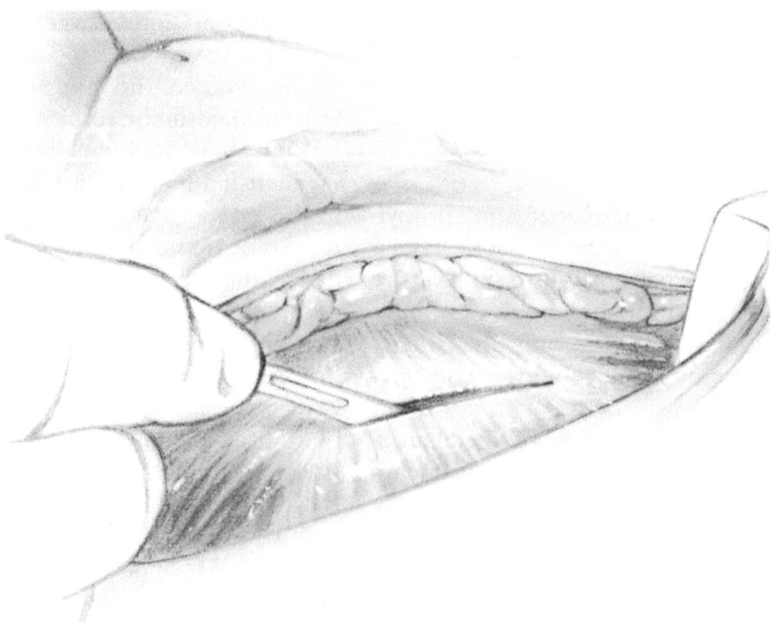

Fig. 19-2

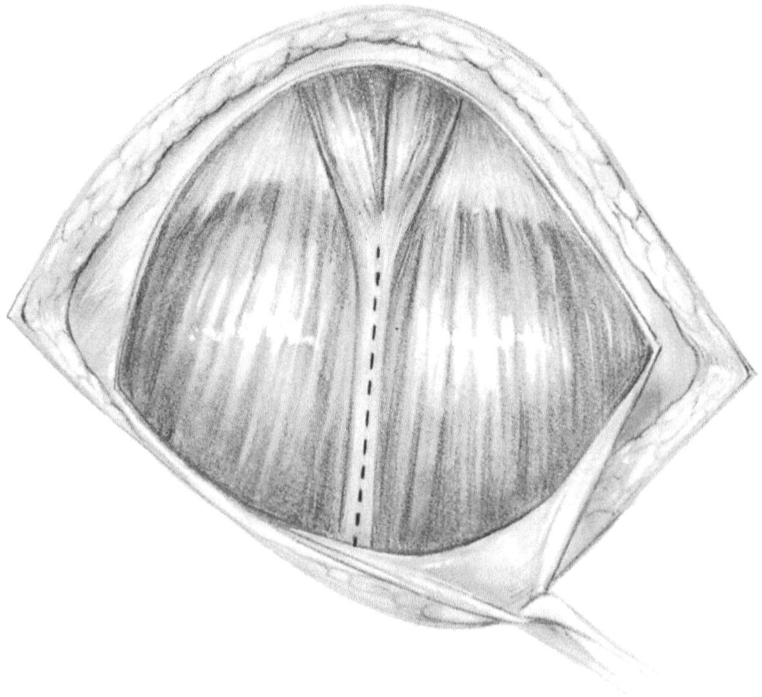

Fig. 19–3

damage to the presacral veins. Inspect the presacral area for hemostasis, which should be perfect before the procedure is continued.

## Application of Mesh

Fit a section of Prolene mesh measuring 5 × 10 cm or 5 × 12 cm into place overlying the lower rectum. The upper margin of the mesh should lie over the rectum at a point 4–5 cm below the sacral promontory. Using a small Mayo needle, insert three interrupted sutures of 2-0 Prolene or Tevdek into the right margin of the mesh and attach the mesh to the sacral periosteum along a line about 1–2 cm to the right of the mid-sacral line. Use the same technique to insert three interrupted sutures in the left lateral margin of the mesh and through the sacral fascia and periosteum **(Fig. 19–4a)**. Tie none of these sutures yet, but apply a hemostat to each of them temporarily. After all six sutures have been inserted, have the assistants draw them taut. Then insert two fingers between the rectum and sacrum to check the tension of the mesh, thereby ensuring that there will be no constriction of the rectum **(Fig. 19–4b)**. Now tie all six sutures. Use additional sutures of 4-0 atraumatic Prolene or Tevdek to attach both the proximal and distal margins of the mesh to the underlying rectum, so there is no possibility of the rectum sliding forward underneath the mesh.

Because there is a significant incidence of severe constipation and narrowing of the lumen by the mesh, Nicosia and Bass described fixation of the mesh to the presacral fascia using sutures or a fascial stapler. The mesh is then *partially* wrapped around and sutured to the rectum, leaving the anterior third of the rectal circumference free to dilate as necessary **(Figs. 19–5, 19–6)**.

## Closure of Pelvic Peritoneum

Irrigate the pelvic cavity. Close the incision in the pelvic peritoneum with a continuous suture of 2-0 atraumatic PG **(Fig. 19–7)**.

## Wound Closure

To close the Pfannenstiel incision, grasp the peritoneum with hemostats and approximate it with a continuous 2-0 atraumatic PG suture. Use several sutures of the same material loosely to approximate the rectus muscle in the midline. Close the transverse incision in the rectus sheath and external oblique aponeurosis with interrupted sutures of atraumatic 2-0 PG. Close the skin with a continuous 4-0 PG subcuticular suture.

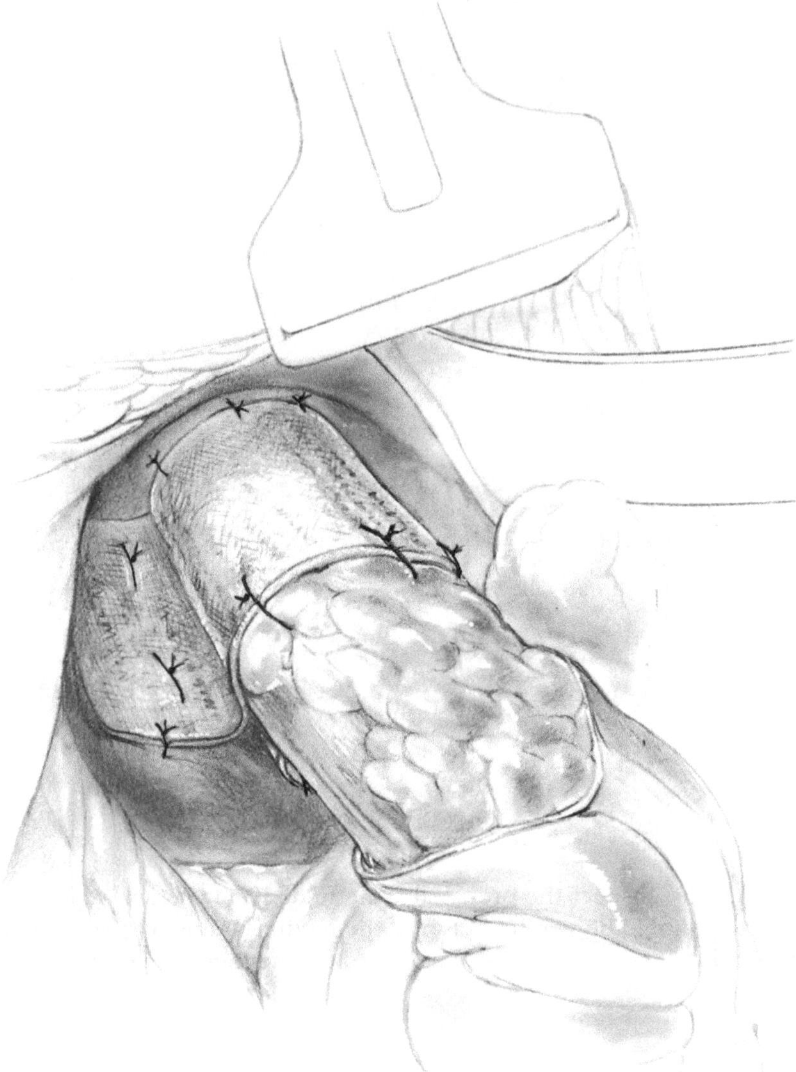

Fig. 19–4a

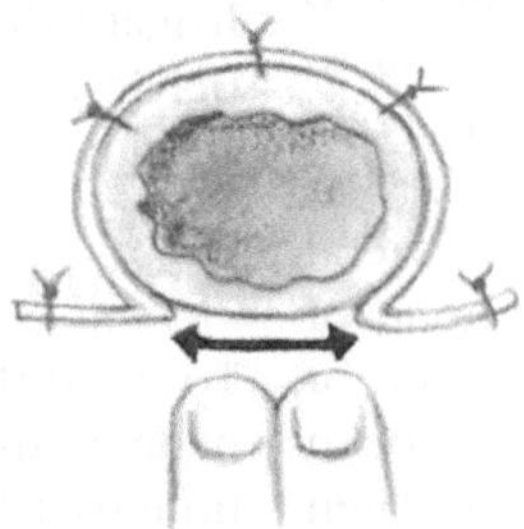

Fig. 19–4b

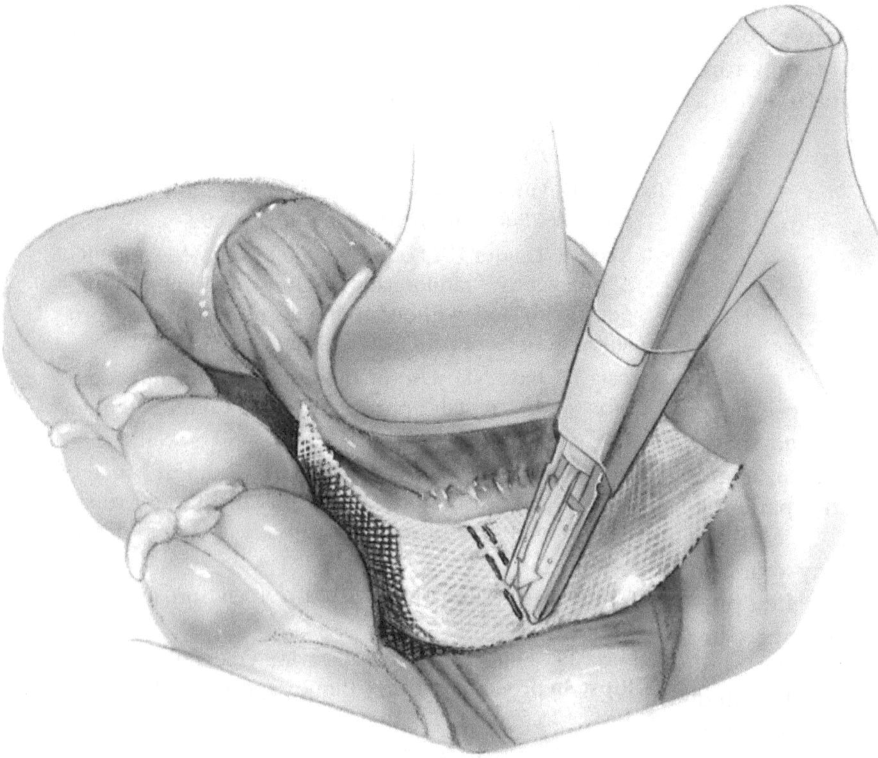

Fig. 19-5

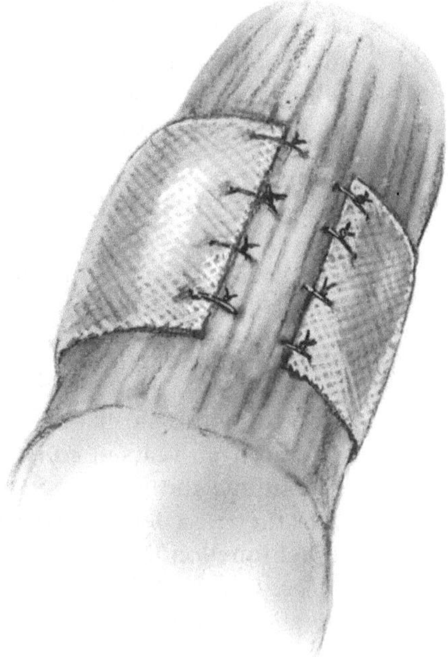

Fig. 19-6

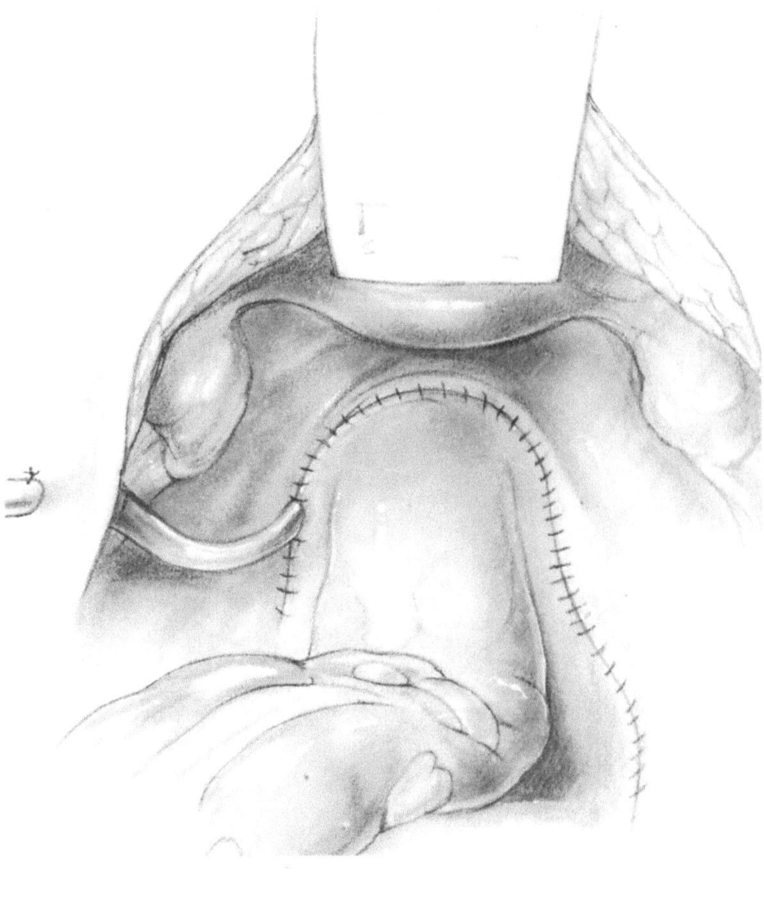

Fig. 19-7

Generally, no pelvic drains are necessary. If hemostasis is not perfect, bring a 6mm Silastic catheter out from the presacral space through a puncture wound in the lower abdomen and attach it to a closed-suction device (Fig. 19-5).

## POSTOPERATIVE CARE

Nasogastric suction is not necessary.

## COMPLICATIONS

Most patients who have a complete prolapse have suffered from years of *constipation*. They may have to continue the use of laxatives, although in some cases there is a definite improvement in the patient's bowel function following the operation.

*Fecal incontinence*—the result of many years of dilatation of the anal sphincters due to repeated prolapse—is also common among these patients. Correction of the prolapse does not automatically eliminate incontinence. This condition is alleviated over time in more than 30% of patients who are placed on a regimen of high fiber and muscle-strengthening exercises, occasionally supplemented with biofeedback.

## REFERENCES

Corman ML. Rectal prolapse: surgical techniques. Surg Clin North Am 1988;68:1255.

Cuschieri A, Shimi SM, Vander Velpen G, Banting S, Wood RA. Laparoscopic prosthesis fixation rectopexy for complete rectal prolapse. Br J Surg 1994;81:138.

Eu KW, Seow-Choen F. Functional problems in adult rectal prolapse and controversies in surgical treatment. Br J Surg 1997;84:904.

Jacobs LK, Lin YJ, Orkin BA. The best operation for rectal prolapse. Surg Clin North Am 1997;77:49.

McKee RF, Lauder JC, Poon FW, Aitchison MA, Finlay IG. A prospective randomized study of abdominal rectopexy with and without sigmoidectomy in rectal prolapse. Surg Gynecol Obstet 1992;174:145.

Nicosia JF, Bass NM. Use of the fascial stapler in proctopexy for rectal prolapse. Dis Colon Rectum 1987;30:900.

Prasad ML, Pearl RK, Abcarian H, et al. Perineal proctectomy, posterior rectopexy, and postanal levator repair for the treatment of rectal prolapse. Dis Colon Rectum 1986;29:547.

Ripstein CB. Surgical care of massive rectal prolapse. Dis Colon Rectum 1965;8:34.

Roberts PL, Schoetz DJ Jr, Coller JA, Veidenheimer MC. Ripstein procedure: Lahey Clinic experience. Arch Surg 1988;123:554.

Tobin SA, Scott IH. Delorme operation for rectal prolapse. Br J Surg 1994;81:1681.

Watts JD, Rothenberger DA, Buls JG, et al. The management of procidentia, 30 years experience. Dis Colon Rectum 1985;28:96.

Yoshioka K, Hyland G, Keighley MR. Anorectal function after abdominal rectopexy: parameters of predictive value in identifying return of continence. Br J Surg 1989;76:64.

# Part II

## Anus, Rectum, and Pilonidal Region

# 20 Concepts in Surgery of the Anus, Rectum, and Pilonidal Region

Amanda M. Metcalf

Successful management of anorectal disease depends on a clear understanding of what symptoms can be attributed to various conditions.[1,2] In addition, consideration must be given to the impact of other aspects of colorectal physiology on function and healing. The perianal skin and lower aspect of the anal canal is richly innervated by sensory fibers. External hemorrhoids are venous plexuses located below the dentate line and covered with squamous epithelium. Internal hemorrhoids are submucosal vascular tissue containing blood vessels, smooth muscle, and connective tissue that are normally located above the dentate line. They are covered with transitional epithelium. Chronic straining is thought to cause excessive engorgement of the vascular cushions and disruption of the smooth muscle and connective tissue. This disruption allows the vascular cushions and the overlying mucosa to slide down the anal canal and prolapse during straining. Repetitive straining promotes further prolapse.

Internal hemorrhoids are classified by their extent of prolapse down the anal canal during straining. Second-degree internal hemorrhoids are those that prolapse down the anal canal during straining and spontaneously reduce. Third-degree internal hemorrhoids prolapse with straining and require manual reduction. Fourth-degree hemorrhoids cannot be reduced.

The pressure generated in the anal canal to keep it closed during periods of inattention or sleep is called the resting anal tone. Approximately half of the normal resting anal tone is contributed by the internal anal sphincter, which is a continuation of the circular muscle of the rectum **(Fig. 20–1)**. The lower edge of the internal sphincter and the groove between the internal and external sphincter can be palpated approximately 1 cm below the dentate line. The remainder of the resting anal tone is provided by the external sphincter muscles and the puborectalis. The external anal sphincters encircle the lower portion of the anal canal, and the puborectalis surrounds the posterior and lateral portions of the upper anal canal. The puborectalis, which is continuous with the levator ani muscles that form the pelvic diaphragm, is best palpated posteriorly and is often referred to as the anorectal ring.

The maximum pressure that can be generated in the anal canal is produced by the voluntary contraction of the external sphincters and the puborectalis. It is called the maximum voluntary squeeze and can be maintained for only a short time. Contraction of the striated sphincteric mechanism is also caused as a reflex in response to coughing or sneezing. Continence depends on the interaction between the anal sphincters, the type of challenge (solid, liquid, gas), and the compliance of the rectum. The compliance of the rectum can be thought of as its ability to act as a reservoir. Decreased compliance of the rectum produces urgent calls to stool at low intrarectal volumes. Common causes of decreased rectal compliance include radiation proctitis, inflammatory bowel disease, rectal resection, and irritable bowel syndrome. Patients with incontinence often have abnormalities in more than one area. Patients with a sphincter injury may have a good control of formed stool but be incontinent with liquid stool. Subtle abnormalities in sphincter function and continence may be unmasked by anal surgery. This can occur even with procedures that are usually not associated with changes in continence, such as a partial lateral internal sphincterotomy. Therefore it is extremely important to determine any abnormalities in bowel function that would predispose individuals to impaired continence postoperatively. Historical information regarding bowel habits and symptoms of minor sphincter dysfunction such as seepage, pruritus, or incontinence of flatus should be noted and documented.

Anal fissures are posterior or anterior midline epithelial defects or ulcers in the anal canal. Anal fissures are caused by the trauma of defecation and should never extend above the level of the dentate line or out onto the anal verge. The biomechanics of the anal canal are such that most fissures occur in

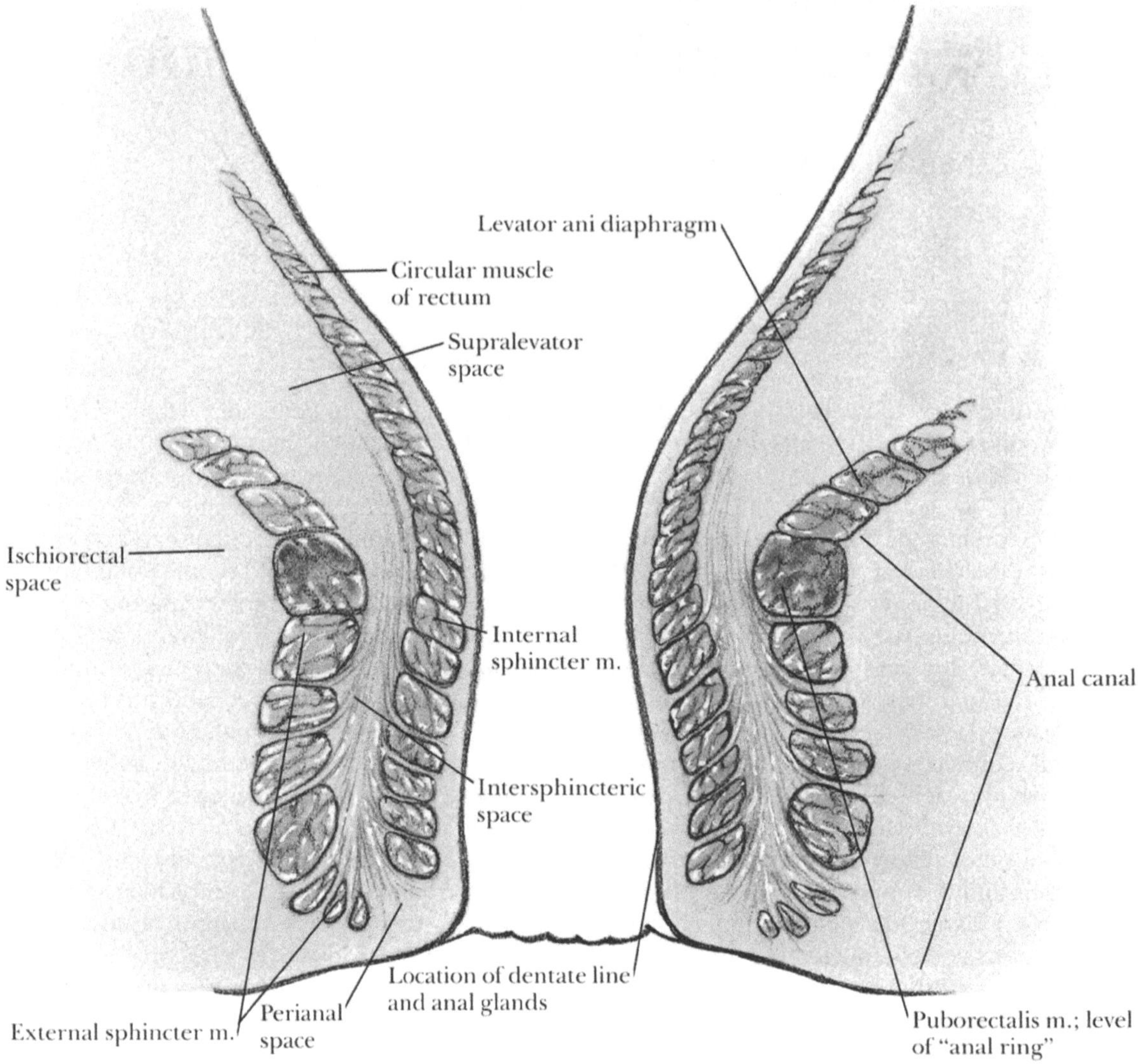


Fig. 20–1

the midline posteriorly or, less commonly, anteriorly. Painful anal fissures are associated with spasm of both the internal and external sphincters. Despite this spasm, it should be possible to see an anal fissure by gently spreading the skin of the anal verge and lower anal canal. Decreased resting anal tone in association with an anal fissure or an anal fissure in a patient with diarrhea suggests the diagnosis of Crohn's disease. Other possibilities are viral infection, such cytomegalovirus or herpes in an immunocompromised host. In either of these situations, the ulcer commonly appears unusually broad or deep. Current theory regarding the etiology of typical anal fissures is that the spasm of the sphincteric mechanism results in decreased blood flow to the lining of the anal canal, and that the resultant relative ischemia produces poor healing.

Perianal infections may present as obviously indurated, erythematous areas adjacent to the anus. They may also present more subtly with complaints of discomfort in the perineum or buttock and minimal physical findings. Most perianal infections are caused by enteric flora and originate in anal glands. Perianal infections caused by skin organisms are more likely to be manifestations of other processes such as folliculitis or hidradenitis suppurativa. The anal glands thought to be the origin of most perianal infections empty into the anal crypts at the level of the dentate line. The function of these glands is obscure. Only a small proportion of the anal glands traverse the internal sphincter into the intersphincteric space and can therefore serve as a source of infection. Infection in the intersphincteric space can spread directly caudad to the perianal skin or can penetrate the external sphincter or puborectalis to produce infection in the ischiorectal fossa. Midline anal glands posteriorly towad the coccyx can produce horseshoe abscesses, as potential perianal spaces communicate posteriorly.

Fistulas that result from perianal abscesses have been classified according to their relation to the sphincteric mechanism by Parks and others (1976). A type 1 fistula is intersphincteric **(Fig. 20–2)** and extends from its origin through the intersphincteric space to the perianal skin. A type 2 fistula is transsphincteric **(Fig. 20–3)** and extends through the external sphincter into the ischiorectal space to the skin of the buttocks. A type 3 fistula is suprasphincteric **(Fig. 20–4)**. It travels cephalad in the intersphincteric space, encircles the puborectalis, and then perforates the levator ani, continuing to the perianal skin. A type 4 fistula is extrasphincteric **(Fig. 20–5)**. Only rarely related to cryptoglandular infection, it usually originates from an intraabdominal source that has caused an infection in the pelvis. Conditions that could cause this type of fistula include diverticulitis, Crohn's disease, and foreign body perforation of the rectum. Fistulas caused by cryptoglan-

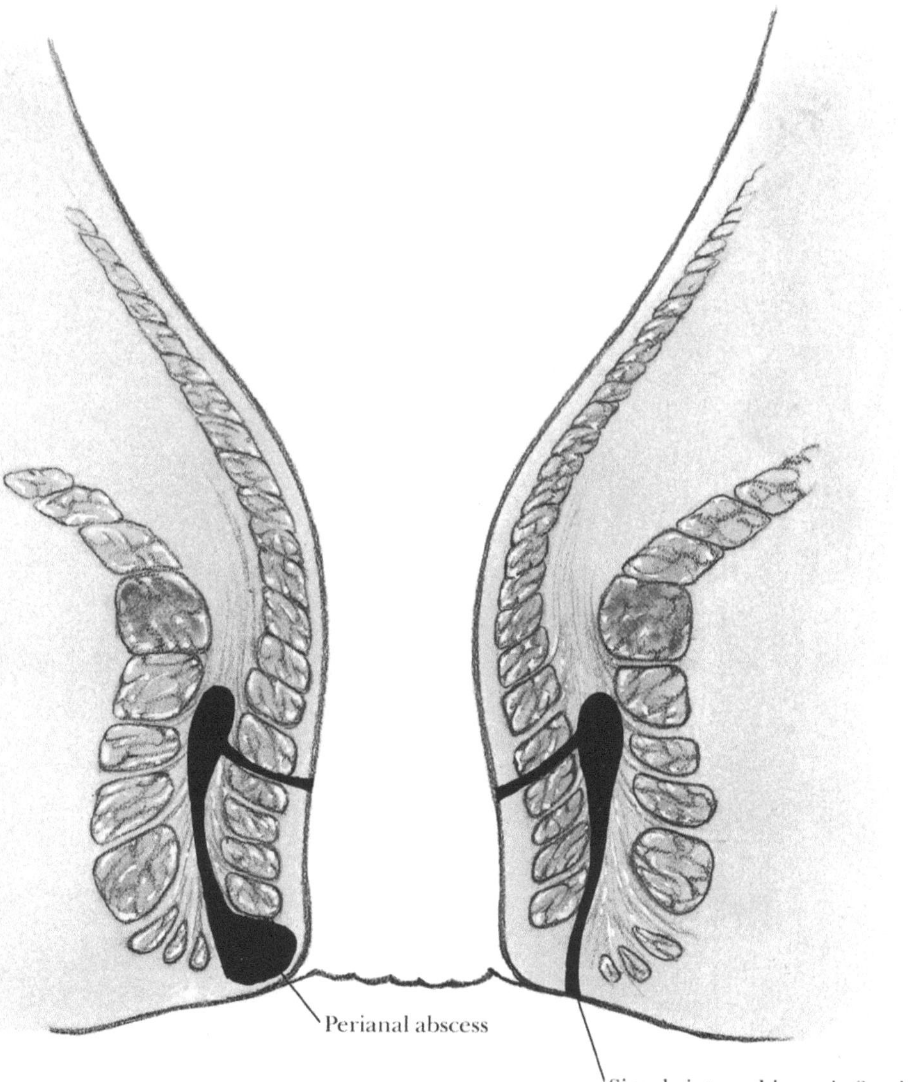


Fig. 20–2

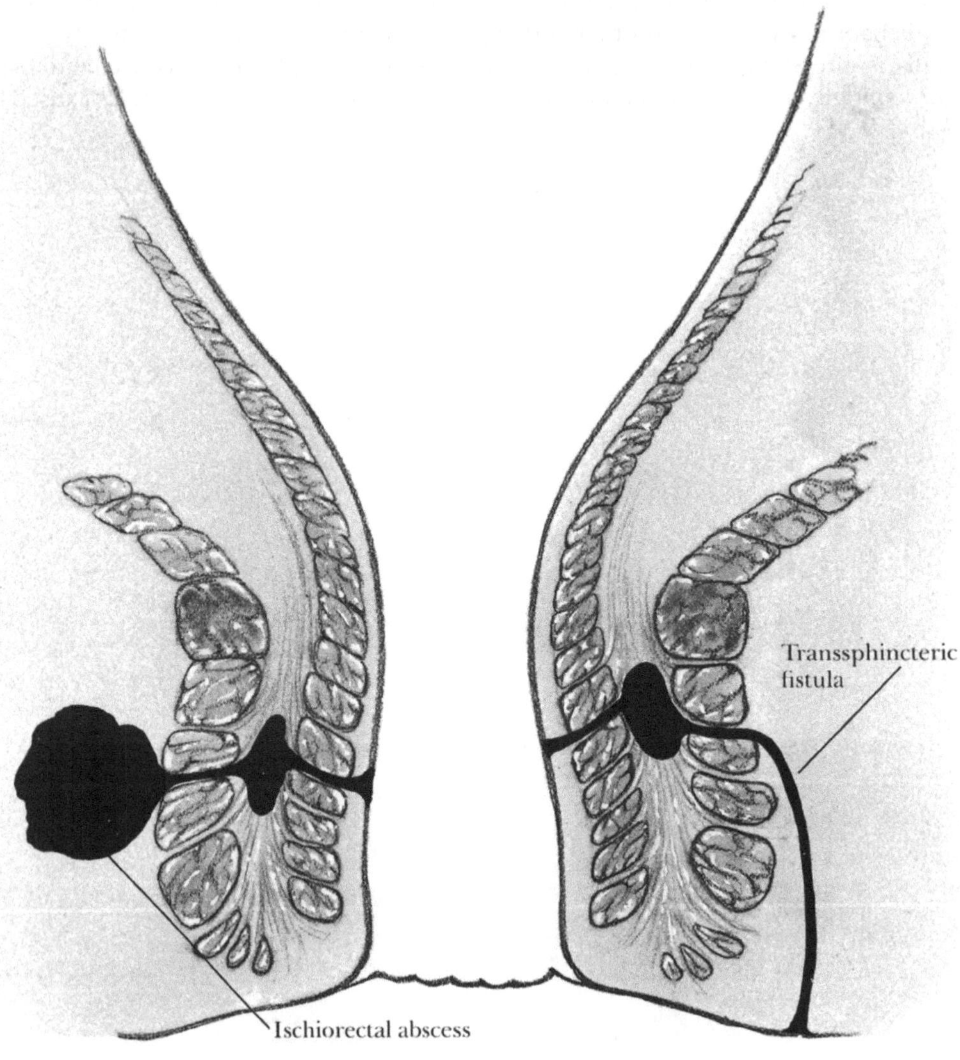


Fig. 20-3. Transphincteric fistula and ischiorectal abscess.

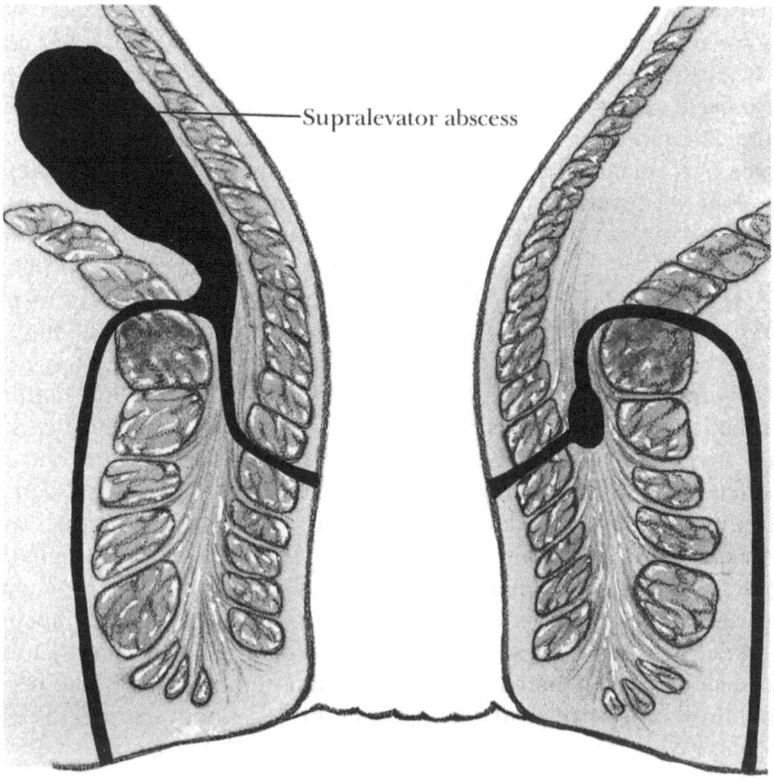


Fig. 20-4. Suprasphincteric fistulas.

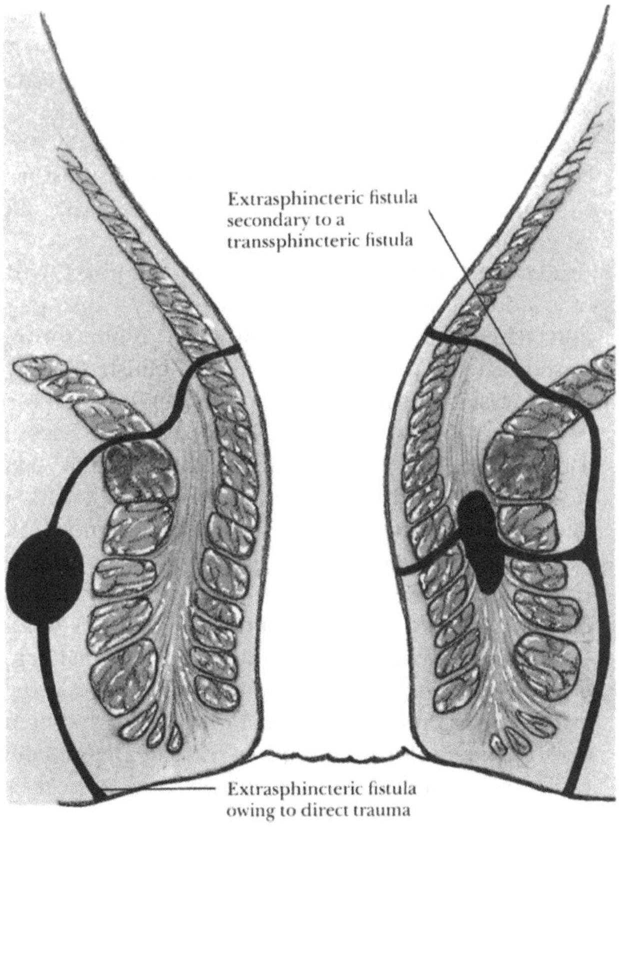


Fig. 20-5. Extrasphincteric fistulas.

dular infection therefore always surround a portion of the internal sphincter and a variable portion of the external sphincter. Because there is a relative deficiency of sphincter muscle anteriorly owing to the absence of the puborectalis, anterior fistulas encompass a relatively larger percentage of the sphincter mechanism than do posterior fistulas.

## CLINICAL CONDITIONS: SYMPTOMS AND MANAGEMENT CONCEPTS

The most common symptom of *internal hemorrhoids* is painless rectal bleeding. The bleeding can vary in quantity and frequency, but generally the quantity is fairly predictable for a given patient. It is not usually of significant amount to produce anemia unless the patient is coagulopathic or the internal hemorrhoids are grade 3 or larger. In general, internal hemorrhoids cause an unpleasant pressure sensation while they are prolapsed, which resolves with reduction of the prolapse. Internal hemorrhoids that do not prolapse should not cause pain. The amount of hemorrhoidal prolapse a patient has is best assessed while the patient is on the commode. The patient is asked to strain on the commode; and then, while still straining, is asked to lean forward to allow the examiner to visualize the perineum.

Irritation of the perianal skin produces an itching or burning sensation. These symptoms are independent of any underlying venous plexuses or redundant skin and are therefore not a symptom of external hemorrhoids. Internal hemorrhoids contribute to these symptoms only when they are chronically prolapsed and in this state increase perianal moisture. Chronically prolapsed internal hemorrhoids should be readily visible at the anal orifice.

*External hemorrhoids* become engorged with blood during a Valsalva maneuver. They cause pain only when they become thrombosed. When thrombosed, they appear as firm, painful, bluish skincovered masses on the anal verge. Although discomfort is maximal for the first 48–72 hours, residual discomfort persists for 7 days, and the "lump" may take several weeks to resolve. Within the first 72 hours of occurrence, excision of the thrombosed hemorrhoid relieves more pain than it causes. The converse is true after this time interval. As previously discussed, discomfort from internal hemorrhoids occurs when they remain prolapsed after straining. If internal hemorrhoids are acutely prolapsed and not reduced, they cause engorgement and edema of the external hemorrhoidal complex on the ipsilateral side. Eventually, both components may thrombose and appear as firm, painful, nonreducible masses, the inner covered with mucosa and the outer with squamous epithelium. When thrombosis has already occurred, treatment should be dictated by the time interval since onset: If less than 72 hours, hemorrhoidectomy is reasonable; if more than 72 hours, conservative management with stool softeners and analgesics is appropriate.

Over the years many treatments have been proposed for symptomatic internal hemorrhoids and have enjoyed brief surges of popularity. Among the nonsurgical techniques, only rubber band ligation has truly withstood the test of time.

Hemorrhoid banding is the treatment of choice for prolapsing symptomatic internal hemorrhoids. It is easily performed in the outpatient setting, requires no anesthetic, and is associated with few complications. With this technique, a strangulating rubber band is placed on the redundant rectal mucosa above the hemorrhoid. This procedure not only removes some of the redundant mucosa but also produces fixation of residual mucosa to the submucosa in the region of the banding. The residual vascular cushion in this location is fixed in the anal canal and does not prolapse with straining.

Hemorrhoidectomy should be reserved for patients who have failed banding, have large grade 3 or grade 4 hemorrhoids, or have smaller hemorrhoids associated with other anal pathology that requires operative intervention.

*Anal fissures* usually cause painful rectal bleeding. Reducing the anal canal pressure medically or by dividing a portion of the internal sphincter increases anal canal blood flow and promotes healing of the anal fissure. Medical therapy of an anal fissure should almost always precede surgical therapy. Stool bulking agents such as psyllium seed or methylcellulose in quantities sufficient to provide bulky soft stools reliably are the mainstays of medical therapy. Stool softeners and other laxatives should be avoided, as the resultant stool is so soft it does not dilate the anal canal. Dilute nitroglycerine ointment (0.2%) applied to the anus before and after bowel movements has been advocated by some as an adjunct to bulking agents to decrease pain and promote healing. Persistence of a painful anal fissure for 6 weeks on good medical therapy or development of a complication such as infection constitute an indication for surgical therapy. Surgical therapy is not indicated for a painless anal fissure.

*Perianal abscesses* require surgical drainage unless spontaneous rupture has produced adequate drainage. Because most perianal infections caused by cryptoglandular infections result in an anal fistula, it is helpful to drain the abscess through an incision as close to the anus as possible. This minimizes the length of a subsequent fistulotomy wound. Small abscesses that are easily visible on inspection and are not associated with systemic signs or symptoms can often be drained under local anesthesia. Ischiorectal fossa abscesses that present with ill-defined areas of induration and are associated with fever and leukocytosis are probably best drained under regional or general anesthesia. Whatever technique is used, it is imperative to have close follow-up examinations of the patient to document resolution of the problem. This is especially true in patients with diabetes, who are prone to developing necrotizing fascitis in an incompletely drained perianal abscess.

A *fistula-in-ano* can be diagnosed by failure of the drainage wound to heal completely or by abscess recurrence after apparently complete healing. A recurrent abscess may occur years after the original infection. A typical fistula tract can often by palpated subcutaneously as a fibrous cord between the external opening and the anal orifice. The origin of the fistula in the anal canal (primary opening) is most easily found when there is an active external (secondary) opening. If the site of the primary opening cannot be identified, a fistulotomy should not be performed. A fistulotomy always impairs sphincter function to some degree. Because the puborectalis is not present anteriorly, an anterior fistulotomy is more likely to result in a perceptible alteration in continence than a posterior fistulotomy of an equivalent amount of muscle. The amount of sphincter division that can be tolerated by the patient depends on the baseline sphincter function, the usual consistency of their stools, and the compliance of their rectum. A young patient with infrequent predictable stools tolerates far more sphincter division than does the elderly patient with irritable bowel syndrome and frequent erratic stools. No patient is continent if the entire anorectal ring is divided, regardless of his or her bowel habits. A history of diarrhea in association with a perianal fistula mandates preoperative evaluation for inflammatory bowel disease.

*Delayed wound healing* after anal surgery can be frustrating to both patient and surgeon. The single best agent to promote healing in the anal canal without stenosis after anal surgery is a bulky, soft, formed stool. Psyllium seed preparations or methylcellulosebased agents should be prescribed postoperatively for most patients. The use of constipating analgesics should be minimized. Altered bowel consistency, whether too hard or too loose, delays wound healing. Delayed wound healing is also seen in patients who have undergone irradiation, have diabetes or inflammatory bowel disease, or who have compromised immune systems.

*Pilonidal disease* is not an anorectal disease in the purest sense. Its association with anorectal disease is only by proximity. Pilonidal disease is a term used to describe infections that originate in the gluteal cleft. It is currently thought to be an acquired rather than a congenital disorder. The precise sequence of events is debated, but there is agreement that the shape of the gluteal cleft and its effect on loose hair in this region leads to penetration of hair underneath the skin. This leads to formation of chronic subcutaneous abscesses that contain hair. Multiple infectious episodes create multiple openings along the midline and lateral to it that can mimic other anal conditions. The variety of operations that have been described for this condition suggest that there is no solitary infallible procedure for cure. Current trends are toward less radical surgery. Avoidance of a midline wound, removal of the foreign material from the abscess cavity, and removal of hair in the region of the gluteal cleft by shaving or tweezing seem to be important elements for obtaining a healed wound.

## REFERENCES

Beck DE, Wexner SD. Fundamentals of Anorectal Surgery, 2nd ed. Philadelphia, Saunders, 1998.

Gordan PH, Nivatvongs S. Principles and Practice of Surgery for Colon, Rectum and Anus, 2nd ed. St. Louis, Quality, 1999.

Parks AG, Hardcastle JD, Gordon PH. A classification of fistula-in-ano. Br J Surg 1976;63:1.

# 21 Rubber Band Ligation of Internal Hemorrhoids

## INDICATIONS

Symptomatic (bleeding or prolapsed) internal hemorrhoids situated above the area in the anal canal, which is innervated by sensory nerves

## PITFALLS AND DANGER POINTS

Applying a rubber band in an area supplied by sensory nerves

## OPERATIVE STRATEGY

To avoid postoperative pain, apply the rubber band to a point *at least 5-6mm above the dentate line*. In some patients a margin of 5-6mm is not sufficient to avoid pain. These patients can be identified by pinching the mucosa at the site of the proposed application of the band. If the patient has pain when the mucosa is pinched, apply the band at a higher level where the mucosa is not sensitive or abandon the rubber-banding procedure.

If the patient has severe pain after the rubber band has been applied, remove the rubber band immediately using fine-tipped forceps and sharp pointed scissors. If this removal is delayed until several hours after the application, surrounding edema often makes the procedure difficult if not impossible without anesthesia and without causing bleeding.

## OPERATIVE TECHNIQUE

Perform sigmoidoscopy to rule out other possible sources of rectal bleeding. With the patient in the knee-chest position, insert a fenestrated anoscope (e.g., Hinkel-James type) that permits the internal hemorrhoid to protrude into the lumen of the anoscope. A lighted anoscope is a great convenience. Inspect the circumference of the anal canal. Try to identify the hemorrhoid that caused the bleeding. If this is not possible, identify the largest internal hemorrhoid. Insert the curved Allis tissue forceps into the anoscope and pinch the mucosa around the base of the hemorrhoid to identify an insensitive area. Ask the assistant to hold the anoscope in a steady position. Now inspect the McGivney rubber band applicator. Be sure that two rubber bands have been inserted into their proper position on the drum of the applicator. Ask the patient to strain. With the left hand pass the drum up to the *proximal* portion of the hemorrhoid. Insert the angled tissue forceps through the drum.

When grasping the rectal mucosa, be sure to grasp it along the cephalad surface of the hemorrhoid at point A (not point B) in **Figure 21–1**. If this is done, the rubber band does not encroach on the sensitive tissue at the dentate line. Draw the mucosa into the drum and simultaneously press the drum against the wall of the rectum **(Fig. 21–2)**. When the McGivney applicator is in the proper position, compress the handle of the applicator. Remove the tissue forceps and the McGivney applicator from the anoscope. The result should be a round purple mass of hemorrhoid about the size of a cherry and strangulated by the two rubber bands at its base.

Tchirkow et al. (1982) recommended injecting 1-2ml of a local anesthetic (we use 0.25% bupivacaine or lidocaine with epinephrine 1:200,000), using a 25-gauge needle, into the banded hemorrhoid. This maneuver appears to lessen some of the postoperative discomfort and may accelerate sloughing of the strangulated mass.

Nivatvongs and Goldberg (1982) advocate applying the band to redundant rectal mucosa just proximal to the hemorrhoid. Insert the slotted anoscope and ask the patient to strain. The redundant rectal mucosa just *proximal to the hemorrhoid* bulges into the slot of the anoscope. Apply the band to this mucosa as detailed above.

In general, only one hemorrhoid is treated at each office visit. Have the patient return in about 3 weeks for the second application. Rarely are more than

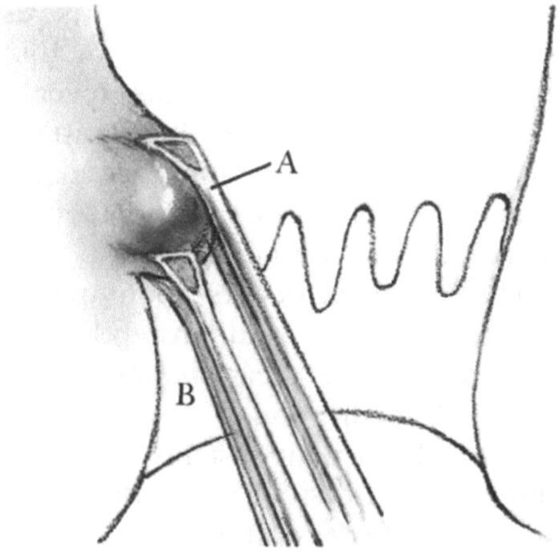


Fig. 21-1

three applications necessary. Applying two or three bands at one sitting often causes significant discomfort.

## POSTOPERATIVE CARE

Inform the patient that postoperatively he or she may feel a vague discomfort in the area of the rectum accompanied by mild tenesmus, especially for 1-2 days after the procedure. Prescribe mild nonconstipating analgesic medication. Apprehensive patients do well if this medication is supplemented by a tranquilizer such as diazepam.

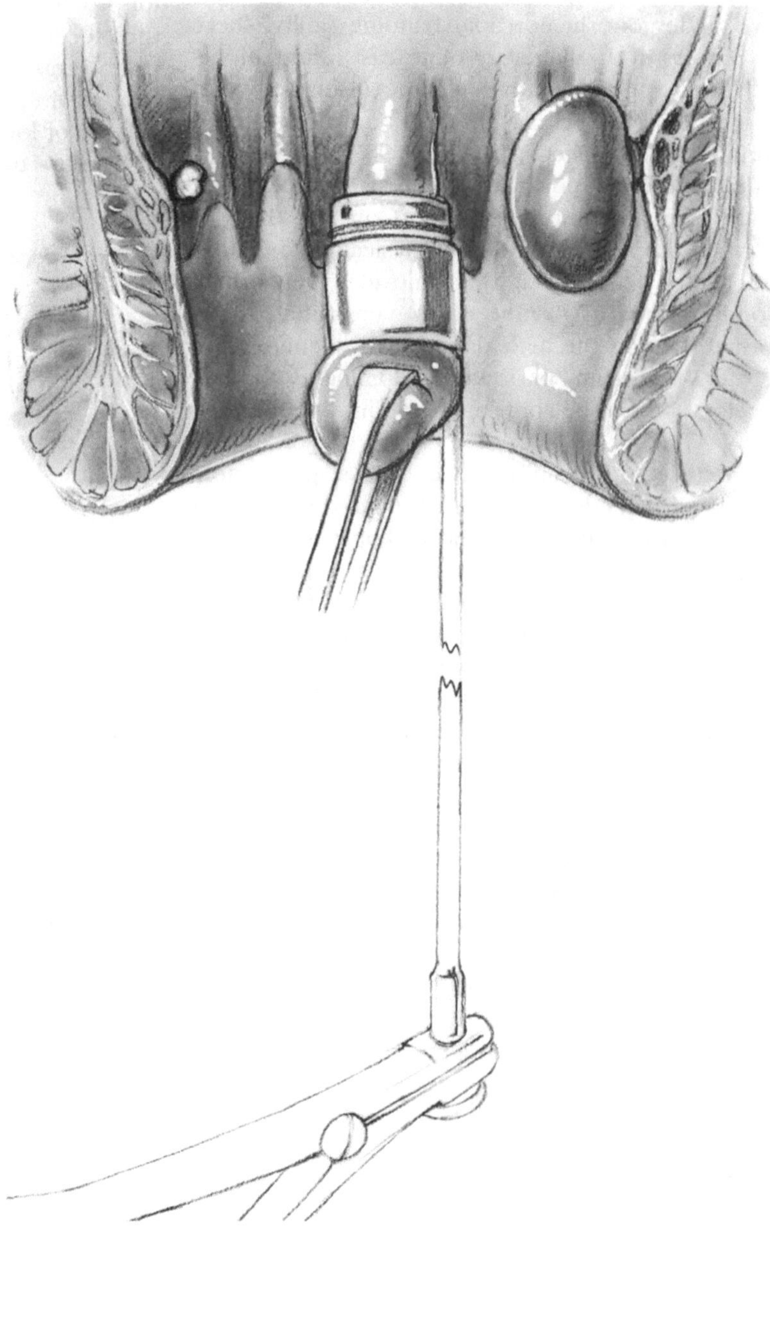

Fig. 21-2

Warn the patient prior to the procedure that on rare occasions sometime between the 7th and 10th postoperative days, when the slough separates, there may be active bleeding into the rectum. A serious degree of bleeding requiring hospitalization occurs in no more than 1–2% of cases.

Prescribe a stool softener such as Colace. For constipated patients, Senokot-S (two tablets nightly) helps to keep the stool soft and stimulates colonic peristalsis.

Patients may return to their regular occupation when they so desire.

## COMPLICATIONS

*Sepsis.* Even though tens of thousands of patients have undergone hemorrhoid banding safely, there are reports in the literature of at least nine patients with serious postoperative pelvirectal sepsis, five of whom died (Clay et al., 1986; O'Hara; Russell and Donohue, 1980; Shemesh et al., 1987). The typical patient suffering postbanding sepsis complains of rectal pain and urinary retention on the third of fourth postoperative day. The physical examination and leukocyte count at this time may be normal. Blood cultures in all nine cases were found to be normal. During the next day or two edema of the rectum, perineum, or lower abdominal wall may develop and can be confirmed by computed tomography (CT).

Proctoscopic examination at this stage demonstrates marked edema of the rectum and necrosis at the sites of banding; fever and leukocytosis are also notable at this time, and death is not far off. At autopsy, marked rectal and pelvic edema, sometimes phlegmonous, is common, occasionally accompanied by a small rectal or pelvic abscess. Shemesh et al. theorized that following band ligation transmural ischemic necrosis of the tissue enclosed in the band allowed egress of bowel bacteria into the surrounding pelvic soft tissues. Although the blood cultures were all negative in the reported cases, postmortem bacterial cultures revealed coliform bacteria and, in one case, *Clostridium perfringens, Clostridium sporogenes*, and *Bacteroides* (O'Hara).

All the patients who survived this complication were treated as soon as they presented with pain and urinary symptoms. Intensive, early treatment with intravenous antibiotics aimed at clostridia, other anaerobes, and gram-negative rods is essential. Patients who undergo banding must be told that if they experience urinary symptoms, fever, or pain 1–4 days after the procedure they must promptly return to the surgeon for hospital admission to receive immediate antibiotic treatment, even if physical signs at that time are negligible.

*Pain.* If *severe* pain occurs upon application of the band, remove the band promptly before the patient leaves the office. Treat a *mild* degree of vague discomfort with medication.

*Bleeding.* If the patient sustains a mild degree of blood spotting in the stool when the slough separates a week or 10 days after the banding, treat it expectantly. If the patient has lost more than a few hundred milliliters, admit the patient to the hospital for proctoscopy. Suction out all the clots and identify the bleeding point. In some cases the bleeding point can be grasped with Allis tissue forceps and a rubber band again applied to the area. Alternatively, under general or local anesthesia, use either electrocautery or a suture to control the bleeding.

## REFERENCES

Barron J. Office ligation treatment of hemorrhoids. Dis Colon Rectum 1963;6:109.

Clay LD III, White JJ Jr, Davidson JT, et al. Early recognition and successful management of pelvic cellulitis following hemorrhoidal banding. Dis Colon Rectum 1986;29:579.

Lee HH, Spencer RJ, Beart RW Jr. Multiple hemorrhoidal bandings in a single session. Dis Colon Rectum 1994;37:37.

Nivatvongs S, Goldberg SM. An improved technique of rubber band ligation of hemorrhoids. Am J Surg 1982;144:379.

O'Hara VS. Fatal clostridial infection following hemorrhoidal banding. Dis Colon Rectum 1980;23:570.

Rudd WWH. Ligation of hemorrhoids as an office procedure. Can Med Assoc J 1973;108:56.

Russell TR, Donohue JH. Hemorrhoidal banding: a warning. Dis Colon Rectum 1985;28:291.

Shemesh EL, Kodner IJ, Fry RD, et al. Severe complication of rubber band ligation of internal hemorrhoids. Dis Colon Rectum 1987;30:199.

Tchirkow G, Haas PA, Fox TA Jr. Injection of a local anesthetic solution into hemorrhoidal bundle following rubber band ligation. Dis Colon Rectum 1982;25:62.

# 22 Hemorrhoidectomy

## INDICATIONS

Persistent bleeding or protrusion

Symptomatic second- and third-degree (combined internal-external) hemorrhoids

Symptomatic hemorrhoids combined with mucosal prolapse

Strangulation of internal hemorrhoids

Early stage of acute thrombosis of external hemorrhoid

## CONTRAINDICATIONS

Portal hypertension

Inflammatory bowel disease

Anal malignancy

## PREOPERATIVE PREPARATION

Advise patients to discontinue aspirin and other nonsteroidal antiinflammatory agents.

A sodium phosphate packaged enema (Fleet) is adequate cleansing for most patients.

Sigmoidoscopy, colonoscopy, or both are done as indicated by the patient's symptoms.

Routine preoperative blood coagulation profile (partial thromboplastin time, prothrombin time, platelet count) in performed.

Preoperative shaving of the perianal area is preferred by some surgeons but is not necessary.

## PITFALLS AND DANGER POINTS

Narrowing the lumen of the anus, thereby inducing anal stenosis

Trauma to sphincter

Failing to identify associated pathology (e.g., inflammatory bowel disease, leukemia, portal hypertension, coagulopathy, squamous carcinoma of the anus)

Failure to manage postoperative bowel function

## OPERATIVE STRATEGY

### Avoiding Anal Stenosis

The most serious error when performing hemorrhoidectomy is failure to leave adequate bridges of mucosa and anoderm between each site of hemorrhoid excision. If a minimum of 1.0–1.5 cm of viable anoderm is left intact between each site of hemorrhoid resection, the risk of developing anal stenosis is minimized. Preserving viable anoderm is much more important than is removal of all external hemorrhoids and redundant skin.

One method of preventing anal stenosis is to insert a large anal retractor, such as the Fansler or large Ferguson, after resecting the hemorrhoids. If the incisions in the mucosa and anoderm ("closed hemorrhoidectomy") can be sutured with the retractor in place, anal stenosis should not occur if good bowel function is maintained postoperatively.

### Achieving Hemostasis

Traditionally, surgeons have depended on mass ligature of the hemorrhoid "pedicle" for achieving hemostasis. This policy ignores the fact that small arteries penetrate the internal sphincter and enter the operative field. Also, numerous vessels are divided when incising the mucosa to dissect the pedicle. In fact, the concept of a "pedicle" as being the source of a hemorrhoidal mass is large erroneous. A hemorrhoidal mass is not a varicose vein situated at the termination of the portal venous system. It is a vascular complex with multiple channels fed by many small vessels. Therefore it is important to control bleeding from each vessel as it is transected during the operation. A convenient method for accomplishing this goal is careful, accurate application of coagulating electrocautery. As pointed out by Goldberg and associates (1980), much of the bleeding comes from the mucosal incision. Therefore it is well to achieve perfect hemostasis before suturing the defect following hemorrhoid excision.

## Associated Pathology

Even though hemorrhoidectomy is a minor operation, a complete history and physical examination are necessary to rule out important systemic diseases such as leukemia. Leukemic infiltrates in the rectum can cause severe pain and can mimic hemorrhoids and anal ulcers. Operating erroneously on an undiagnosed acute leukemia patient is fraught with the dangers of bleeding, failure to heal, and sepsis. Crohn's disease must also be ruled out by history, local examination, and sigmoidoscopy, as well as biopsy in doubtful situations.

Another extremely important condition sometimes overlooked during the course of hemorrhoidectomy is squamous cell carcinoma of the anus. It may resemble nothing more than a small ulceration on what appears to be a hemorrhoid. Any hemorrhoid that demonstrates a break in the continuity of the overlying mucosa should be suspected of being a carcinoma, as should any ulcer of the anoderm, except for the classic anal fissure located in the posterior commissure. Before scheduling hemorrhoidectomy, biopsy all ulcerations and atypical lesions of the anal canal.

# OPERATIVE TECHNIQUE

## Closed Hemorrhoidectomy

### *Local Anesthesia*

#### *Choosing an Anesthetic Agent*

A solution of 0.5% lidocaine (maximum dosage 80 ml) or 0.25% bupivacaine (maximum dosage 80 ml), combined with epinephrine 1:200,000 and 150–300 units of hyaluronidase is effective and has extremely low toxicity. Because perianal injection of these agents is painful, premedicate the patient 1 hour before the operation with an intramuscular injection of some combination of narcotic and sedative (e.g., Demerol and a barbiturate, or Innovar, 1–2 ml). Alternatively, give diazepam in a dose of 5–10 mg intravenously just before the perianal injection.

#### *Techniques of Local Anesthesia*

With the technique originally introduced by Kratzer (1974), the anesthetic agent is placed in a syringe with a 25-gauge needle. The needle should be at least 5 cm in length. Initiate the injection at a point 2–3 cm lateral to the middle of the anus. Inject 10–15 ml of the solution in the *subcutaneous* tissues surrounding the right half of the anal canal including the area of the anoderm at the anal verge. Warn the patient that this injection may be quite painful. Repeat this maneuver through a needle puncture site to the left of the anal canal. After placing a slotted anoscope in the anal canal, insert the needle into the tissues just underneath the anoderm and into the plane between the submucosa and the internal sphincter 3–4 cm deep into the anal canal **(Fig. 22–1)**. If the injection creates a wheal in the mucosa similar to that seen in the skin after an intradermal injection, the needle is

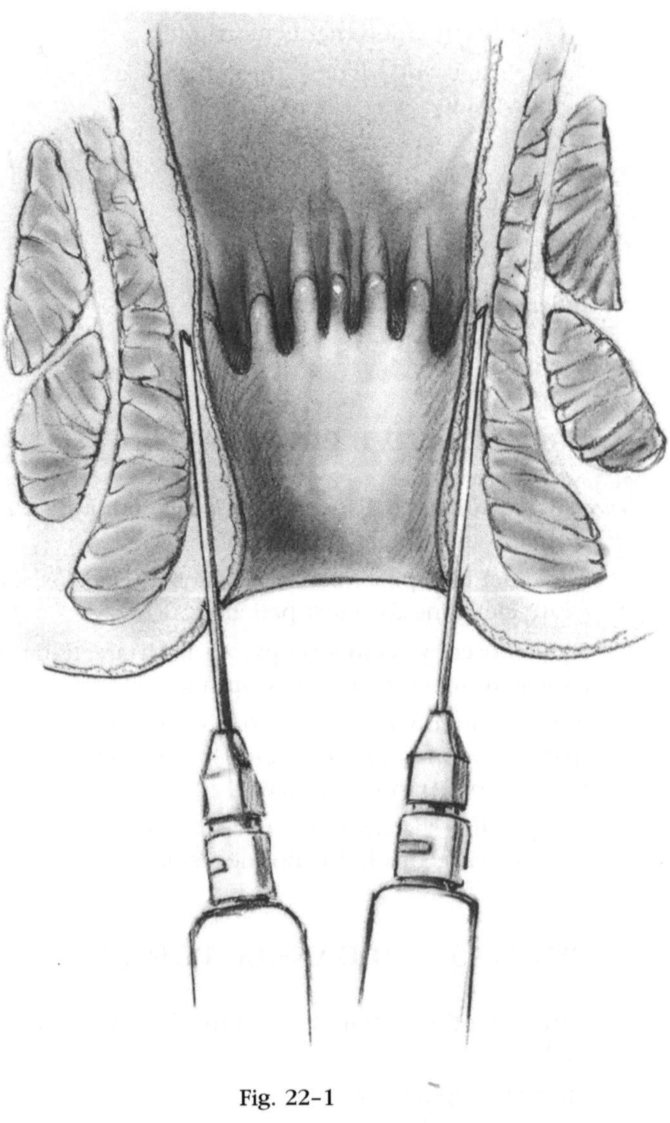

Fig. 22–1

in a too-shallow position. An injection into the proper submucosal plane produces no visible change in the overlying mucosa. Inject 3–4 ml of anesthetic solution during the course of withdrawing the needle. Make similar injections in each of the four quadrants until the subdermal and submucosal tissues of the anal canal have been surrounded with anesthetic agent. It should require no more than 30–40 ml of anesthetic solution. Satisfactory relaxation of the sphincters is achieved without the need to inject solution directly into the muscles or to attempt to block the inferior hemorrhoidal nerve in the ischiorectal space. Wait 5–10 minutes for complete relaxation and anesthesia.

In 1982, Nivatvongs described a technique to minimize pain. It consisted, first, of inserting a small anoscope into the anal canal. Make the first injection into the *submucosal* plane 2 mm *above* the dentate line. Because of the difference in sensory innervation of the mucosa above the dentate line, injection here does not produce acute pain. Inject 2–3 ml of anesthetic solution and then an equal amount of solution in each of the remaining three quadrants of the anus. Remove the anoscope and insert a well lubricated index finger into the anal canal. Use the tip of the index finger to massage the anesthetic agent from the submucosal area down into the tissues underneath the anoderm. Repeat this maneuver with respect to each of the four injection sites. By spreading the anesthetic agent distally, this maneuver serves to anesthetize the highly sensitive tissues of the anoderm just distal to the dentate line. When this has been accomplished, make another series of injections 2 mm *distal* to the dentate line. Inject 2–3 ml of solution underneath the anoderm and the subcutaneous tissues in the perianal region through four sites, one in each quadrant of the anus. Then use the index finger again to massage the tissues of the anal canal to spread the anesthetic solution circumferentially around the anal and perianal area. In some cases additional anesthetic agent is necessary for complete circumferential anesthesia. An average of 20–25 ml of solution is required. Nivatvongs stated that this technique provides excellent relaxation of the sphincters and permits operation such as hemorrhoidectomy to be accomplished without general anesthesia. For a lateral sphincterotomy, it is not necessary to anesthetize the entire circumference of the anal canal when using this technique. Inject only the area of the sphincterotomy.

### Intravenous Fluids

Because local anesthesia has few systemic effects, it is not necessary to administer a large volume of intravenous fluid during the operation. If large volumes of fluid are administered intraoperatively, the bladder becomes rapidly distended. In the presence of general anesthesia or even heavy sedation during local anesthesia, the patient is not sufficiently alert to have the desire to void. By the time the patient is alert, the bladder muscle has been stretched and may be too weak to empty the bladder, especially if the patient also has anal pain and some degree of prostatic hypertrophy. This can cause postoperative urinary retention, requiring catheterization. All of this can be prevented by avoiding general anesthesia and heavy premedication and by limiting the dosage of intravenous fluids to 100–200 ml during and after hemorrhoidectomy.

### Positioning the Patient

We prefer to place the patient in the semiprone jackknife position with either a sandbag or rolled-up sheet under the hips and a small pillow to support the feet. It is not necessary to shave the perianal area; if the buttocks are hirsute, shave this area. Then apply tincture of benzoin. When this solution has dried, apply wide adhesive tape to the buttock and attach the other end of the adhesive strap to the operating table. In this fashion lateral traction is applied to each buttock, affording excellent exposure of the anus.

### Incision and Dissection

Gently dilate the anal canal so it admits two fingers. Insert a bivalve speculum such as the Parks retractor or a medium-size Hill-Ferguson retractor. One advantage of using the medium Hill-Ferguson retractor is that it approximates the diameter of the normal anal canal. If the defects remaining in the mucosa and anoderm can be sutured closed with the retractor in place following hemorrhoid excision, no narrowing of the anal canal occurs. Each of the hemorrhoidal masses can be identified by rotating the retractor and applying countertraction to the skin of the opposite wall of the anal canal. Generally, three hemorrhoidal complexes are excised: one in the left midlateral position, another in the right anterolateral position, and the third in the right posterolateral location. Avoid placing incisions in the anterior or posterior commissures. Grasp the most dependent portion of the largest hemorrhoidal mass in a Babcock clamp. Then make an incision in the anoderm outlining the distal extremity of the hemorrhoid **(Fig. 22–2)** using a No. 15 (Bard Parker) scalpel. If the hemorrhoidal mass is unusually broad (>1.5 cm), do not excise all of the anoderm and mucosa overlying the hemorrhoid. If each of the hemorrhoidal masses is equally

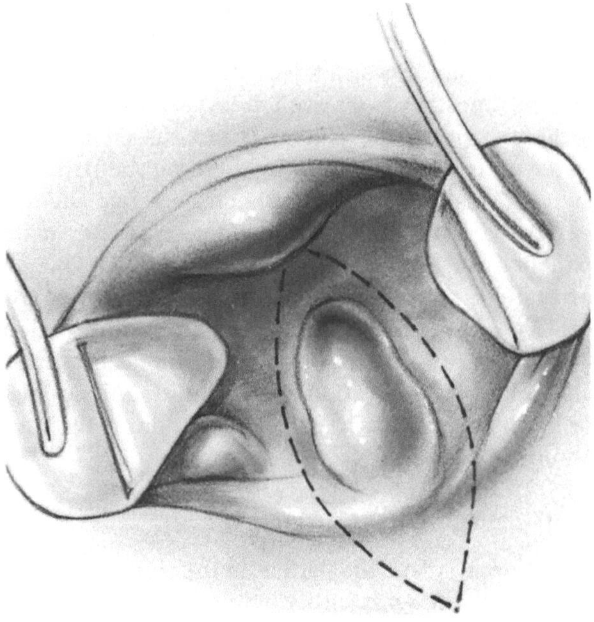

Fig. 22-2

broad, excising all of the anoderm and mucosa overlying each of the hemorrhoids results in inadequate tissue bridges between the sites of hemorrhoid excision. In such a case incise the mucosa and anoderm overlying the hemorrhoid in an elliptical fashion. Then initiate a submucosal dissection using small, pointed scissors to elevate the mucosa and anoderm from the portion of the hemorrhoid that remains in a submucosal location. Carry the dissection of the hemorrhoidal mass down to the internal sphincter muscle **(Fig. 22–3)**. After incising the mucosa and anoderm, draw the hemorrhoid away from the sphincter, using blunt dissection as necessary, to demonstrate the lower border of the internal sphincter. This muscle has whitish muscle fibers that run in a transverse direction. A thin bridge of fibrous tissue is often seen connecting the substance of the hemorrhoid to the internal sphincter. Divide these fibers with a scissors. Dissect the hemorrhoidal mass for a distance of about 1–2 cm above the dentate line where it can be divided with the electrocoagulator **(Fig. 22–4)**. Remove any residual internal hemorrhoids from underneath the adjacent mucosa. Achieve complete hemostasis, primarily with careful electrocoagulation. It is not necessary to clamp and suture the hemorrhoidal "pedicle," although many surgeons prefer to do so **(Fig. 22–5)**. It is helpful to remove all the internal hemorrhoids, but we do not attempt to extract fragments of external hemorrhoids from underneath the anoderm, as this step does not appear necessary. Most of these small external hemorrhoids disappear spontaneously following interna hemorrhoidectomy.

After complete hemostasis has been achieved, insert an atraumatic 5-0 Vicryl suture into the apex of the hemorrhoidal defect. Tie the suture and then close the defect with a continuous locking suture taking 2- to 3-mm bites of mucosa on each side **(Fig. 22–6)**. Also include a small bit of the underlying internal sphincter muscle with each pass of the needle. This maneuver serves to force the mucosa to adhere to the underlying muscle layer and thereby helps prevent mucosal prolapse and recurrent hemorrhoids. Continue the suture line until the entire defect has been closed. Now repeat the same dissection for each of the other two hemorrhoidal masses. Close each of the mucosal defects by the same technique **(Fig. 22–7)**. Be certain not to constrict the lumen of the anal canal. The rectal lumen should admit a Fanster or a large Ferguson rectal retractor after the suturing is completed. To avoid anal stenosis remember that the ellipse of mucosaanoderm excised with each hemorrhoidal mass must be relatively narrow. Also remember that if the tissues are sutured under tension, the suture line will undoubtedly break down.

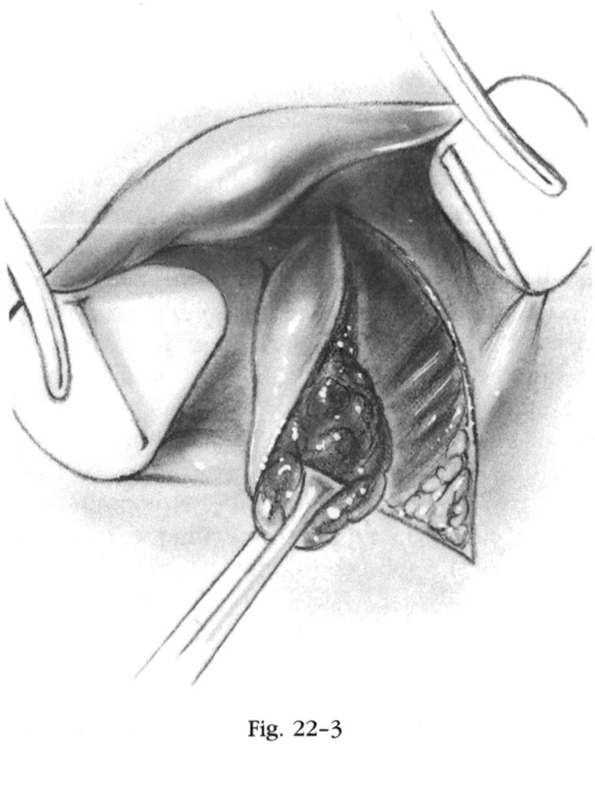

Fig. 22-3

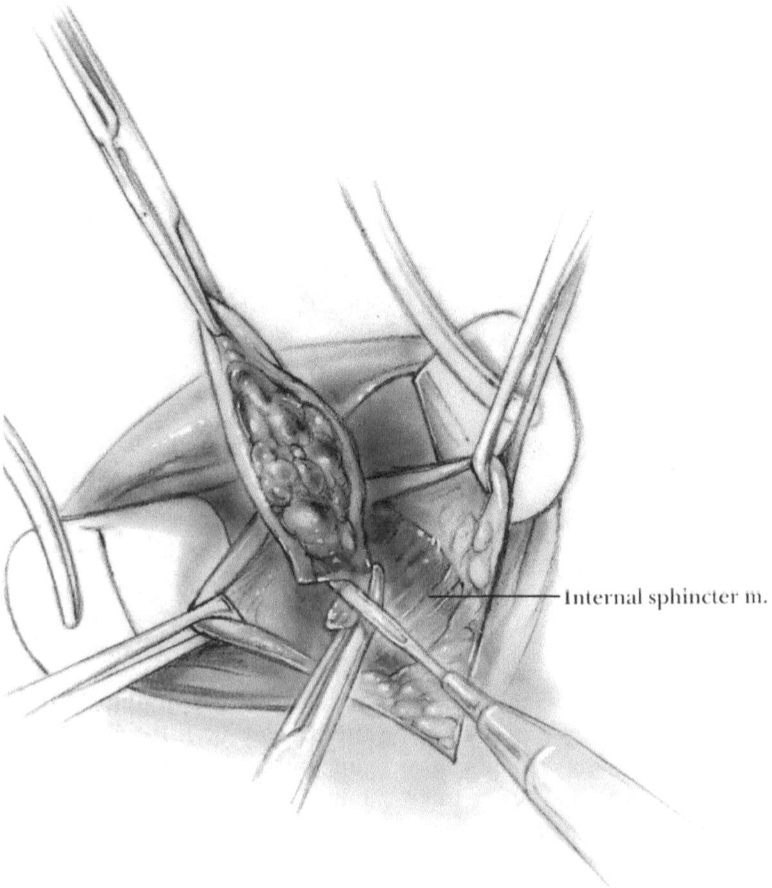


Fig. 22-4

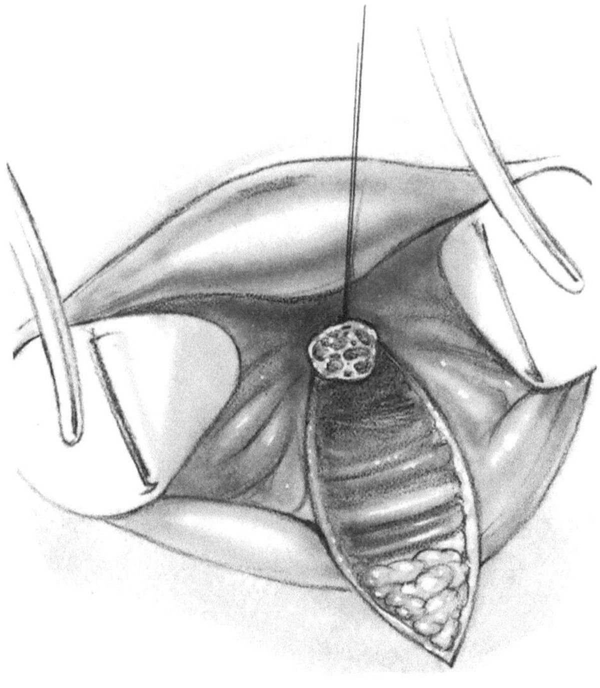

Fig. 22-5

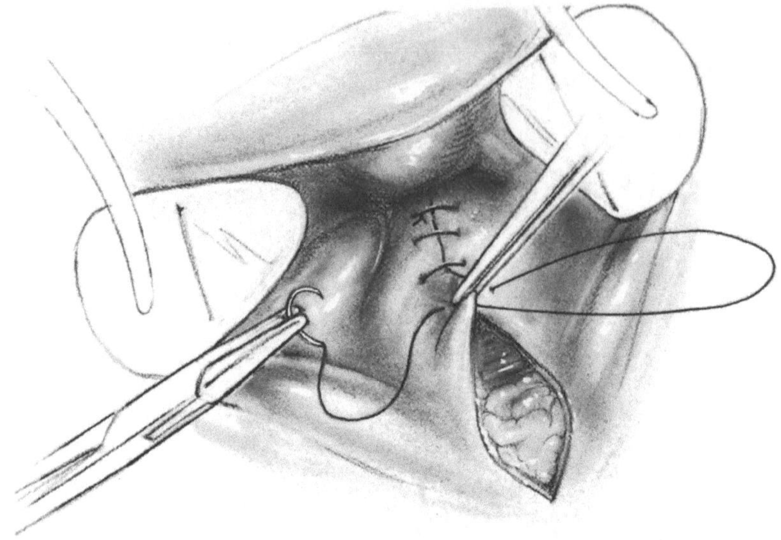

Fig. 22-6

A few patients have some degree of anal stenosis in addition to hemorrhoids. Under these conditions, rather than forcibly dilating the anal canal at the onset of the operation, perform a partial lateral internal sphincterotomy to provide adequate exposure for the operation. This is also true for patients who have a concomitant chronic anal fissure.

For surgeons who prefer to keep the skin unsutured for drainage, modify the above operative procedure by discontinuing the mucosal suture line at the dentate line, leaving the defect in the anoderm unsutured. It is also permissible not to suture the mucosal defects at all after hemorrhoidectomy (see above).

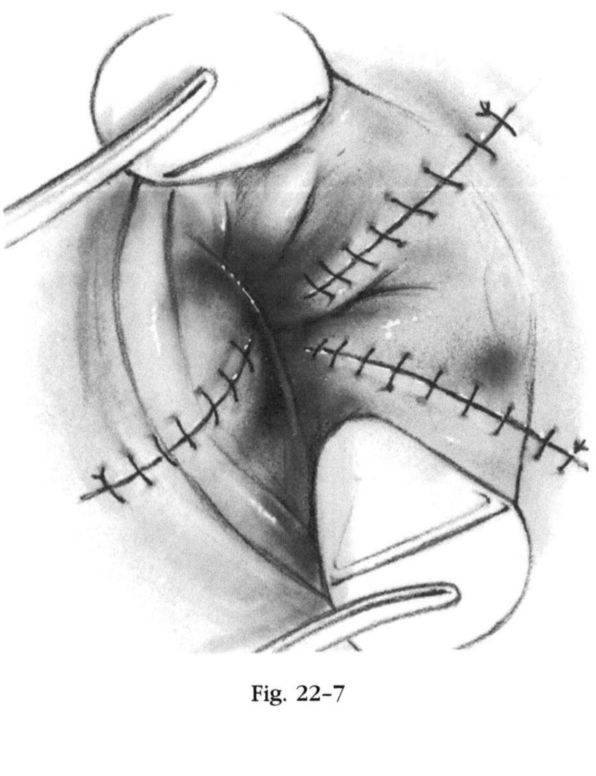

Fig. 22-7

## Radical Open Hemorrhoidectomy

### *Incision*

Radical open hemorrhoidectomy is restricted to patients who no longer have three discrete hemorrhoidal masses but in whom all of the hemorrhoids and prolapsing rectal mucosa seem to have coalesced into an almost circumferential mucosal prolapse. For these patients the operation excises the hemorrhoids, both internal and external, the redundant anoderm, and prolapsed mucosa from both the left and right lateral portions of the anus, leaving 1.5 cm bridges of intact mucosa and anoderm at the anterior and posterior commissures. With the patient in the prone position, as described above for closed hemorrhoidectomy, outline the incision on both sides of the anus as shown in **Figure 22–8**.

### *Excising the Hemorrhoidal Masses*

Elevate the skin flap together with the underlying hemorrhoids by sharp and blunt dissection until the lower border of the internal sphincter muscle has been unroofed **(Fig. 22–9)**. This muscle can be identified by its transverse whitish fibers. Now elevate the anoderm above and below the incision to enucleate adjacent hemorrhoids that have not been included

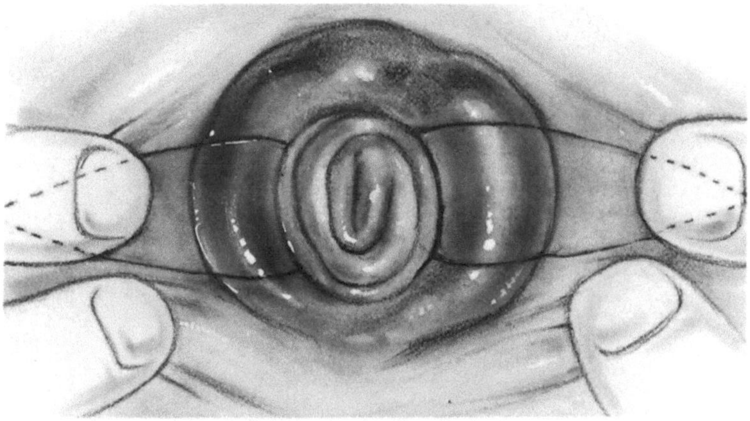

Fig. 22-8

in the initial dissection **(Fig. 22–10)**. This maneuver permits removal of almost all the hemorrhoids and still allows an adequate bridge of anoderm in the anterior and posterior commissures.

After the mass of hemorrhoidal tissue with overlying mucosa has been mobilized to the level of the normal location of the dentate line, amputate the mucosa and hemorrhoids with electrocautery at the level of the dentate line. This leaves a free edge of rectal mucosa. Suture this mucosa to the underlying internal sphincter muscle with a continuous 5-0 atraumatic Vicryl suture, as illustrated in **Figure 22–11**, to recreate the dentate line at its normal location. Do not bring the rectal mucosa down to the area that is normally covered by anoderm or skin, as it would result in continuous secretion of mucus, which would irritate the perianal skin.

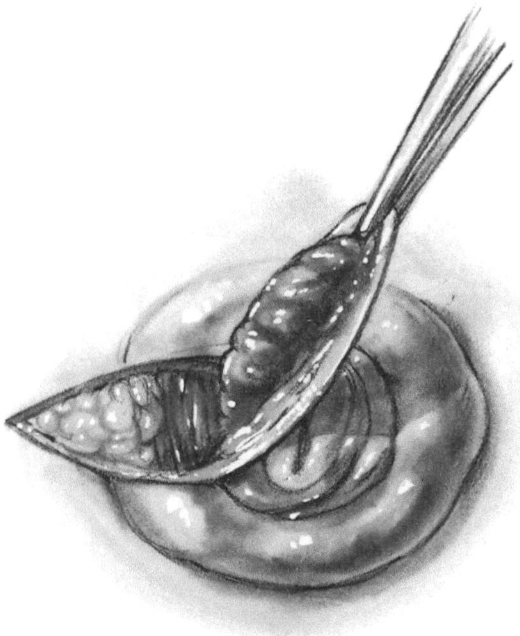

Fig. 22-9

Execute the same dissection to remove all of the hemorrhoidal tissue between 1 and 5 o'clock on the right side and reattach the free cut edge of rectal mucosa to the underlying internal sphincter muscle, as depicted in **Figure 22–12**. There may be some redundant anoderm together with some external hemorrhoids at the anterior or posterior commissure of the anus. Do not attempt to remove every last bit of external hemorrhoid as it would jeopardize the viability of the anoderm in the commissures. Unless viable bridges, about 1.5 cm each in width, are preserved in the anterior and posterior commissures, the danger of a postoperative anal stenosis far outweighs the primarily cosmetic ill effect of leaving behind a skin tag or an occasional external hemorrhoid.

Ensure that hemostasis is complete using electrocautery and occasional suture-ligatures of fine PG or chromic catgut. Some surgeons also insert a small piece of rolled-up Gelfoam into the anus at the completion of the procedure. This roll, which should not be more than 1 cm in thickness, serves to apply gentle pressure and to encourage coagulation of minor bleeding points that may have been overlooked. The Gelfoam need not be removed, as it dissolves when the patient starts having sitz baths postoperatively. Apply a sterile dressing to the perianal area.

Anal packing with anything more substantial than the 1 cm roll of soft Gelfoam should not be necessary, as hemostasis with electrocautery should be meticulous. Large gauze or other rigid packs are

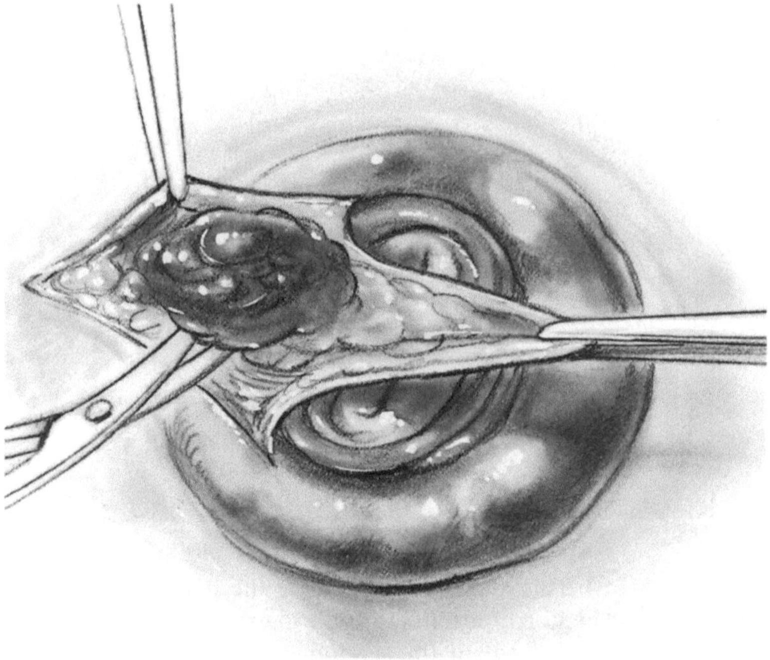

Fig. 22–10

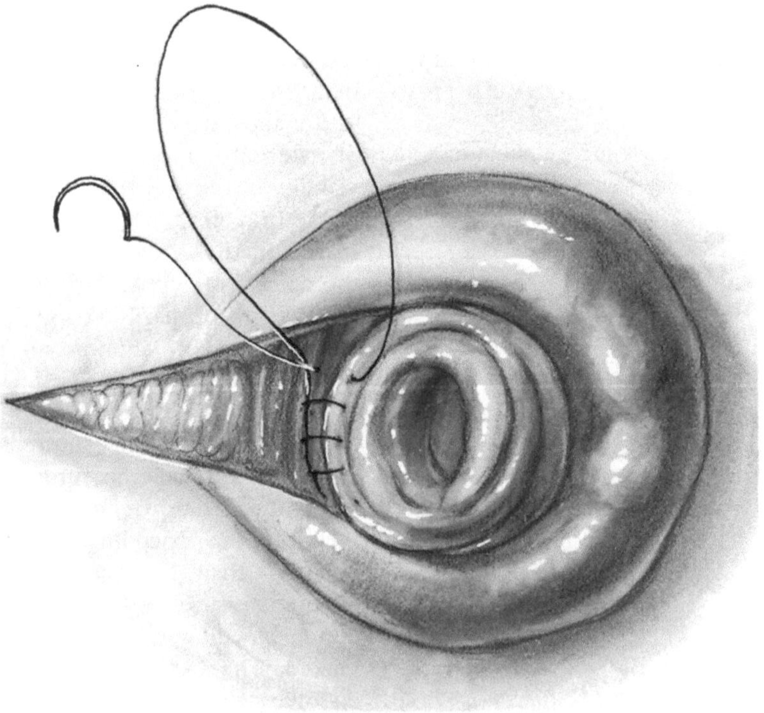

Fig. 22–11

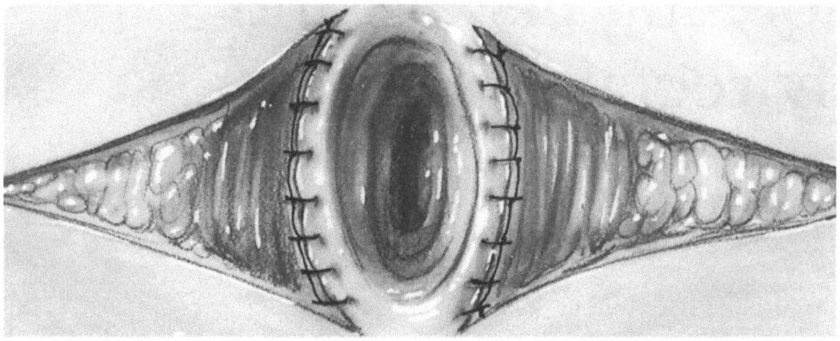

Fig. 22-12

associated with increased postoperative pain and urinary retention.

## POSTOPERATIVE CARE

Encourage ambulation the day of operation. Prescribe analgesic medication preferably of a nonconstipating type such as Darvocet.

Prescribe Senokot-S, Metamucil, or mineral oil while the patient is in the hospital. After discharge, limit the use of cathartics because passage of a well formed stool is the best guarantee the anus will not become stenotic. In patients with severe chronic constipation, dietary bran and some type of laxative or stool softener is necessary following discharge from the hospital.

Order warm sitz baths several times a day, especially following each bowel movement.

Discontinue intravenous fluids as soon as the patient returns to his or her room and initiate a regular diet and oral fluids as desired.

If the patient was hospitalized for the hemorrhoidectomy, he or she is generally discharged on the first or second postoperative day. Most patients tolerate hemorrhoidectomy in the ambulatory outpatient setting.

## COMPLICATIONS

*Serious bleeding* during the postoperative period is rare if complete hemostasis has been achieved in the operating room. However, if bleeding is brisk, the patient should probably be returned to the operating room to have the bleeding point suture-ligated. Most patients who experience major bleeding after discharge from the hospital have experienced a minor degree of bleeding before discharge. About 1% of patients present with hemorrhage severe enough to require reoperation for hemostasis, generally 8–14 days following operation. If the bleeding is slow but continues or if no bleeding site is identified, the patient should be evaluated for coagulopathy, including that caused by platelet dysfunction.

If for some reason the patient is not returned to the operating room for the control of bleeding, it is possible to achieve at least temporary control by inserting a 30 ml Foley catheter into the rectum. The Foley balloon is then blown up, and downward traction is applied to the catheter. Reexploration of the anus for surgical control of bleeding is far preferable.

*Infection* occurs but is rare.

*Skin tags* follow hemorrhoidectomy in 6–10% of cases. Although no treatment is required, for cosmetic purposes a skin tag may be excised under local anesthesia as an office procedure when the operative site has healed completely.

## REFERENCES

Corman ML. Hemorrhoids. In Colon and Rectal Surgery, 3rd ed. Philadelphia, Lippincott, 1993, pp 54–115.

Ferguson JA, Heaton JR. Closed hemorrhoidectomy. Dis Colon Rectum 1959;2:176.

Goldberg SM, Gordon PH, Nivatvongs, S. Essentials of Anorectal Surgery. Philadelphia, Lippincott, 1980.

Kratzer GL. Improved local anesthesia in anorectal surgery. Am Surg 1974;40:609.

Mazier WP. Hemorrhoids, fissures, and pruritus ani. Surg Clin North Am 1994;74:1277.

Nivatvongs S. An improved technique of local anesthesia for anorectal surgery. Dis Colon Rectum 1982;25:259.

Thomson WHF. The nature of hemorrhoids. Br J Surg 1975;162:542.

# 23 Anorectal Fistula and Pelvirectal Abscess

## INDICATIONS

Drainage of anorectal abscess is indicated *as soon as the diagnosis is made*. There is no role for conservative management because severe sepsis can develop and spread before fluctuance and typical physical findings appear. This is especially true in diabetic patients.

Recurrent or persistent drainage from a perianal fistula calls for repair.

Weak anal sphincter muscles are a relative *contraindication* to fistulotomy, especially in the unusual cases in which the fistulotomy must be performed through the anterior aspect of the anal canal. Absence of the puborectalis muscle in the anterior area of the canal causes inherent sphincter weakness in this location. This category of case is probably better suited for treatment by inserting a seton or by an advancement flap, especially in women.

## PREOPERATIVE PREPARATION

Cathartic the night before operation and saline enema on the morning of operation

Preoperative anoscopy and sigmoidoscopy

Colonoscopy, small bowel radiography series, or both when Crohn's enteritis or colitis is suspected

Antibiotic coverage with mechanical bowel preparation if an advancement flap is contemplated

## PITFALLS AND DANGER POINTS

Failure to diagnose anorectal sepsis and to perform early incision and drainage

Failure to diagnose or control Crohn's disease

Failure to rule out anorectal tuberculosis or acute leukemia

Induction of fecal incontinence by excessive or incorrect division of the anal sphincter muscles

## OPERATIVE STRATEGY

### Choice of Anesthesia

Because palpation of the sphincter mechanism is a key component of the surgical procedure, a light general anesthetic is preferable to a regional anesthetic.

### Localizing Fistulous Tracts

#### *Goodsall's Rule*

When a fistulous orifice is identified in the perianal skin posterior to a line drawn between 3 o'clock and 9 o'clock, the internal opening of the fistula is almost always found in the posterior commissure in a crypt approximately at the dentate line. Goodsall's rule also states that if a fistulous tract is identified anterior to the 3 o'clock/9 o'clock line, its internal orifice is likely to be located along the course of a line connecting the orifice of the fistula to an imaginary point exactly in the middle of the anal canal. In other words, a fistula draining in the perianal area at 4 o'clock in a patient lying prone is likely to have its internal opening situated at the dentate line at 4 o'clock. There are exceptions to this rule. For instance, a horseshoe fistula may drain anterior to the anus but continue in a posterior direction and terminate in the posterior commissure.

If the external fistula opening is more than 3 cm from the anal verge, be suspicious of unusual pathology. Look for Crohn's disease, tuberculosis, or other disease processes such as hidradenitis suppurativa or pilonidal disease.

#### *Physical Examination*

First, attempt to identify the course of the fistula in the perianal area by palpating the associated fibrous tract. Second, carefully palpate the region of the dentate line. The site of origin is often easier to feel than it is to see. Next, insert a bivalve speculum into the anus and try to identify the internal opening by gentle probing at the point indicated by Goodsall's rule. If the internal opening is not readily apparent, do not make any false passages. The most accurate method for identifying the direction of the tract is gently to insert a blunt malleable probe, such as a lacrimal duct probe, into the fistula with the index finger in the rectum. In this fashion it may be possible to identify the internal orifice by palpating the probe with the index finger in the anal canal.

## Injection of Dye or Radiopaque Material

On rare occasions injection of a blue dye may help identify the internal orifice of a complicated fistula. Some surgeons have advocated the use of milk or hydrogen peroxide instead of a blue dye. These agents allow one to perform multiple injections without the extensive tissue staining that follows the use of blue dye. Injection of a radiopaque liquid followed by radiographic studies can be valuable for the extrasphincteric fistulas leading high up into the rectum, but it does not appear to be helpful for the usual type of fistula.

Endorectal sonography and computed tomography (CT) or magnetic resonance imaging (MRI) fistulography are more modern techniques for evaluating complex fistulas. However, they do not reveal enough detail to identify the site of origin of the fistula precisely.

## Preserving Fecal Continence

As mentioned in the discussion above, the puborectalis muscle (anorectal ring) must function normally to preserve fecal continence following fistulotomy. Identify this muscle accurately before dividing the anal sphincter muscles during the course of a fistulotomy. Use local anesthesia with sedation or general anesthesia for the fistulotomy. If the fistulous tract can be identified with a *probe preoperatively*, the surgeon's index finger in the anal canal can identify the anorectal ring without difficulty, especially if the patient is asked to tighten the voluntary sphincter muscles.

If there is any doubt about the identification of the anorectal ring (the proximal portion of the anal canal), do not complete the fistulotomy; rather, insert a heavy silk or braided polyester ligature through the remaining portion of the tract. Tie the ligature loosely with five or six knots without completing the fistulotomy. When the patient is examined in the awake state, it is simple to determine whether the upper border of the seton has encircled the anorectal ring or there is sufficient puborectalis muscle (1.5 cm or more) above the seton to complete the fistulotomy by dividing the muscles enclosed in the seton at a later stage. If no more than half of the external sphincter muscles in the anal canal have been divided, fecal continence should be preserved in patients with formed stools and a normally compliant rectum. An exception would be those patients who had a weak sphincter muscle prior to operation.

## Fistulotomy Versus Fistulectomy

When performing surgery to cure an anal fistula, most authorities are satisfied that incising the fistula along its entire length constitutes adequate therapy. Others have advocated excision of the fibrous cylinder that constitutes the fistula, leaving only surrounding fat and muscle tissue behind. The latter technique leaves a large open wound, however, which takes much longer to heal. Moreover, much more bleeding is encountered during a fistulectomy than a fistulotomy. Hence there is no evidence to indicate that excising the wall of the fistula has any advantages.

## Combining Fistulotomy with Drainage of Anorectal Abscess

For patients with an acute ischiorectal abscess, some have advocated that the surgical procedure include a fistulotomy simultaneous with drainage of the abscess. After the pus has been evacuated, a search is made for the internal opening of the fistulous tract and then the tract is opened. This combination of operations is contraindicated for two reasons. First, many of our patients who undergo simple drainage of an abscess never develop a fistula. It is likely that the internal orifice of the anal duct has become occluded before the abscess is treated. These patients do not require a fistulotomy. Second, acute inflammation and edema surrounding the abscess make accurate detection and evaluation of the fistulous tract extremely difficult. There is great likelihood that the surgeon will create false passages that may prove so disabling to the patient that any time saved by combining the drainage operation with a fistulotomy is insignificant. We presently drain many anorectal abscesses in the office under local anesthesia, in part because this method removes the temptation to add a fistulotomy to the drainage procedure.

# OPERATIVE TECHNIQUE

## Anorectal and Pelvirectal Abscesses

### *Perianal Abscess*

When draining an anorectal abscess it is important to excise a patch of overlying skin so the pus drains freely. The typical perianal abscess is located fairly close to the anus, and often drainage can be performed under local anesthesia. Packing is rarely necessary and may impede drainage.

A Malecot catheter can be placed in the cavity and sewn in place in patients with recurrent abscesses or Crohn's disease in whom continued problems may be anticipated. After 10 days, ingrowth of tissue keeps the Malecot in place without sutures. This serves as a temporizing procedure prior to fistulotomy in patients without Crohn's disease. It may be used as a permanent solution for the difficult Crohn's patient with perianal fistula disease.

### *Ischiorectal Abscess*

The ischiorectal abscess is generally larger than the perianal abscess, develops at a greater distance from the anus, and may be deep-seated. Fluctuance on physical examination may be a late sign. Early drainage under general anesthesia is indicated. Make a cruciate incision over the apex of the inflamed area close to the anal verge so any resulting fistula is short. Excise enough of the overhanging skin to permit free drainage and evacuate the pus. Explore the abscess for loculations.

### *Intersphincteric Abscess*

Many physicians fail to diagnose an intersphincteric abscess until the abscess ruptures into the ischiorectal space and forms an ischiorectal abscess. A patient who complains of persistent anal pain should be suspected of harboring an intersphincteric abscess. This is especially true if, on inspecting the anus with the buttocks spread apart, the physician can rule out the presence of an anal fissure. Examination under anesthesia may be necessary to confirm the diagnosis. Digital examination in the unanesthetized patient may indicate at which point in the anal canal the abscess is located. Parks and Thomson (1973) found that 61% of the intersphincteric abscesses occurred in the posterior quadrant of the anal canal. In half their patients a small mass could be palpated in the anal canal with the index finger inside the canal and the thumb just outside. Occasionally an internal opening draining a few drops of pus is identified near the dentate line. A patient may have both an anal fissure and an intersphincteric abscess.

Under local or general anesthesia, carefully palpate the anal canal. Then insert a bivalve speculum and inspect the circumference of the anus to identify a possible fissure or an internal opening of the intersphincteric abscess. After identifying the point on the circumference of the anal canal that is the site of the abscess, perform an internal sphincterotomy by the same technique as described in Chapter 24 for an anal fissure. Place the internal sphincterotomy directly over the site of the intersphincteric abscess. Explore the cavity, which is generally small, with the index finger. If the abscess has been properly unroofed, simply reexamine the area daily with an index finger for the first week or so postoperatively. Uneventful healing can be anticipated unless the abscess has already penetrated the external sphincter muscle and created an undetected extension in the ischiorectal space.

### *Pelvirectal Supralevator Abscess*

An abscess above the levator diaphragm is manifested by pain (gluteal and perineal), fever, and leukocytosis; it often occurs in patients with diabetes or other illnesses. Pus can appear in the supralevator space by extension upward from an intersphincteric fistula, penetration through the levator diaphragm of a transsphincteric fistula, or direct extension from an abscess in the rectosigmoid area. When there is obvious infection in the ischiorectal fossa secondary to a *transsphincteric* fistula, manifested by local induration and tenderness, make an incision at the dependent point of the ischiorectal infection **(Fig. 23–1)**. The incision must be large enough to explore the area with the index finger. It may be necessary to incise the levator diaphragm from below and to enlarge this opening with a long Kelly hemostat to provide adequate drainage of the supralevator abscess. After thoroughly irrigating the area, insert gauze packing.

In pelvirectal abscesses arising from an *intersphincteric* fistula, one is often able to palpate the fluctuant abscess by inserting the index finger high up in the rectum. Aspirate the region of fluctuation under general anesthesia. If pus is obtained, make an incision in the rectum with electrocautery and drain the abscess through the rectum (Fig. 23-1).

Under no condition should one drain a supralevator abscess through the rectum if the abscess has its origin in an *ischiorectal* space infection **(Fig. 23–2)**, an error that could result in a high extrasphincteric fistula. Similarly, if the supralevator sepsis has arisen

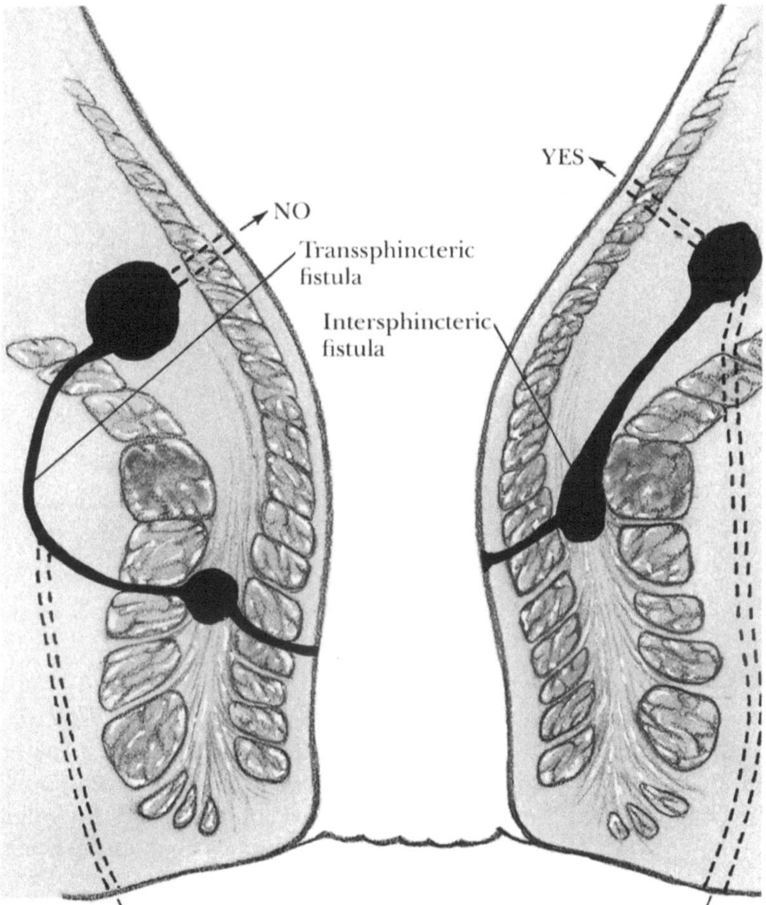
NO
Transsphincteric fistula
YES
Intersphincteric fistula
YES
NO

Fig. 23-1

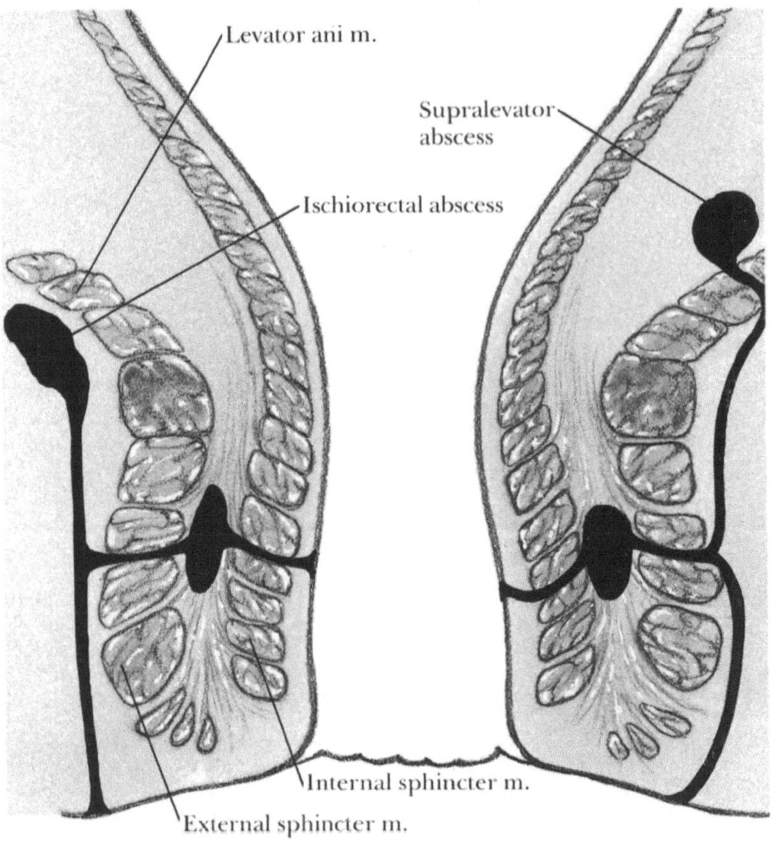


Fig. 23-2. Transsphincteric fistulas (with high blind tracks).

from an intersphincteric abscess, draining the supralevator infection through the ischiorectal fossa also leads to a high extrasphincteric fistula, and this error should also be avoided **(Fig. 23–3)**.

## Anorectal Fistula

### *Intersphincteric Fistula*

#### *Simple Low Fistula*

When dealing with an unselected patient population, simple low fistula occurs in perhaps half of all patients presenting with anorectal fistulas. Here the injected anal gland burrows distally in the intersphincteric space to form either a perianal abscess or a perianal fistula, as illustrated in Figure 20-2. Performing a fistulotomy here requires only division of the internal sphincter and overlying anoderm up to the internal orifice of the fistula approximately at the dentate line. This divides the distal half of the internal sphincter, rarely producing any permanent disturbance of function.

#### *High Blind Track (Rare)*

With a high blind track fistula the mid-anal infection burrows in a cephalad direction between the circular internal sphincter and the longitudinal muscle fibers of the upper canal and lower rectal wall to form a small *intramural* abscess above the levator diaphragm **(Fig. 23–4)**. This abscess can be palpated by digital examination. The infection will probably heal if the primary focus is drained by excising a 1 × 1 cm square of internal sphincter at the site of the internal orifice of this "fistula." Parks et al. (1976) stated that even if the entire internal sphincter is divided while laying open this high blind track by opening the internal sphincter from the internal orifice of the track to the upper extension of the track, little disturbed continence develops because the edges of the sphincter are held together by the fibrosis produced as the track develops.

#### *High Track Opening into Rectum (Rare)*

With a high track opening into the rectum, a probe inserted into the internal orifice continues upward

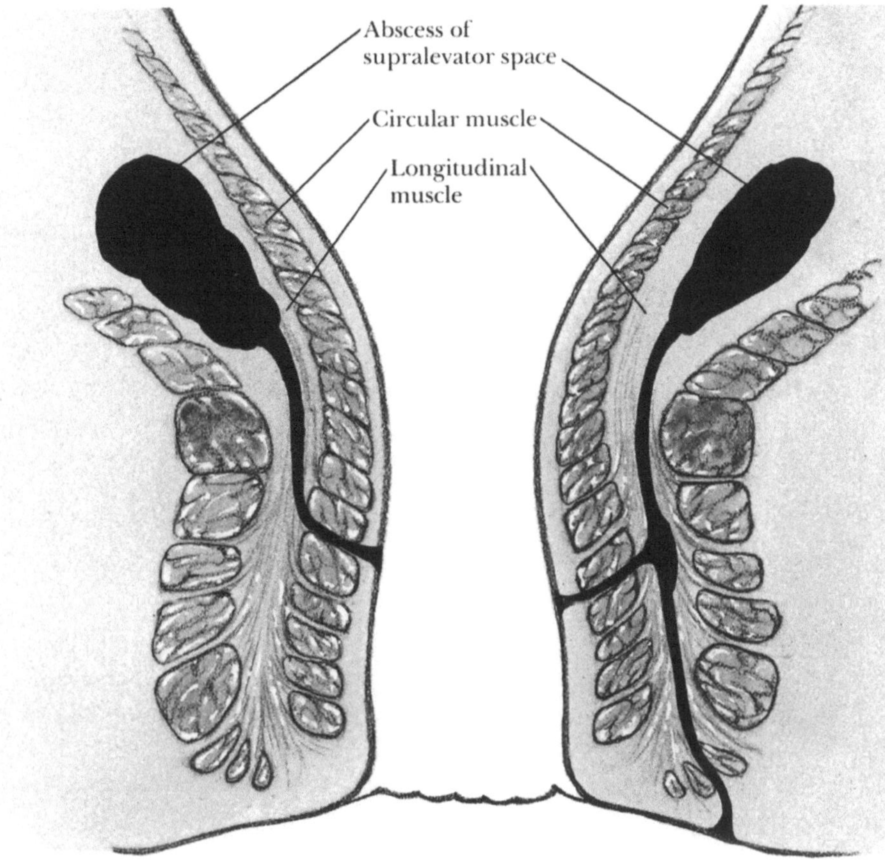


Fig. 23-3. High intersphincteric track fistulas (with supralevator abcesses).

between the internal sphincter and the longitudinal muscle of the rectum. The probe opens into the rectum at the upper end of the fistula (Fig. 23-4). If by palpating the probe the surgeon recognizes that this fistula is quite superficial and is located deep only to the circular muscle layer, the tissue overlying the probe can be laid open without risk. On the other hand, if the probe goes deep to the *external* sphincter muscle prior to reentering the rectum (see Fig. 20-5), it constitutes a type of extrasphincteric fistula that is extremely difficult to manage (see below). If there is any doubt about the true nature of this type of fistula, refer the patient to a specialist.

### *High Track with No Perineal Opening (Rare)*

An unusual intersphincteric fistula is the high track fistula with no perineal opening. The infection begins in the mid-anal intersphincteric space and burrows upward in the rectal wall, reentering the lower rectum through a secondary opening above the anorectal ring **(Fig. 23-5)**. There is no downward spread of the infection and no fistula in the perianal skin. To treat this fistula it is necessary to lay the track open from its internal opening in the mid-anal canal up into the lower rectum. Parks and associates emphasized that the lowermost part of the track in the mid-anal canal must be excised because it contains the infected anal gland, which is the primary source of the infection. Leaving it behind may result in a recurrence. If a fistula of this type presents in the acute phase, it resembles a "submucous abscess," but this is an erroneous term because the infection is indeed deep not only to the mucosa but also to the circular muscle layer (Fig. 23-5). This type of abscess is drained by incising the overlying mucosa and circular muscle of the rectum.

### *High Track with Pelvic Extension (Rare)*

With a high track fistula with pelvic extension the infection spreads upward in the intersphincteric space, breaks through the longitudinal muscle, and enters the pelvis (supralevator) (Fig. 23-3). To treat

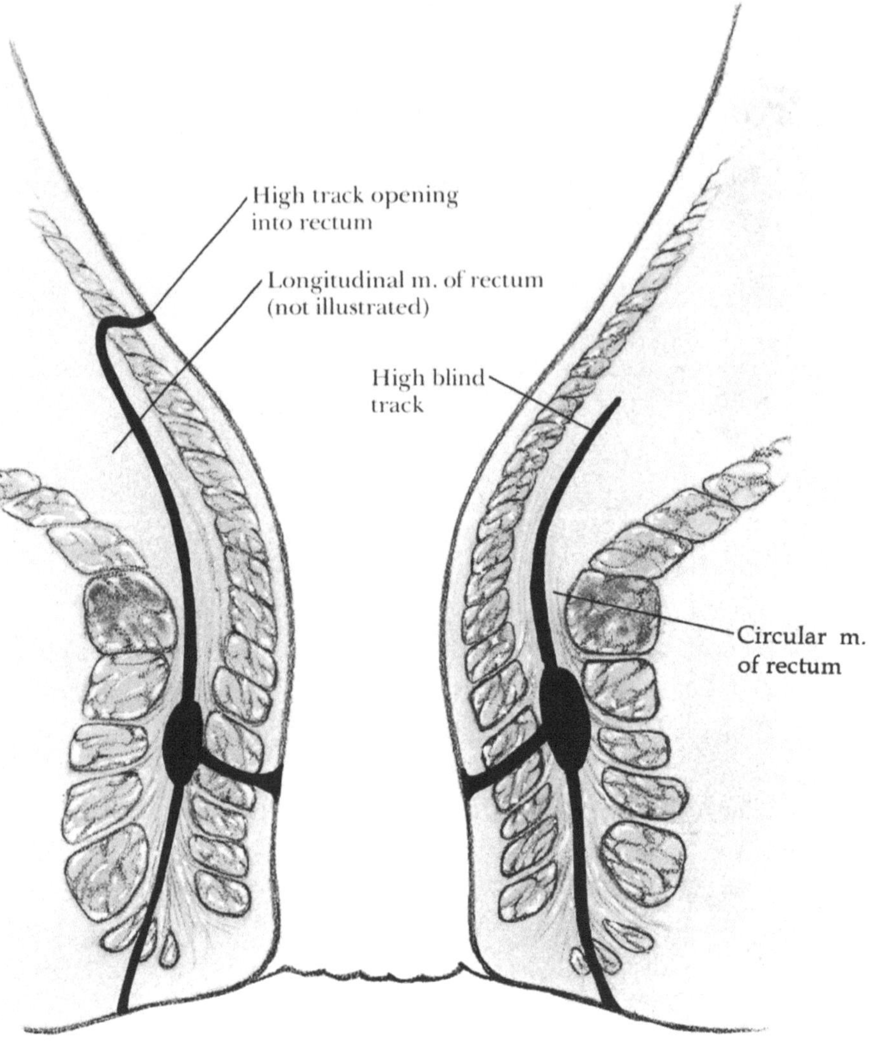


Fig. 23-4. High intersphincteric fistulas.

it, open the fistulous track by incising the internal sphincter together with the overlying mucosa or anoderm up into the rectum for 1-3 cm. Drain the pelvic collection through this incision, with the drain exiting into the rectum.

## *High Track Secondary to Pelvic Disease (Rare)*

As mentioned above, the intersphincteric plane "is a natural pathway for infection from the pelvis to follow should it track downward" (Parks et al.). This type of fistula **(Fig. 23–6)** does not arise from anal disease and does not require perianal surgery. Treatment consists of removing the pelvic infection by abdominal surgery.

## ***Transsphincteric Fistula***

### *Uncomplicated Fistula*

As illustrated in Figure 20-3, the fairly common uncomplicated transsphincteric fistula arises in the intersphincteric space of the mid-anal canal, with the infection then burrowing laterally directly through the external sphincter muscle. There it may form either an abscess or a fistulous track down through the skin overlying the ischiorectal space. If a probe is passed through the fistulous opening in the skin and along the track until it enters the rectum at the internal opening of the fistula, all of the overlying tissue may be divided without serious functional disturbance because only the distal half of the internal

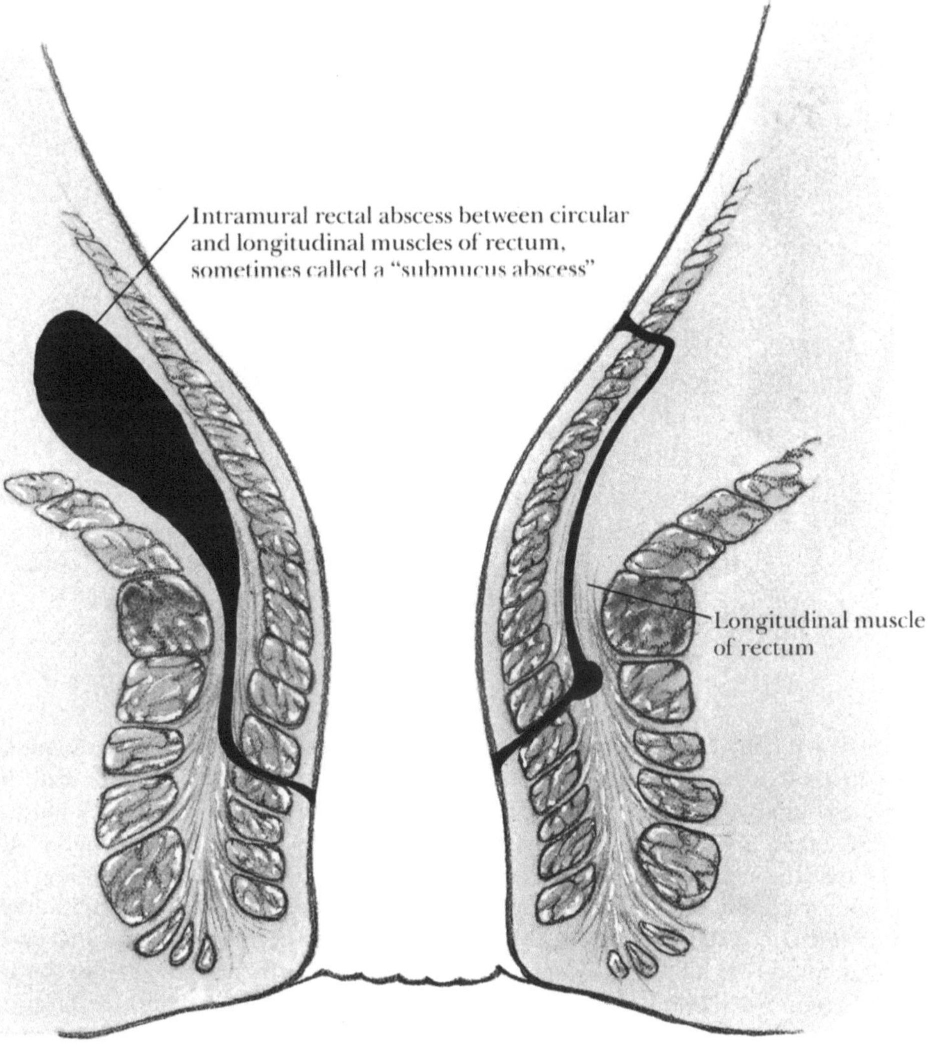


Fig. 23-5. High intersphincteric fistula (or abscess) with no perineal openings.

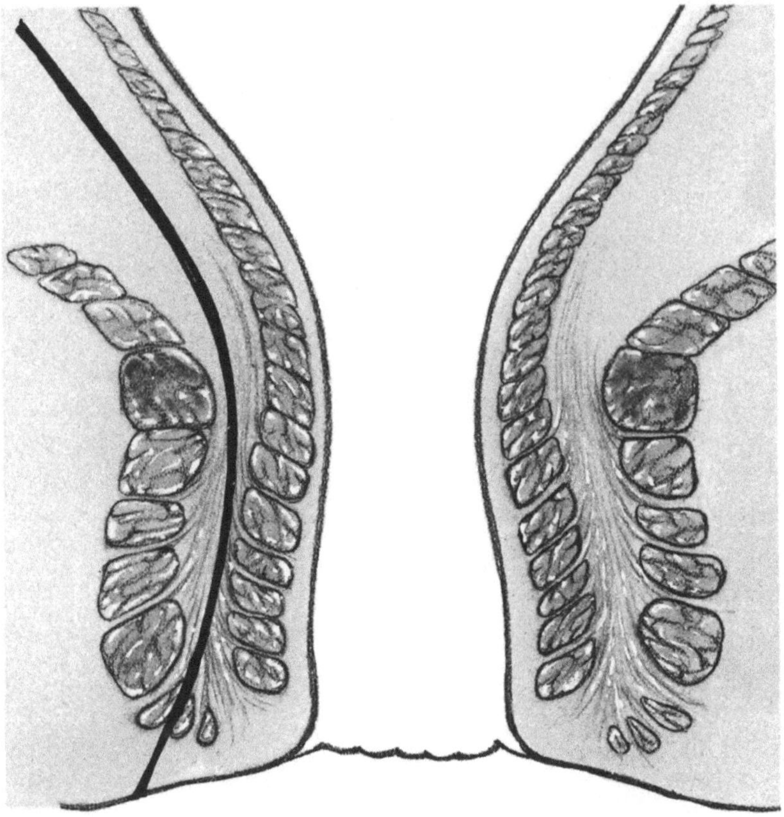

Fig. 23-6. High intersphincteric track fistula (*secondary* to pelvic sepsis).

sphincter and the distal half of the external sphincter has been transected. Occasionally one of these fistulas crosses the external sphincter closer to the puborectalis muscle than is shown here. In this case, if there is doubt that the entire puborectalis can be left intact, the external sphincter should be divided in two stages. Divide the distal half during the first stage and insert a seton through the remaining fistula, around the remaining muscle bundle. Leave it intact for 2-3 months before dividing the remainder of the sphincter.

## *High Blind Track*

The fistula with high blind track burrows through the external sphincter, generally at the level of the mid-anal canal. The fistula then not only burrows downward to the skin but also in a cephalad direction to the apex of the ischiorectal fossa (Fig. 23-2).

Occasionally it burrows through the levator ani muscles into the pelvis. Parks et al. pointed out that when a probe is passed into the external opening, it generally goes directly to the upper end of the blind track and that the internal opening in the midanal canal may be difficult to delineate by such probing. Occasionally there is localized induration in the mid-anal canal to indicate the site of the infected anal gland that initiated the pathologic process. Probing this area should reveal the internal opening. By inserting the index finger into the anal canal, one can often feel, above the anorectal ring, the induration that is caused by the supralevator extension of the infection. The surgeon can often feel the probe in the fistula with the index finger. The probe may feel close to the rectal wall. Parks emphasized that it is dangerous to penetrate the wall of the rectum with this probe or to try to drain this infection through the upper rectum. If it is done, an extrasphincteric fistula would be created with grave implications for the patient. The proper treatment for this type of fistula, even with a supralevator extension, is to transect the mucosa, internal sphincter, external sphincter, and perianal skin from the mid-anal canal down to the orifice of the track in the skin of the buttock. The upper extension heals with this type of drainage.

### *Suprasphincteric Fistula (Extremely Rare)*

The suprasphincteric fistula originates, as usual, in the mid-anal canal in the intersphincteric space, where its internal opening can generally be found. The fistula extends upward in the intersphincteric plane above the puborectalis muscle into the supralevator space, where it often causes a supralevator abscess. The fistula then penetrates the levator diaphragm and continues downward in the ischiorectal space to its external orifice in the perineal skin (Fig. 20-4). This type of supralevator infection must not be drained through an incision in the rectum. Parks and Stitz (1958) recommended an internal sphincterotomy from the internal opening of the fistula distally and excision of the abscess in the intersphincteric space, if present. They then divide the lower 30-50% of the external sphincter muscle and continue this incision laterally until the lower portion of the fistulous track has been opened down to its external opening in the skin. This maneuver leaves the upper half of the external and internal sphincter muscles and the puborectalis muscle intact. Insert a seton of heavy braided nylon through the fistula as it surrounds the muscles. Tie the seton with five or six knots but keep the loop in the seton loose enough so it does not constrict the remaining muscles at this time. Insert a drain into the supralevator abscess, preferably in the intersphincteric space between the seton and the remaining internal sphincter muscle. Once adequate drainage has been established, remove this drain, as the heavy seton prevents the lower portion of the wound from closing prematurely. Parks does not remove these setons for at least 3 months. It is often necessary to return the patient to the operating room 10-14 days following the initial operation to examine the situation carefully and to ascertain that no residual pocket of infection has remained undrained. Examination under anesthesia may be necessary on several occasions before complete healing has been achieved. In most cases, after 3 months or more has passed the supralevator infection has healed completely, and it is not necessary to divide the muscles enclosed in the seton. In these cases simply remove the seton and permit the wound to heal spontaneously. If after 3-4 months there is lingering infection in the upper reaches of the wound, it is possible to divide the muscles contained in the seton because the longstanding fibrosis prevents significant retraction and the muscle generally heals with restoration of fecal continence.

Alternatively, an advancement flap to close the internal opening of the fistula may save these patients multiple operations. It also avoids sphincter division.

### *Extrasphincteric Fistula (Extremely Rare)*

#### *Secondary to Transsphincteric Fistula*

In an unusual situation, a transsphincteric fistula, after entering the ischiorectal fossa, travels not only downward to the skin of the buttocks but also in a cephalad direction, penetrating the levator diaphragm into the pelvis and then through the entire wall and mucosa of the rectum (Fig. 20-5). If this fistula were to be completely laid open surgically, the entire internal and entire external sphincter together with part of the levator diaphragm would have to be divided. The result would be total fecal incontinence. The proper treatment here consists of a temporary diverting colostomy combined with simple laying open of the portion of the fistula that extends from the mid-anal canal to the skin. After the defect in the rectum heals, the colostomy can be closed.

The extrasphincteric fistula may also be treated by fashioning an advancement flap. With this procedure it is often unnecessary to create a temporary colostomy.

#### *Secondary to Trauma*

A traumatic fistula may be caused by a foreign body penetrating the perineum, the levator ani muscle, and the rectum. A swallowed foreign body such as a fish bone may also perforate the rectum above the anorectal ring and be forced through the levator diaphragm into the ischiorectal fossa. An infection in this space may then drain out through the skin of the perineum to form a complete extrasphincteric fistula. In either case, treatment consists of removing any foreign body, establishing adequate drainage, and sometimes performing a temporary colostomy. It is not necessary to divide any sphincter muscle because the anal canal is not the cause of the patient's pathology.

#### *Secondary to Specific Anorectal Disease*

Conditions such as ulcerative colitis, Crohn's disease, and carcinoma may produce unusual and bizarre fistulas in the anorectal area. They are not usually amenable to local surgery. The primary disease must be remedied, often requiring total proctectomy.

#### *Secondary to Pelvic Inflammation*

A diverticular abscess of the sigmoid colon, Crohn's disease of the terminal ileum, or perforated pelvic appendicitis may result in perforation of the levator diaphragm, with the infection tracking downward to the perineal skin. To make the proper diagnosis, a radiographic sinogram is performed by injecting an aqueous iodinated contrast medium into the fistula. This procedure may demonstrate a supralevator entrance into the rectum. Therapy for this type of fistula consists of eliminating the pelvic sepsis by abdominal surgery. There is no need to cut any of the anorectal sphincter musculature.

### *Technical Hints for Performing Fistulotomy*

#### *Position*

We prefer the prone position, with the patient's hips elevated on a small pillow. The patient should be under regional or local anesthesia with sedation.

#### *Exploration*

In accordance with Goodsall's rule, search the suspected area of the anal canal after inserting a Parks bivalve retractor. The internal opening should be located in a crypt near the dentate line, most often in the posterior commissure. If an internal opening has been identified, insert a probe to confirm this fact. Then insert a probe into the external orifice of the fistula. With a simple fistula, in which the probe goes directly into the internal orifice, simply make a scalpel incision dividing all of the tissues superficial to the probe. A grooved directional probe is helpful for this maneuver.

With complex fistulas the probe may not pass through the entire length of the track. In some cases gentle maneuvering with variously sized lacrimal probes may be helpful. If these maneuvers are not successful, Goldberg and associates suggested injecting a dilute (1:10) solution of methylene blue dye into the external orifice of the fistula. Then incise the tissues over a grooved director along that portion of the track the probe enters easily. At this point it is generally easy to identify the probable location of the fistula's internal opening. For fistulas in the posterior half of the anal canal, this opening is located in the posterior commissure at the dentate line. If a patient has multiple fistulas, including a horseshoe fistula, the multiple tracks generally enter into a single posterior track that leads to an internal opening at the usual location in the posterior commissure of the anal canal. In patients with multiple complicated fistulas, fistulograms obtained by radiography or magnetic resonance imaging help delineate the pathology.

#### *Marsupialization*

When fistulotomy results in a large gaping wound, Goldberg and associates suggested marsupializing the wound to speed healing: Suture the outer walls of the laid-open fistula to the skin with a continuous absorbable suture. Curet all of the granulation tissue away from the wall of the fistula that has been laid open.

## POSTOPERATIVE CARE

Administer a bulk laxative such as Metamucil daily. For the first bowel movement, an additional stimulant, such as Senokot-S (two tablets) may be necessary.

The patient is placed on a regular diet.

For patients who have had operations for fairly simple fistulas, warm sitz baths two or three times daily may be initiated beginning on the first postoperative day, after which no gauze packing may be necessary.

For patients who have complex fistulas, light general anesthesia may be required for removal of the first gauze packing on the second or third postoperative day.

During the early postoperative period, check the wound every day or two to be sure that healing takes place in the depth of the wound before any of the more superficial tissues heal together. Later check the patient once or twice weekly.

When a significant portion of the external sphincter has been divided, warn the patient that for the first week or so there will be some degree of fecal incontinence.

In the case of the rare types of fistula with high extension and a deep wound, Parks and Sitz recommended that the patient be taken to the operating room at intervals for careful examination under anesthesia.

Perform a weekly anal digital examination and dilatation, when necessary, to avoid an anal stenosis secondary to the fibrosis that takes place during the healing of a fistula.

## COMPLICATIONS

Urinary retention

Postoperative hemorrhage

Fecal incontinence

Sepsis including cellulitis and recurrent abscess

Recurrent fistula

Thrombosis of external hemorrhoids

Anal stenosis

## REFERENCES

Eisenhammer S. A new approach to the anorectal fistulous abscess based on the high intermuscular lesion. Dis Colon Rectum 1976;19:487.

Garcia-Aguilar J, Belmonte C, Wong WD, Goldberg SM, Madoff RD. Anal fistula surgery: factors associated with recurrence and incontinence. Dis Colon Rectum 1996;39:723.

Goldberg SM, Gordon PH, Nivatvongs S. Essentials of Anorectal Surgery. Philadelphia, Lippincott, 1980.

Kodner IJ, Mazor A. Shemesh EI, et al. Endorectal advancement flap repair of rectovaginal and other complicated anorectal fistulas. Surgery 1993; 114:682.

McCourtney JS, Finlay IG. Setons in the surgical management of fistula in ano. Br J Surg 1995;82:448.

Parks AG, Stitz RW. The treatment of high fistula-in-ano. Dis Colon Rectum 1958;106:595.

Parks AG, Thomson JPS. Intersphincter abscess. BMJ 1973;2:337.

Parks AG, Hardcastle JD, Gordon PH. A classification of fistula-in-ano. Br J Surg 1976;63:1.

Rosen L. Anorectal abscess-fistulae. Surg Clin North Am 1994;74:1293.

# 24 Lateral Internal Sphincterotomy for Chronic Anal Fissure

## INDICATIONS

Painful chronic anal fissure not responsive to medical therapy

## PREOPERATIVE PREPARATION

Many patients with anal fissure cannot tolerate a preoperative enema because of excessive pain. Consequently, a mild cathartic the night before operation constitutes the only preoperative care necessary.

## PITFALLS AND DANGER POINTS

Injury to external sphincter

Inducing fecal incontinence by overly extensive sphincterotomy

Bleeding, hematoma

## OPERATIVE STRATEGY

Accurate identification of the lower border of the internal sphincter is essential to successful completion of an internal sphincterotomy. Insert a bivalve speculum (e.g., Parks retractor) into the anal and open the speculum for a distance of about two fingerbreadths to place the internal sphincter on stretch. Feel for a distinct groove between the subcutaneous external sphincter and the lower border of the tense internal sphincter. This groove accurately identifies the lower border of the internal sphincter. Optionally, the surgeon may make a radial incision through the mucosa directly over this area to identify visually the lower border of the internal sphincter (we have not found this step necessary).

## OPERATIVE TECHNIQUE

### Anesthesia

A light general or local anesthesia is satisfactory for this procedure.

### Closed Sphincterotomy

Place the patient in the lithotomy position. (The prone position is also satisfactory.) Insert a Parks retractor with one blade placed in the anterior aspect and the other in the posterior aspect of the anal canal. Open the retractor about two fingerbreadths. Now, at the right or left lateral margin of the anal canal, palpate the groove between the internal and external sphincter. Once this has been clearly identified, insert a No. 11 scalpel blade into this groove **(Fig. 24–1)**. During this insertion keep the flat portion of the blade parallel to the internal sphincter. When the blade has reached the level of the dentate line (about 1.5 cm), rotate the blade 90° so its sharp edge rests against the internal sphincter muscle **(Fig. 24–2)**. Insert the left index finger into the anal canal opposite the scalpel blade. Then, with a gentle sawing motion transect the lower portion of the internal sphincter muscle. There is a gritty sensation while the internal sphincter is being transected, followed by a sudden "give" when the blade has reached the mucosa adjacent to the surgeon's left index finger. Remove the knife and palpate the area of the sphincterotomy with the left index finger. Any remaining muscle fibers are ruptured by lateral pressure exerted by this finger. In the presence of bleeding, apply pressure to this area for at least 5 minutes. It is rarely necessary to make an incision in the mucosa to identify and coagulate a bleeding point.

An alternative method of performing the subcutaneous sphincterotomy is to insert a No. 11 scalpel blade between the mucosa and the internal sphincter. Then turn the cutting edge of the blade so it faces laterally; cut the sphincter in this fashion. This

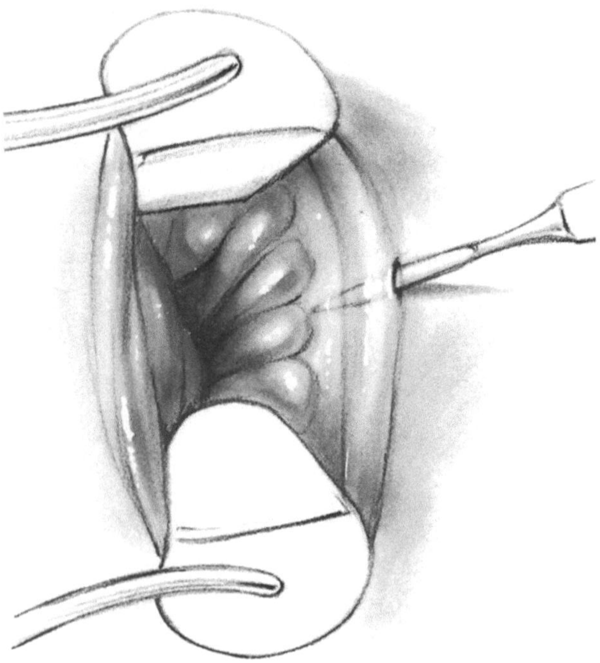

Fig. 24-1

approach has the disadvantage of possibly lacerating the external sphincter if excessive pressure is applied to the blade. Do not suture the tiny incision in the anoderm.

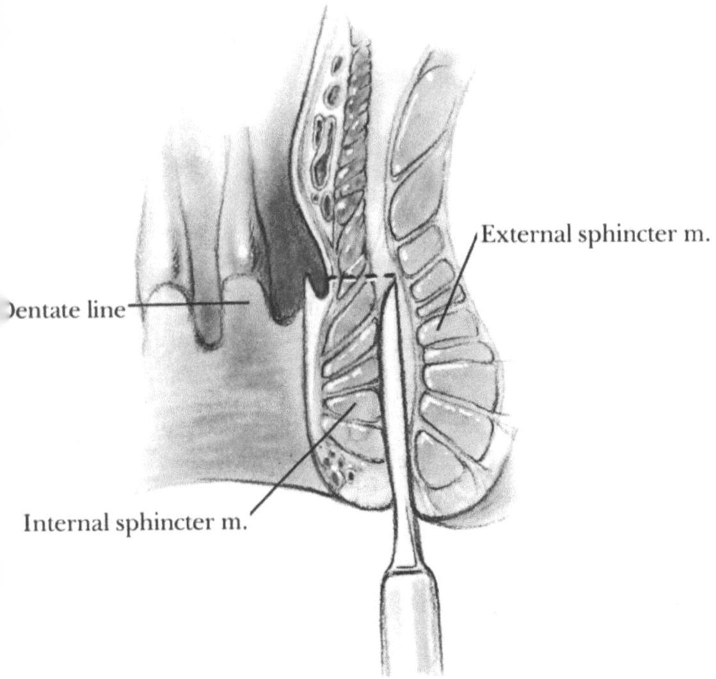


Fig. 24-2

## Open Sphincterotomy

For an open sphincterotomy a radial incision is made in the anoderm just distal to the dentate line and is carried across the lower border of the internal sphincter in the midlateral portion of the anus. Then the lower border of the internal sphincter and intersphincteric groove are identified. The fibers of the internal sphincter have a whitish hue. Divide the lower portion of the internal sphincter up to a point level with the dentate line. Achieve hemostasis with electrocautery, if necessary. Leave the skin wound and apply a dressing.

## Removal of the Sentinel Pile

If the patient has a sentinel pile more than a few millimeters in size, simply excise it with a scissors. Leave the skin defect unsutured. Nothing more elaborate need be done.

If in addition to the chronic anal fissure the patient has symptomatic internal hemorrhoids that require surgery, hemorrhoidectomy may be performed simultaneously with the lateral internal sphincterotomy. If the patient has large internal hemorrhoids, and hemorrhoidectomy is not performed simultaneously, the hemorrhoids may prolapse acutely after sphincterotomy, although it is not common.

# POSTOPERATIVE CARE

Apply a simple gauze dressing to the anus and remove it the following morning.

Discharge the patient the same day. Generally, there is dramatic relief of the patient's pain promptly after sphincterotomy.

Have the patient continue taking the bulk laxative (e.g., psyllium) that was initiated prior to surgery.

Prescribe a mild analgesic in case the patient has some discomfort at the operative site.

# COMPLICATIONS

Hematoma or bleeding (rare)

Perianal abscess (rare)

Flatus and fecal soiling

Some patients complain that they have less control over the passage of flatus following sphincterotomy than they had before operation, or they may have some fecal soiling of their underwear; but generally these complaints are temporary, and the problems rarely last more than a few weeks.

## REFERENCES

Abcarian H. Surgical correction of chronic anal fissure: results of lateral internal sphincterotomy vs fissurectomy—midline sphincterotomy. Dis Colon Rectum 1980;23:31.

Eisenhammer S. The evaluation of the internal anal sphincterotomy operation with special reference to anal fissure. Surg Gynecol Obstet 1959;109:583.

Mazier WP. Hemorrhoids, fissures, and pruritus ani. Surg Clin North Am 1994;74:1277.

Notaras MJ. The treatment of anal fissure by lateral subcutaneous internal sphincterotomy: a technique and results. Br J Surg 1971;58:96.

# 25 Anoplasty for Anal Stenosis

## INDICATIONS

Symptomatic fibrotic constriction of the anal canal not responsive to simple dilatation

## PREOPERATIVE PREPARATION

Preoperative saline enema

## PITFALLS AND DANGER POINTS

Fecal incontinence

Slough of flap

Inappropriate selection of patients

## OPERATIVE STRATEGY

Some patients have a tubular stricture with fibrosis involving mucosa, anal sphincters, and anoderm. This condition, frequently associated with inflammatory bowel disease, is not susceptible to local surgery. In other cases of anal stenosis, elevating the anoderm and mucosa in the proper plane frees these tissues from the underlying muscle and permits formation of sliding pedicle flaps to resurface the denuded anal canal subsequent to dilating the stenosis.

Fecal incontinence is avoided by dilating the anal canal gradually to two or three fingerbreadths and performing, when necessary, a lateral internal sphincterotomy. Patients with mild forms of anal stenosis may respond to a simple internal sphincterotomy if there is no loss of anoderm.

## OPERATIVE TECHNIQUE

### Sliding Mucosal Flap

#### *Incision*

With the patient under local or general anesthesia, in the prone position, and with the buttocks retracted laterally by means of adhesive tape, make an incision at 12 o'clock. This incision should extend from the dentate line outward into the anoderm for about 1.5 cm and internally into the rectal mucosa for about 1.5 cm. The linear incision is then about 3 cm in length. Elevate the skin and mucosal flaps for about 1.0–1.5 cm to the right and to the left of the primary incision. Gently dilate the anus **(Fig. 25–1)**.

#### *Internal Sphincterotomy*

Insert the bivalved Parks or a Hill-Ferguson retractor into the anal canal after gently dilating the anus. Identify the groove between the external and internal sphincter muscles. If necessary, incise the distal portion of the internal sphincter muscle, no higher than the dentate line **(Fig. 25–2)**. This should permit dilatation of the anus to a width of two or three fingerbreadths.

#### *Advancing the Mucosa*

Completely elevate the flap of rectal mucosa. Then advance the mucosa so it can be sutured circumferentially to the sphincter muscle **(Fig. 25–3)**. This suture line should fix the rectal mucosa near the normal location of the dentate line. Advancing the mucosa too far results in an ectropion with annoying chronic mucus secretion in the perianal region. Use fine chromic catgut or PG for the suture material. It is not necessary to insert sutures into the perianal skin. In a few cases of severe stenosis it may be necessary to repeat this process and create a mucosal flap at 6 o'clock **(Figs. 25–4, 25–5)**.

Hemostasis should be complete following the use of accurate electrocautery and fine ligatures. Insert a small Gelfoam pack into the anal canal.

### Sliding Anoderm Flap

#### *Incision*

After gently dilating the anus so a small Hill-Ferguson speculum can be inserted into the anal canal, make

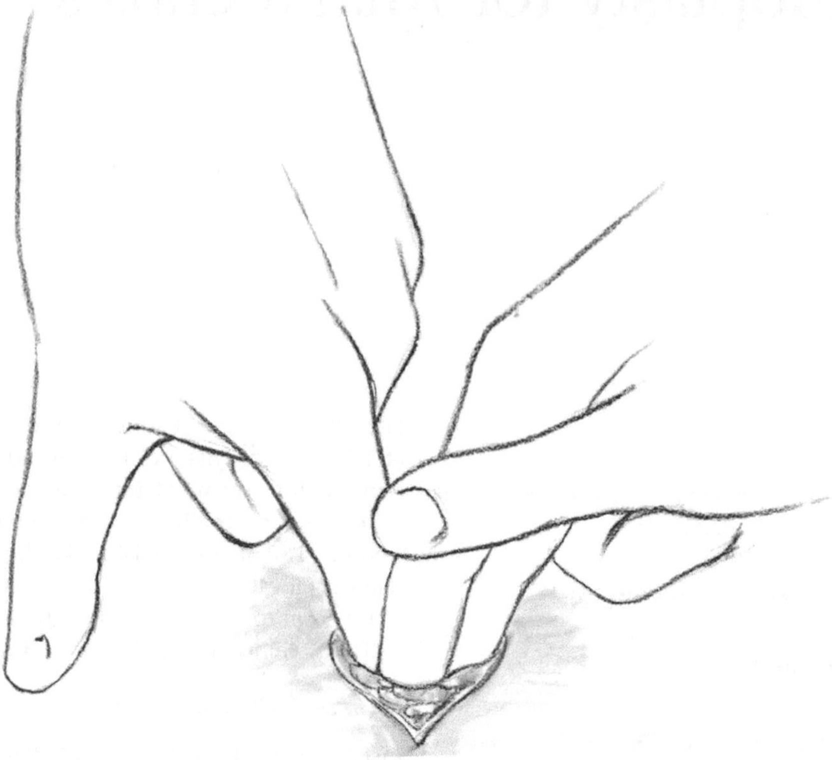

Fig. 25-1

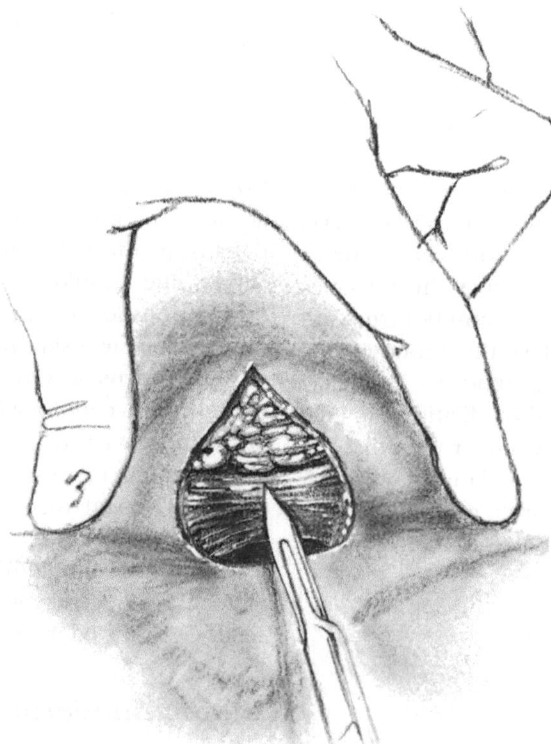

Fig. 25-2

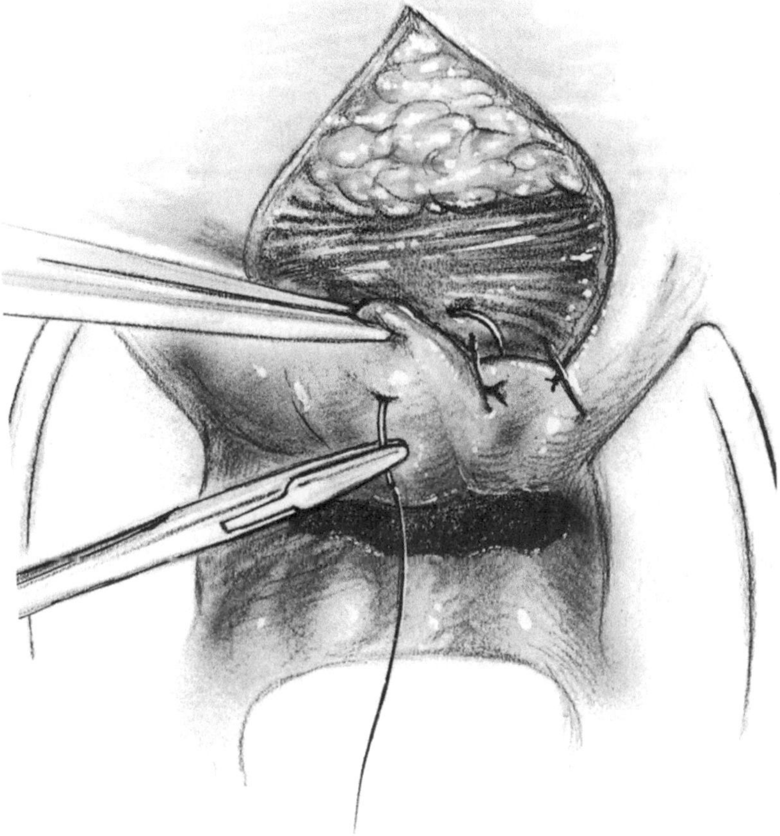

Fig. 25-3

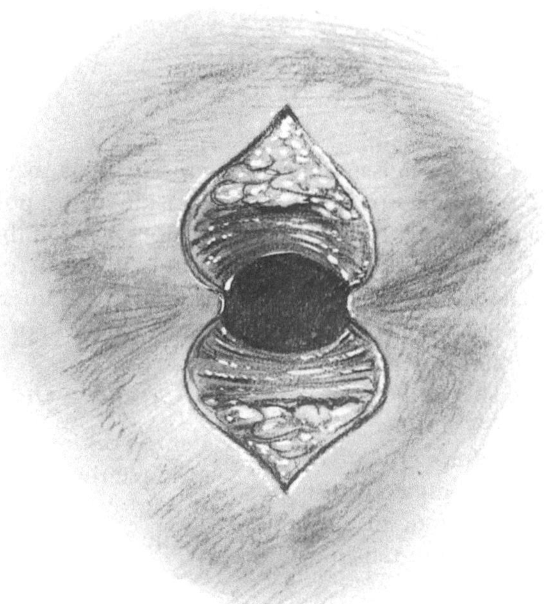

Fig. 25-4

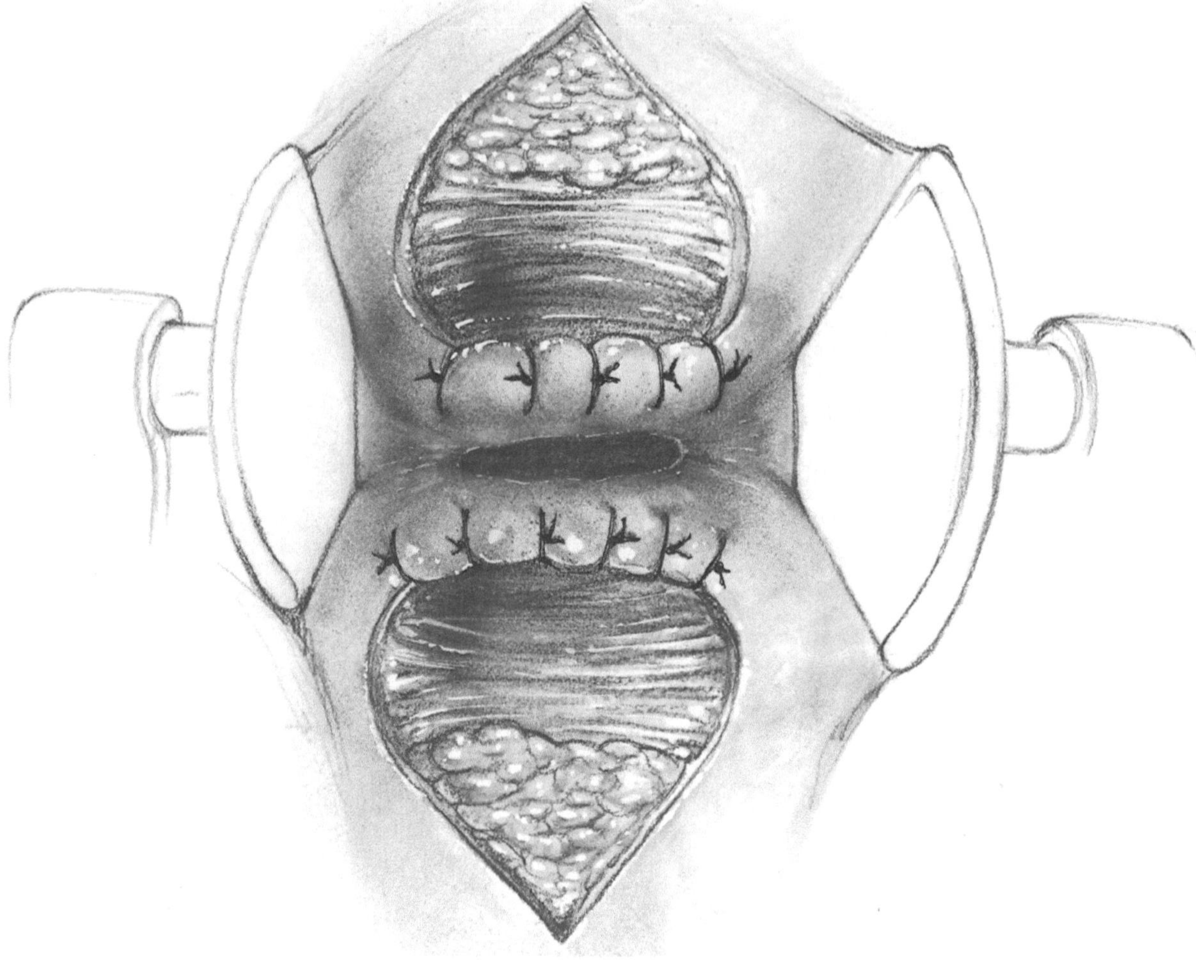

Fig. 25-5

a vertical incision at the posterior commissure, beginning at the dentate line and extending upward in the rectal mucosa for a distance of about 1.5 cm. Then make a Y extension of this incision on to the anoderm as in **Figure 25–6**. Be certain the two limbs of the incision in the anoderm are separated by an angle of at least 90° (angle A in **Fig. 25–7a**). Now by sharp dissection, gently elevate the skin and mucosal flaps for a distance of about 1-2 cm. Take special care not to injure the delicate anoderm during the dissection. When the dissection has been completed, it is possible to advance point A on the anoderm to point B on the mucosa **(Fig. 25–7b)** without tension.

### *Internal Sphincterotomy*

In most cases enlarging the anal canal requires division of the distal portion of the internal sphincter muscle. This may be performed through the same incision at the posterior commissure. Insert a sharp scalpel blade in the groove between the internal and external sphincter muscles. Divide the distal 1.0-1.5 cm of the internal sphincter. Then dilate the anal canal to width of two or three fingerbreadths.

### *Advancing the Anoderm*

Using continuous sutures of 5-0 atraumatic Vicryl, advance the flap of anoderm so point A meets point B (Fig. 25-7b; **Fig. 25–8**) and suture the anoderm to the mucosa with a continuous suture that catches a bit of the underlying sphincter muscle. When the suture line has been completed, the original Y incision in the posterior commissure resembles a V (Fig. 25-7b; **Fig. 25–9**). Insert a small Gelfoam pack into the anal canal.

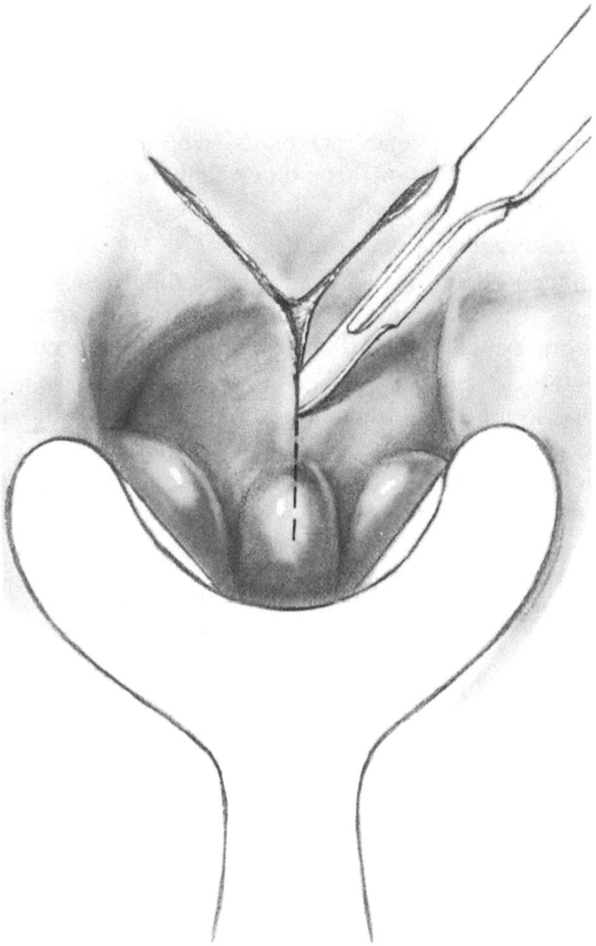

Fig. 25-6

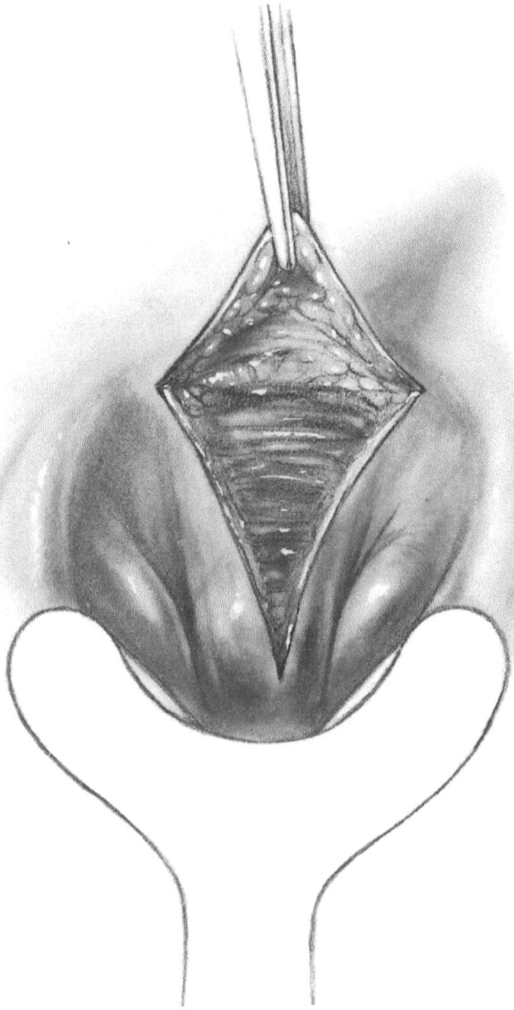

Fig. 25-8

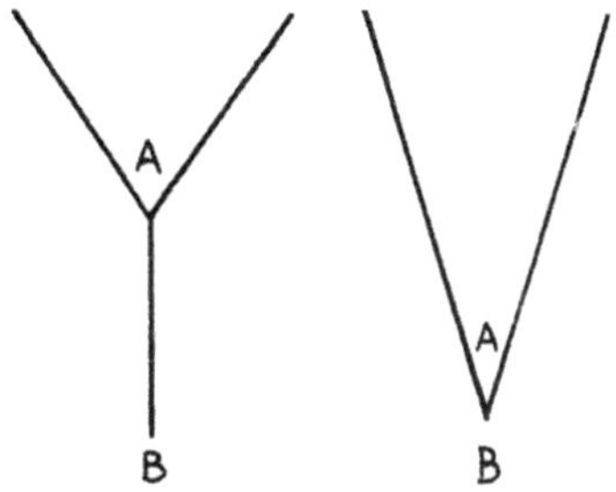


Fig. 25-7ab

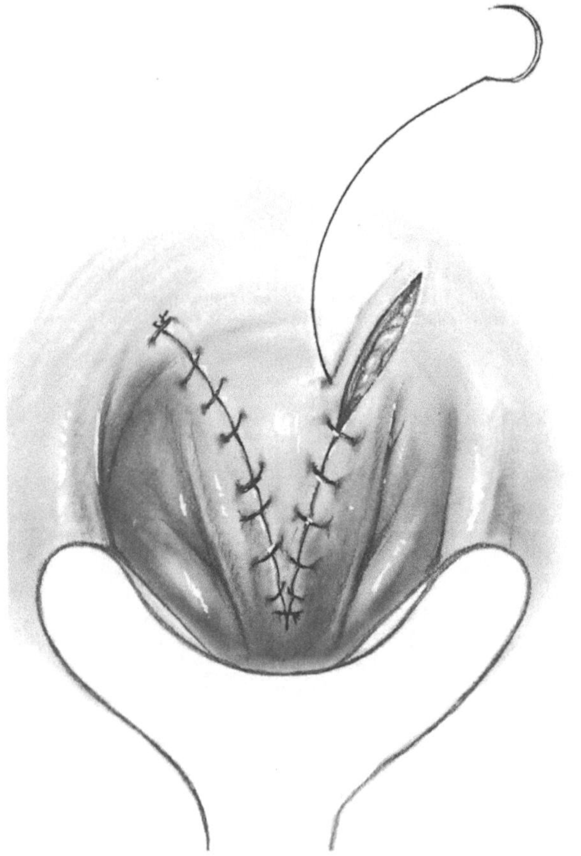

Fig. 25-8

## POSTOPERATIVE CARE

Remove the gauze dressings from the anal wound. It is not necessary to mobilize the Gelfoam because it tends to dissolve in sitz baths, which the patient should start two or three times daily on the day following the operation.

A regular diet is prescribed.

Mineral oil (45 ml) is taken nightly for the first 2–3 days. Thereafter a bulk laxative, such as Metamucil, is prescribed for the remainder of the postoperative period.

Discontinue all intravenous fluids in the recovery room if there has been no postanesthesia complication. This practice reduces the incidence of postoperative urinary retention.

## COMPLICATIONS

Urinary retention

Hematoma

Anal ulcer and wound infection (rare)

## REFERENCE

Khubchandani IT. Anal stenosis. Surg Clin North Am 1994;74:1353.

# 26 Thiersch Operation for Rectal Prolapse

## SURGICAL LEGACY TECHNIQUE

## INDICATIONS

The Thiersch operation is indicated in poor-risk patients who have prolapse of the full thickness of rectum (see Chapter 19). Other perineal operations, including the Delorme procedure, are excellent alternatives in poor-risk patients and have largely supplanted this legacy procedure.

## PREOPERATIVE PREPARATION

Sigmoidoscopy (barium colon enema) is performed.

Because many patients with rectal prolapse suffer from severe constipation, cleanse the colon over a period of a few days with cathartics and enemas.

Initiate an antibiotic bowel preparation 18 hours prior to scheduled operation, as for colon resection (see Chapter 1).

## PITFALLS AND DANGER POINTS

Tying the encircling band too tight so it causes obstruction

Wound infection

Injury to vagina or rectum

Fecal impaction

## OPERATIVE STRATEGY

### Selecting Proper Suture or Banding Material

Lomas and Cooperman (1972) recommended that the anal canal be encircled by a four-ply layer of polypropylene mesh. The band is 1.5 cm in width, so the likelihood it would cut through the tissues is minimized. Labow and associates (1980) used a Dacron-impregnated Silastic sheet (Dow Corning No. 501-7) because it has the advantage of elasticity.

### Achieving Proper Tension of the Encircling Band

Although some surgeons advocate that the encircling band be adjusted to fit snugly around a Hegar dilator, we have not found this technique satisfactory. Achieve proper tension by inserting an index finger into the anal canal while the assistant adjusts the encircling band so it fits snugly around the finger. If the band is too loose, prolapse is not prevented.

## OPERATIVE TECHNIQUE

### Fabricating the Encircling Band of Mesh

Although Lomas and Cooperman preferred Marlex mesh, we believe that Dacron-impregnated Silastic mesh is preferable because of its elasticity. Cut a rectangle of Silastic mesh 1.5 × 20.0 cm. Cut the strip so it is elastic along its longitudinal axis. **Figure 26–1** and subsequent drawings illustrate Lomas and Cooperman's technique of using a tight roll of Marlex; we now use a 1.5 cm strip elasticized Silastic. Except for the nature of the mesh, the surgical technique is unchanged.

### Incision and Position

This operation may be done with the patient in the prone jackknife or the lithotomy position, under general or regional anesthesia. We prefer the prone position. Make a 2 cm radial incision at 10 o'clock starting at the lateral border of the anal sphincter muscle and continue laterally. Make a similar incision at 4 o'clock. Make each incision about 2.5 cm deep.

### Inserting the Mesh Band

Insert a large curved Kelly hemostat or a large right-angle clamp into the incision at 4 o'clock and gently

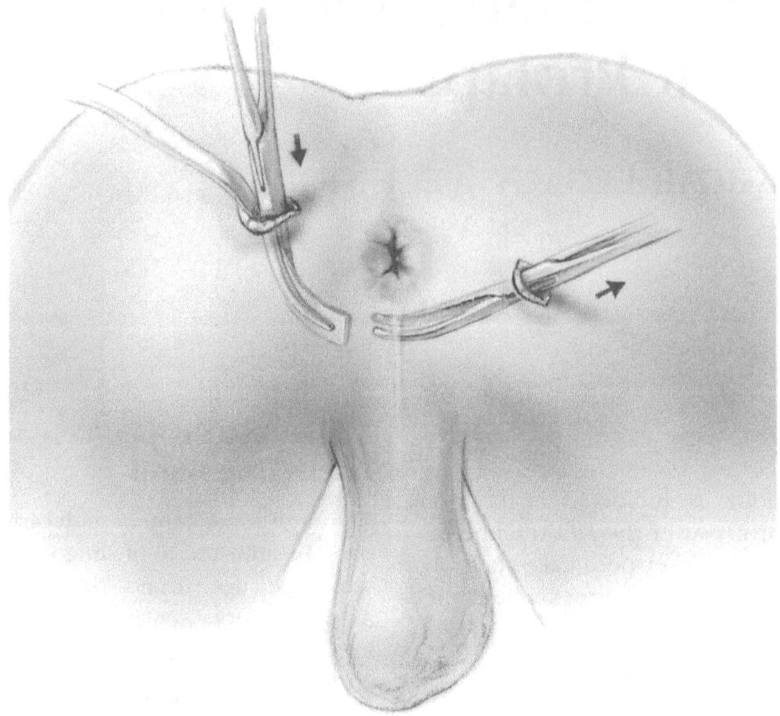

Fig. 26–1

pass the instrument around the external sphincter muscles so it emerges from the incision at 10 o'clock. Insert one end of the mesh strip into the jaws of the hemostat and draw the mesh through the upper incision and extract it from the incision at 4 o'clock. Then pass the hemostat through the 10 o'clock incision around the other half of the circumference of the anal canal until it emerges from the 4 o'clock incision. Insert the end of the mesh into the jaws of the hemostat and draw the hemostat back along this path **(Fig. 26–2)** so it delivers the end of the mesh band into the posterior incision. At this time the entire anal canal has been encircled by the band of mesh, and both ends protrude through the posterior incision. During this manipulation be careful not to penetrate the vagina or the anterior rectal wall. Also, do not permit the mesh to become twisted during its passage around the anal canal. Keep the band flat.

## Adjusting Tension

Apply a second sterile glove on top of the previous glove on the left hand. Insert the left index finger into the anal canal. Apply a hemostat to each end of the encircling band. Ask the assistant to increase the tension gradually by overlapping the two ends of mesh. When the band feels snug around the index finger, ask the assistant to insert a 2-0 Prolene suture to maintain this tension. After the suture has been inserted, recheck the tension of the band. Then remove the index finger and remove the contaminated glove. Insert several additional 2-0 Prolene interrupted sutures or a row of 55 mm linear staples to approximate the two ends of the mesh and amputate the excess length of the mesh band. The patient should now have a 1.5 cm wide band of mesh encircling the external sphincter muscles at the midpoint of the anal canal with sufficient tension to be snug around an index finger in the rectum **(Fig. 26–3)**.

## Closure

Irrigate both incisions thoroughly with a dilute antibiotic solution. Close the deep perirectal fat with interrupted 4-0 PG interrupted sutures in both incisions. Close the skin with interrupted or continuous subcuticular sutures of the same material **(Fig. 26–4)**. Apply collodion over each incision.

Fig. 26–2

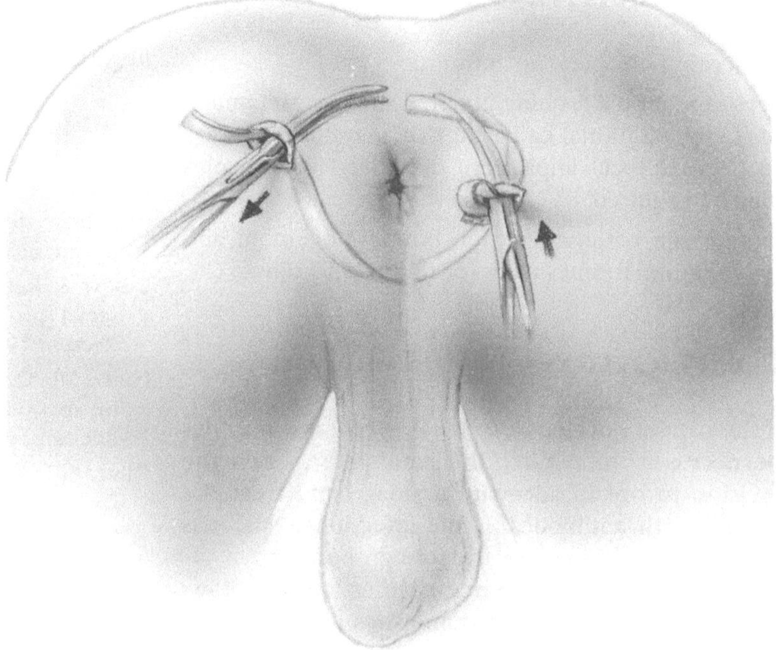

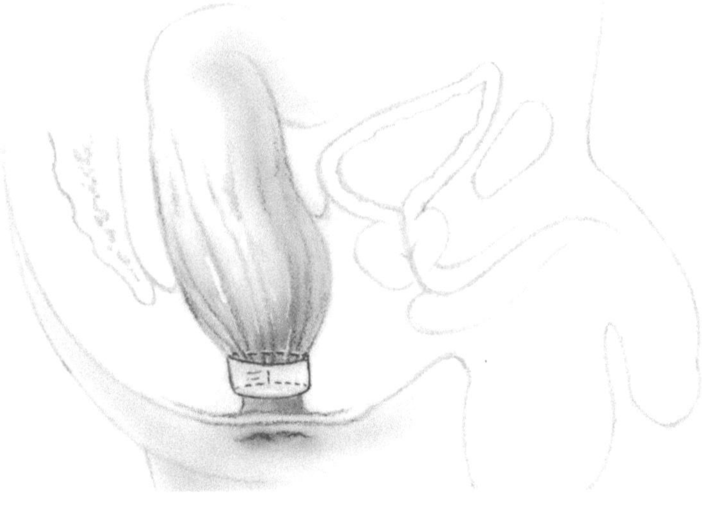

Fig. 26–3

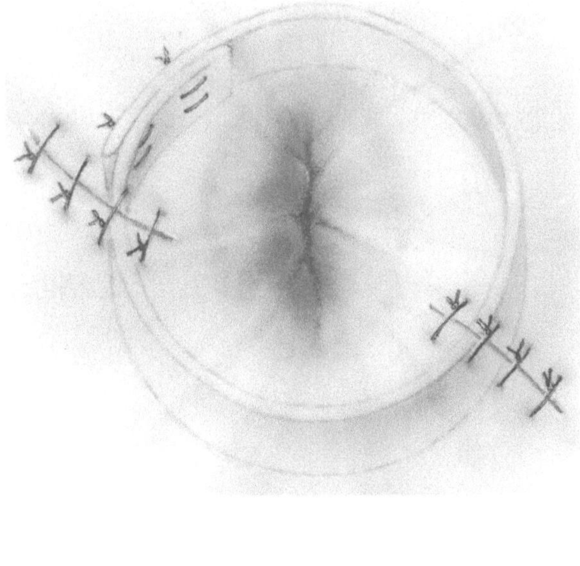

Fig. 26–4

## POSTOPERATIVE CARE

Prescribe perioperative antibiotics.

Prescribe a bulk-forming laxative such as Metamucil plus any additional cathartic that may be necessary to prevent fecal impaction. Periodic Fleet enemas may be required.

Initiate sitz baths after each bowel movement and two additional times daily for the first 10 days.

## COMPLICATIONS

If the patient develops a *wound infection* it may not be necessary to remove the band. First, open the incision to obtain adequate drainage and treat the patient with antibiotics. If the infection heals, it is not necessary to remove the foreign body.

Some patients experience *perineal pain* following surgery, but it usually diminishes in time. If the pain is severe and unrelenting, the mesh must be removed. If removal can be postponed for 4-6 months, there may be enough residual perirectal fibrosis to prevent recurrence of the prolapse.

## REFERENCES

Kuijpers HC. Treatment of complete rectal prolapse: to narrow, to wrap, to suspend, to fix, to encircle, to plicate or to resect? World J Surg 1992;15:826.

Labow S, Rubin RJ, Hoexter B, et al. Perineal repair of rectal procidentia with an elastic sling. Dis Colon Rectum 1980;23:467.

Lomas ML, Cooperman H. Correction of rectal procidentia by use of polypropylene mesh (Marlex). Dis Colon Rectum 1972;15:416.

Oliver GC, Vachon D, Eisenstat TE, Rubin RJ, Salvati EP. Delorme's procedure for complete rectal prolapse in severely debilitated patients: an analysis of 41 cases. Dis Colon Rectum 1994;37:461.

Williams JG, Rothenberger DA, Madoff RD, Goldberg SM. Treatment of rectal prolapse in the elderly by perineal rectosigmoidectomy. Dis Colon Rectum 1992;35:830.

# 27 Operations for Pilonidal Disease

## INDICATIONS

Recurrent symptoms of pain, swelling, and purulent drainage

## PITFALLS AND DANGER POINTS

Unnecessarily radical excision

## OPERATIVE STRATEGY

### Acute Pilonidal Abscess

If an adequate incision can be made and all of the granulation tissue and hair are removed from the cavity, a cure is accomplished in a number of patients with acute abscesses.

### Marsupialization

During marsupialization a narrow elliptical incision is used to unroof the length of the pilonidal cavity. Do not excise a significant width of the overlying skin—only enough to remove the sinus pits. If this is accomplished, one can approximate the lateral margin of the pilonidal cyst wall to the subcuticular layer of the skin with interrupted sutures. At the conclusion of the procedure, no subcutaneous fat is visible in the wound. Healing of exposed subcutaneous fat tends to be slow. On the other hand, the fibrous tissue lining the pilonidal cyst contracts fairly rapidly, producing approximation of the marsupialized edges of skin over a period of only several weeks. There is no need to excise a width of skin more than 0.8–1.0 cm. Conservative skin excision is followed by more rapid healing. Of course, all granulation tissue and hair must be curetted away from the fibrous lining of the pilonidal cyst.

### Excision with Primary Suture

Allow several months to pass after an episode of acute infection to minimize the bacterial content of the pilonidal complex. Successful accomplishment of primary healing requires that the pilonidal cyst be encompassed by excision of a narrow strip of skin that includes the sinus pits and a patch of subcutaneous fat not much more than 1 cm in width. If this can be achieved without entering the cyst, closing the relatively shallow, narrow wound is not difficult. Perform the dissection with electrocautery. Hemostasis must be perfect to ensure complete excision of the cyst and any sinus tracts without unnecessary contamination of the wound. If this technique has been successful, postoperative convalescence is quite short.

It is not necessary to carry the dissection down to the sacrococcygeal ligaments to ensure successful elimination of the pilonidal disease. In essence, the surgeon is simply excising a chronic granulomas surrounded by a fibrous capsule and covered by a strip of skin containing the pits that constituted the original portal of entry of infection and hair into the abscess.

Primary healing requires good wound architecture. If a large segment of subcutaneous fat is excised, simply approximating the skin over a large deadspace may result in temporary healing, but eventually the wound is likely to separate. Unless the surgeon is willing to construct extensive sliding skin flaps or a Z-plasty, excision with primary closure should be restricted to patients in whom wide excision is not necessary.

## OPERATIVE TECHNIQUE

Although it is possible to excise the midline sinus pits and to evacuate the pus and hair through this incision under local anesthesia, often the abscess points in an area away from the gluteal cleft and complete extraction of the hair prove to be too painful to the patient. Consequently, in most cases simply evacuate the pus during the initial drainage procedure and postpone a definitive operation until the infection has subsided.

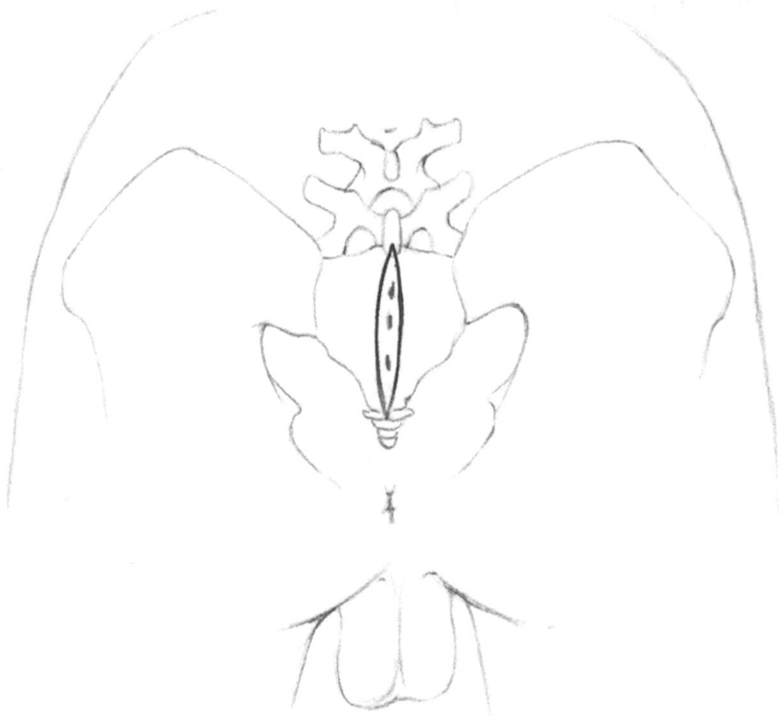

Fig. 27-1

Infiltrate the skin overlying the abscess with 1% lidocaine containing 1:200,000 epinephrine. Make a scalpel incision of sufficient size to evacuate the pus and necrotic material. Whenever possible, avoid making the incision in the midline. If it is possible to extract the loose hair in the abscess, do so; otherwise, simply insert loose gauze packing.

## Marsupialization

First described by Buie in 1944, marsupialization begins by inserting a probe or grooved director into the sinus. Then incise the skin overlying the probe with a scalpel. Do not carry the incision beyond the confines of the pilonidal cyst. If the patient has a tract leading in a lateral direction, insert the probe into the lateral sinus and incise the skin over it. Now excise no more than 1–3 cm of the skin edges on each side to include the epithelium of all of the sinus pits along the edge of the skin wound **(Fig. 27–1)**. This maneuver exposes a narrow band of subcutaneous fat between the lateral margins of the pilonidal cyst and the epithelium of the skin. Achieve complete hemostasis by carefully electrocauterizing each bleeding point.

After unroofing the pilonidal cyst, remove all granulation tissue and hair, if present, using dry gauze, the back of a scalpel handle, or a large curet to wipe clean the posterior wall of the cyst **(Fig. 27–2)**. Then

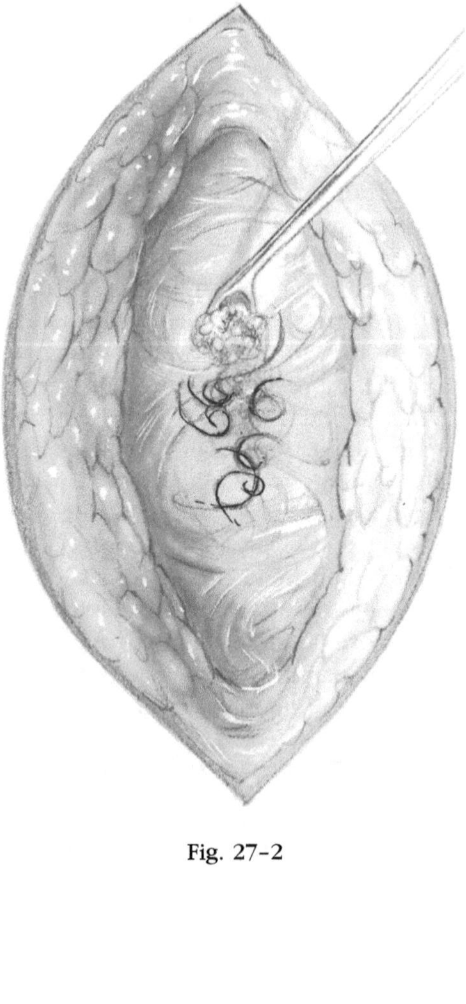

Fig. 27-2

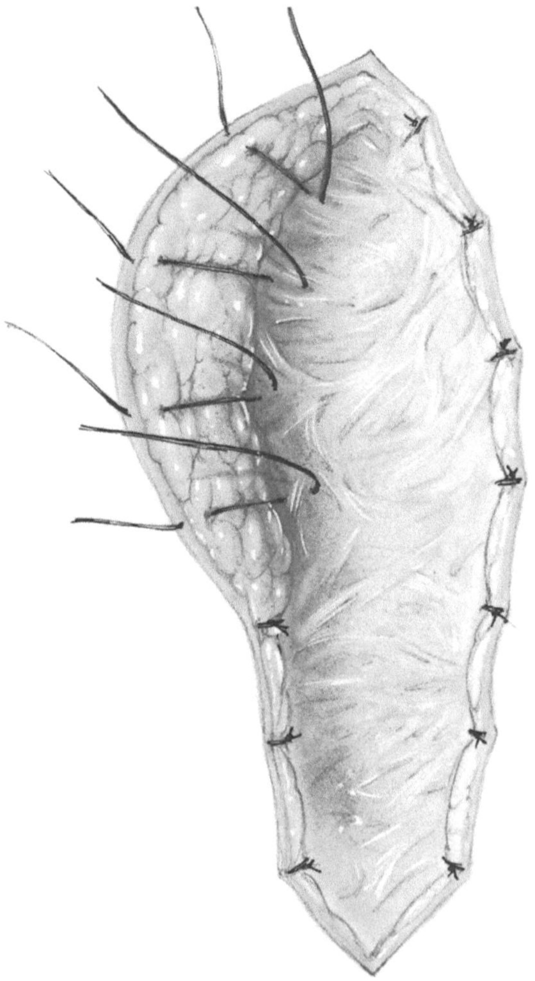

Fig. 27-3

approximate the subcuticular level of the skin to the lateral margin of the pilonidal cyst with interrupted sutures of 3-0 or 4-0 PG **(Fig. 27–3)**.

Ideally, at the conclusion of this procedure there is a fairly flat wound consisting of skin attached to the fibrous posterior wall of the pilonidal cyst, with no subcutaneous fat visible. In the rare situation where the pilonidal cyst wall is covered by squamous epithelium, the marsupialization operation is just as effective as in most cases where the wall consists only of fibrous tissue. We usually perform this operation with the patient in the prone position with the buttocks retracted laterally by adhesive straps under local anesthesia, as Abramson advocated for his modification of the marsupialization operation.

## Pilonidal Excision with Primary Suture

For pilonidal excision with primary suture, use regional, general, or local field block anesthesia. Place the patient in the prone position with a pillow under the hips and the legs slightly flexed.

Apply adhesive strapping to each buttock and retract each in a lateral direction by attaching the adhesive tape to the operating table. Before scrubbing, in preparation for the surgery insert a sterile probe into the pilonidal sinus and gently explore the dimensions of the underlying cavity to confirm that it is not too large for excision and primary suture.

After shaving, cleansing, and preparing the area with an iodophor solution, make an elliptical incision only of sufficient length and width to encompass the underlying pilonidal sinus and the sinus pits in the gluteal cleft (Fig. 27-1). In properly selected patients this requires excising a strip of skin no more than 1.0-1.5 cm in width. Deepen the incision on each side of the pilonidal sinus **(Fig. 27–4)**. Use electrocautery for this dissection to achieve complete hemostasis. Otherwise, the presence of blood prevents the

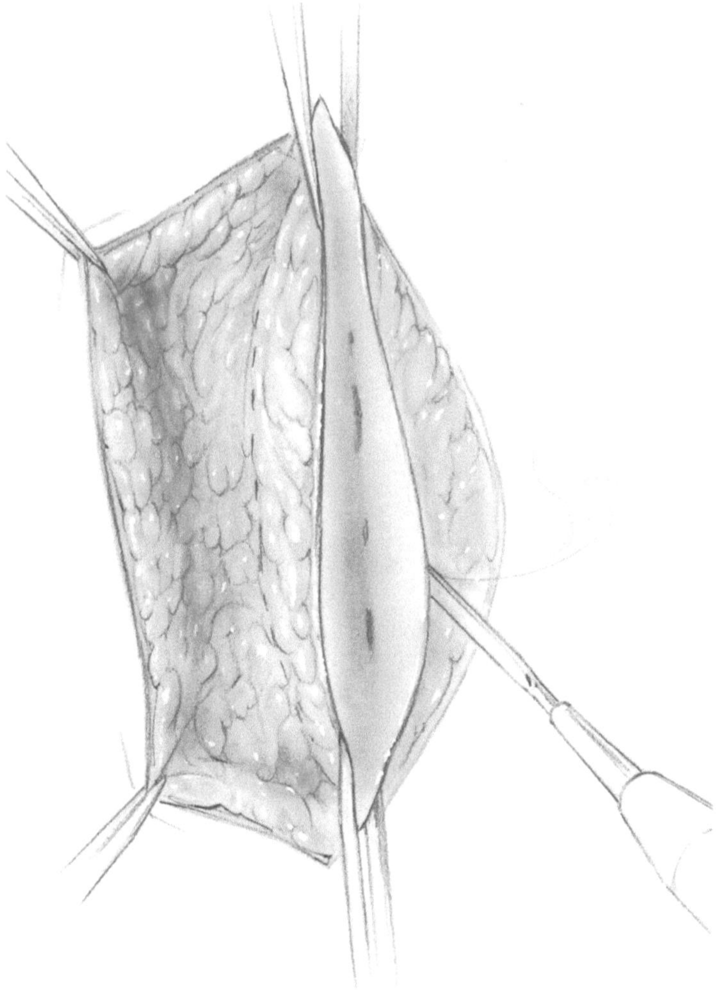

Fig. 27-4

accurate visualization necessary to avoid entering one of the potentially infected pilonidal tracts. Dissect the specimen away from the underlying fat without exposing the sacrococcygeal periosteum or ligaments. Remove the specimen and check for complete hemostasis. The specimen should not measure more than 5.0 × 1.5 × 1.5 cm. It should be possible to approximate the subcutaneous fat with interrupted 3-0 or 4-0 PG sutures without tension **(Fig. 27–5)**. Insert interrupted subcuticular sutures of 4-0 PG **(Fig. 27–6)** or close the skin with interrupted nylon vertical mattress sutures. Avoid leaving any deadspace in the incision. If at some point during the operation the pilonidal cyst has been opened inadvertently, irrigate the wound with a dilute antibiotic solution and complete the operation as planned unless frank pus has filled the wound. In the latter case, simply leave the wound open and insert gauze packing without any sutures. The patient must remain inactive to encourage primary healing.

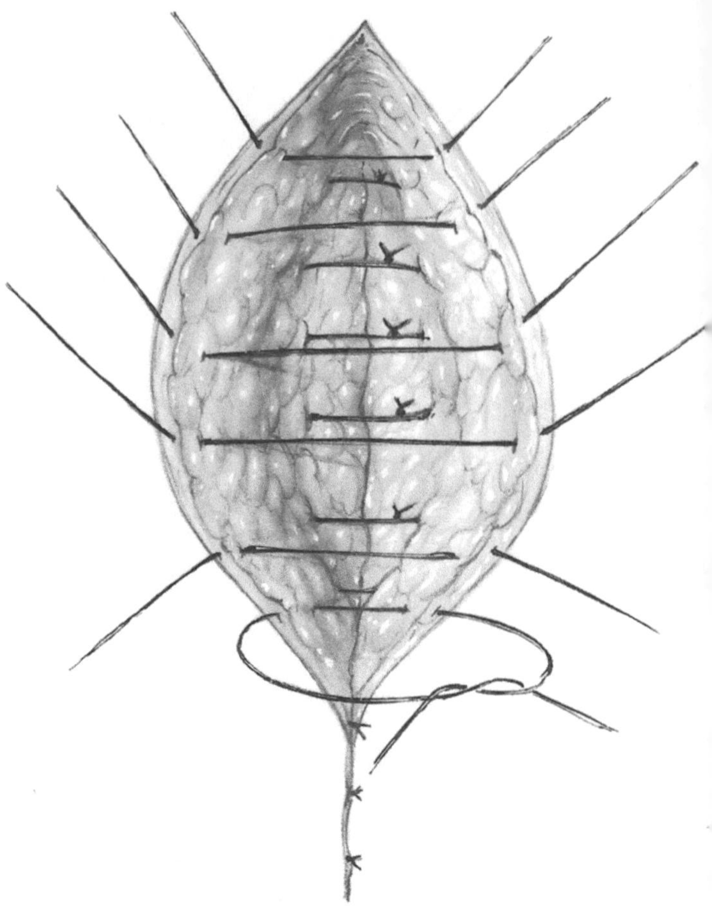

Fig. 27–6

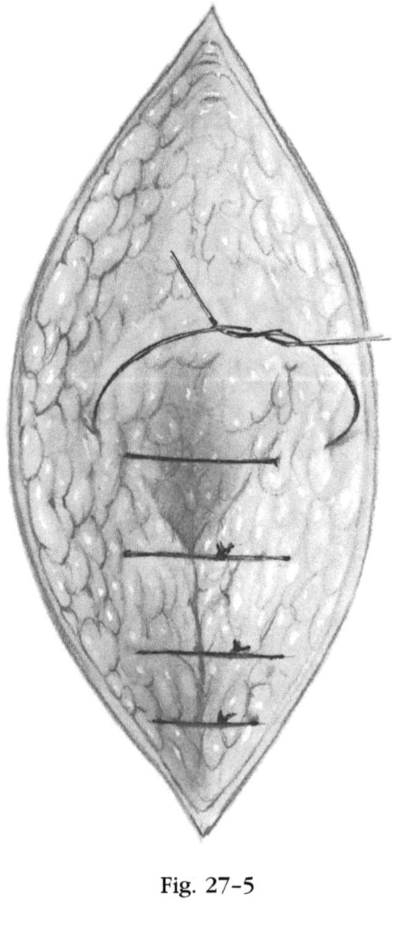

Fig. 27–5

## Excision of Sinus Pits with Lateral Drainage

For Bascom's (1980) modification of Lord and Millar's (1965) operation, only the sinus pits **(Fig. 27–7)** are excised in the mid-gluteal cleft. This may be accomplished with a pointed No. 11 scalpel blade **(Fig. 27–8)** or with the dermatologist's round skin biopsy punches. The latter, available in diameters as large as 5 mm, are simply cork-borers whose ends have been sharpened to a cutting edge. Most of the pits are simply epithelial tubes going down toward the pilonidal cyst for a distance of a few millimeters. Leave unsutured the resulting wounds from the pit excisions.

Insert a probe into the underlying pilonidal cavity to determine its dimensions. Then make a vertical incision parallel to the long axis of the pilonidal cavity. Make this incision about 1.5 cm lateral to the mid-gluteal cleft. Open the pilonidal cyst through

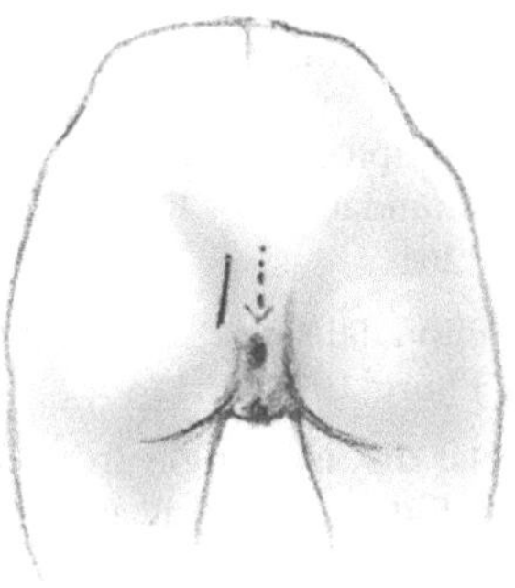

Fig. 27-7

this incision. Curet out all of the granulation tissue and hair. Achieve complete hemostasis with the electrocoagulator. A peanut gauze dissector is also useful for this step. Bascom did not insert drains or packing. Occasionally three or more enlarged follicles (pits) are so close together in the mid-gluteal cleft that individual excision of each follicle is impossible. In this case Bascom simply excised a narrow strip of skin encompassing all of the pits. If the skin defect in the cleft exceeded 7 mm, he sutured it closed. The lateral incision is always left open. In patients who have lateral extensions of their pilonidal disease, each lateral sinus pit is excised. Bascom found that occasionally there was an ingrowth of dermal epithelium into the subcutaneous fat, forming an epithelial tube resembling a thyroglossal duct remnant. These structures resemble pieces of macaroni, and Bascom advised excising these epithelial tubes through the lateral incision.

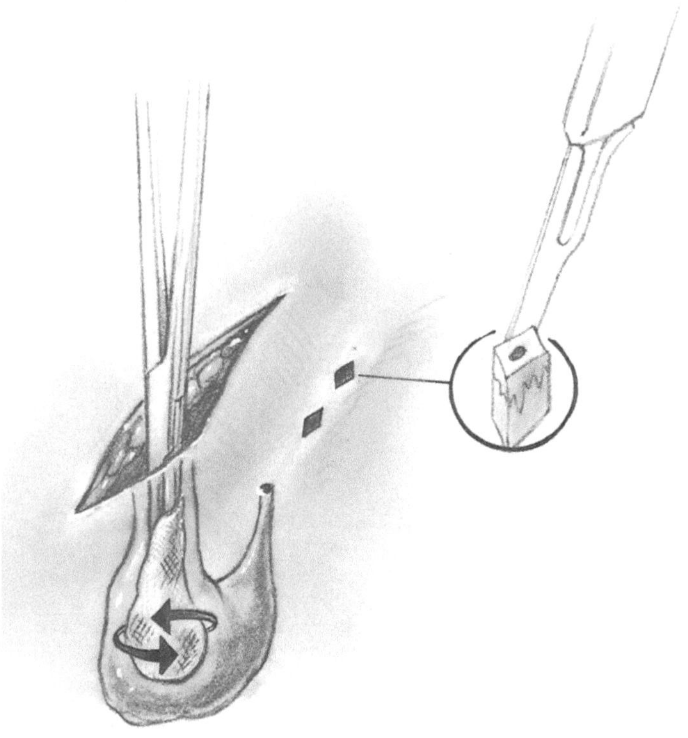

Fig. 27-8

## POSTOPERATIVE CARE

Following drainage of an *acute pilonidal abscess*, remove the gauze packing the next day and have the patient shower daily to keep the gluteal cleft clean and free of any loose hair. Shave the skin for a distance of about 5 cm around the mid-gluteal cleft weekly. In some cases it is possible to use a depilatory cream to achieve the same result. Otherwise, hair finds its way into the pilonidal cavity and acts as a foreign body, initiating a recurrent infection.

Following *excision and primary suture*, remove the gauze dressing on the second day and leave the wound exposed. Initiate daily showering especially after each bowel movement. Observe the patient closely two or three times a week in the office. If evidence of a localized wound infection appears, open this area of the wound and administer appropriate antibiotics, treating the condition the same way you would treat an infection in an abdominal incision. If the infection is extensive, it is then necessary to lay open the entire incision. With good wound architecture, infection is uncommon. Also shave or apply a depilatory cream to the area of the mid-gluteal cleft for the first two to three postoperative weeks or until the wound is completely healed.

If the patient has undergone *pit excision and lateral drainage*, postoperative care is limited to daily showers and weekly observation by the surgeon to remove any hairs that may have invaded the wound. Bascom applied Monsel's solution to granulation tissue. All of his patients have been operated in the ambulatory outpatient setting. No matter what the operative procedure, patients with pilonidal disease require instruction always to avoid accumulation of loose hair in the mid-gluteal cleft. Daily showering with special attention to cleaning this area should prevent recurrence.

## COMPLICATIONS

*Infection* may follow the primary suture operation.

*Hemorrhage* has been reported by Lamke et al. (1974) Of the patients treated by wide excision and packing, 10% experienced postoperative hemorrhage requiring blood transfusion and reoperation. This complication is easily preventable by meticulous electrocoagulation of each bleeding point in the operating room. It is rare following primary suture or marsupialization operations.

Among patients followed for a number of years, pilonidal disease *recurs* in 15% whether treated by primary suture, excision and packing, or marsupialization. Even the radical excision operation does not seem to prevent recurrence. Consequently, it appears that in most cases recurrence is caused by poor hygiene, permitting hair to drill its way into the skin of the mid-gluteal cleft, rather than by inadequate surgery. Most recurrences are in the midline.

There may be a *failure to heal*. Some patients, especially those who have had a radical excision of pilonidal disease that leaves a large midline defect bounded by sacrococcygeal periosteum in its depths and subcutaneous fat around its perimeter, endure healing failure for a period as long as 2 years (Bascom). In some cases it is due to inadequate postoperative care in which the bridging of unhealed cavities has taken place or in which loose hair has found its way into the cavity and produced reinfection. Occasionally, even when postoperative care is conscientious in these patients, there is protracted healing of the residual wound.

## REFERENCES


Abramson DJ. A simple marsupialization technique for treatment of pilonidal sinus; long-term follow-up. Ann Surg 1960;151:261.

Allen-Mersh TG. Pilonidal sinus: finding the right track for treatment. Br J Surg 1990;77:123.

Bascom J. Pilonidal disease: origin from follicles of hairs and results of follicle removal as treatment. Surgery 1980;87:567.

Buie LA. Jeep disease (pilonidal disease of mechanized warfare). South Med J 1944;37:103.

Holm J, Hulten L. Simple primary closure for pilonidal disease. Acta Chir Scand 1970;136:537.

Lamke LO, Larsson J, Nylen B. Results of different types of operation for pilonidal sinus. Acta Chir Scand 1974;140:321.

Lord PH, Millar DM. Pilonidal sinus: a simple treatment. Br J Surg 1965;52:298.

Patey DH, Scarff RW. Pathology of postanal pilonidal sinus: its bearing on treatment. Lancet 1946;2:484.

Surrell JA. Pilonidal disease. Surg Clin North Am 1994;74:1309.

# Index

MIX
Papier aus verantwortungsvollen Quellen
Paper from responsible sources
FSC® C105338

If you have any concerns about our products,
you can contact us on
**ProductSafety@springernature.com**

In case Publisher is established outside the EU,
the EU authorized representative is:
**Springer Nature Customer Service Center GmbH**
**Europaplatz 3, 69115 Heidelberg, Germany**

Printed by Libri Plureos GmbH
in Hamburg, Germany